The Modern Role of β-Blockers (BBs) in Cardiovascular Medicine

The Modern Role of β-Blockers (BBs) in Cardiovascular Medicine

John Malcolm Cruickshank, MD

2010
PEOPLE'S MEDICAL PUBLISHING HOUSE—USA
SHELTON, CONNECTICUT

People's Medical Publishing House–USA
2 Enterprise Drive, Suite 509
Shelton, CT 06484
Tel: 203-402-0646
Fax: 203-402-0854
E-mail: info@pmph-usa.com

PMPH-USA

© 2011 PMPH-USA, Ltd.

All rights reserved. Without limiting the rights under copyright reserved above, no part of this publication may be reproduced, stored in or introduced into a retrieval system, or transmitted, in any form or by any means (electronic, mechanical, photocopying, recording, or otherwise), without the prior written permission of the publisher.

09 10 11 12 13/PMPH/9 8 7 6 5 4 3 2 1

ISBN-13 978-1-60795-108-7
ISBN-10 1-60795-108-8

Printed in China by People's Medical Publishing House of China
Copyeditor/Typesetter: Spearhead Global, Inc.; Cover designer: Mary McKeon

Library of Congress Cataloging-in-Publication Data

Cruickshank, J. M.
 The modern role of β-blockers (BBS) in cardiovascular medicine / John Malcolm Cruickshank.
   p. ; cm.
 Includes bibliographical references and index.
 ISBN-13: 978-1-60795-108-7
 ISBN-10: 1-60795-108-8
 1. Adrenergic beta blockers—Therapeutic use. 2. Cardiovascular system—Diseases—Treatment. 3. Cardiovascular pharmacology. I. Title.
 [DNLM: 1. Adrenergic beta-Antagonists—therapeutic use. 2. Adrenergic beta-Antagonists—pharmacology. 3. Cardiovascular Diseases—drug therapy. QV 150]
 RC684.A35C774 2010
 616.1'06—dc22
                                                            2010026600

Notice: The authors and publisher have made every effort to ensure that the patient care recommended herein, including choice of drugs and drug dosages, is in accord with the accepted standard and practice at the time of publication. However, since research and regulation constantly change clinical standards, the reader is urged to check the product information sheet included in the package of each drug, which includes recommended doses, warnings, and contraindications. This is particularly important with new or infrequently used drugs. Any treatment regimen, particularly one involving medication, involves inherent risk that must be weighed on a case-by-case basis against the benefits anticipated. The reader is cautioned that the purpose of this book is to inform and enlighten; the information contained herein is not intended as, and should not be employed as, a substitute for individual diagnosis and treatment.

Sales and Distribution

Canada
McGraw-Hill Ryerson Education
Customer Care
300 Water St
Whitby, Ontario L1N 9B6
Canada
Tel: 1-800-565-5758
Fax: 1-800-463-5885
www.mcgrawhill.ca

Foreign Rights
People's Medical Publishing House
Suzanne Robidoux, Copyright Sales Manager
International Trade Department
No. 19, Pan Jia Yuan Nan Li
Chaoyang District
Beijing 100021
P.R. China
Tel: 8610-59787337
Fax: 8610-59787336
www.pmph.com/en/

Japan
United Publishers Services Limited
1-32-5 Higashi-Shinagawa
Shinagawa-ku, Tokyo 140-0002
Japan
Tel: 03-5479-7251
Fax: 03-5479-7307
Email: kakimoto@ups.co.jp

United Kingdom, Europe, Middle East, Africa
McGraw Hill Education
Shoppenhangers Road
Maidenhead
Berkshire, SL6 2QL
England
Tel: 44-0-1628-502500
Fax: 44-0-1628-635895
www.mcgraw-hill.co.uk

Singapore, Thailand, Philippines, Indonesia, Vietnam, Pacific Rim, Korea
McGraw-Hill Education
60 Tuas Basin Link
Singapore 638775
Tel: 65-6863-1580
Fax: 65-6862-3354
www.mcgraw-hill.com.sg

Australia, New Zealand
Elsevier Australia
Locked Bag 7500
Chatswood DC NSW 2067
Australia
Tel: 161 (2) 9422-8500
Fax: 161 (2) 9422-8562
www.elsevier.com.au

Brazil
SuperPedido Tecmedd
Beatriz Alves, Foreign Trade Department
R. Sansao Alves dos Santos, 102 | 7th floor
Brooklin Novo
Sao Paolo 04571-090
Brazil
Tel: 55-16-3512-5539
www.superpedidotecmedd.com.br

India, Bangladesh, Pakistan, Sri Lanka, Malaysia
CBS Publishers
4819/X1 Prahlad Street 24
Ansari Road, Darya Ganj,
New Delhi-110002
India
Tel: 91-11-23266861/67
Fax: 91-11-23266818
Email:cbspubs@vsnl.com

People's Republic of China
People's Medical Publishing House
International Trade Department
No. 19, Pan Jia Yuan Nan Li
Chaoyang District
Beijing 100021
P.R. China
Tel: 8610-67653342
Fax: 8610-67691034
www.pmph.com/en/

*This book is dedicated to
my wife and patient secretary,
Moira, and her assistant
and granddaughter, Freya.*

Foreword

Many years have passed since James Black had the original concept of β-blockers (BBs) in the late 1950s (for which he was duly awarded the Nobel Prize for medicine and later Knighted), the first appearance of BBs on the market (for ischemic heart disease) in the early 1960s, and the discovery in 1964 by Brian Prichard that BBs could lower blood pressure.

The β-blocker story, in its entirety, has already been attempted by myself and the present author, John Cruickshank, in the 1st and 2nd editions of the book β-*Blockers in Clinical Practice*. However, the 1200-page 2nd edition appeared in 1994 and, of course, is now well out of date, particularly in the fields of hypertension and heart failure. John Cruickshank has attempted to rectify (and succeeds in rectifying) this situation in the present concise book, *The Modern Role of β-Blockers in Cardiovascular Medicine*. He is passionate on the wrongness of the position (2006) taken up by the U.K. NICE (National Institute for Clinical Excellence) Committee/British Hypertension Society in demoting BBs as first-line agents for the treatment of hypertension and their warnings against the use of the BB/diuretic combination.

John Cruickshank is decidedly well-qualified to write the present concise book on BBs because he has well over 100 publications relating to BBs. He will be particularly remembered for his early work on the ability of BBs to prevent catecholamine-induced myocardial necrosis (associated with either subarachnoid hemorrhage or acute head injury); he was first to demonstrate that BBs (atenolol) could be administered once-daily for 24-hour control of blood pressure; he was a pioneer of the concept of the J-curve phenomenon in treated hypertensive patients with coronary heart disease; he also invented the term, and published on, "the economy-class syndrome" (deep vein thrombosis with pulmonary embolus) as a result of his being a victim (and survived to tell the tale!) owing to his extensive traveling program.

Brian N Prichard
February 2010

Preface

It is 16 years since Brian Prichard and I completed the 1200 page 2nd edition of β-*Blockers in Clinical Practice*. In that time, "much of the proverbial water has gone under the bridge."

The most recent major events have been the deaths of two giants of the world of β-blockers. Brian Prichard (who discovered that propranolol lowered blood pressure) and Sir James Black (who invented β-blockers) died in the spring of 2010 within 2 weeks of each other. These are two massive losses to the medical fraternity. We are indeed lucky that Brian Prichard was able, before his terminal illness ran an unexpectedly rapid course, to write the Foreword to this book.

One major event since the 1994 book, β-*Blockers in Clinical Practice*, was the discovery that β-blockers without intrinsic sympathomimetic activity (ISA; carvedilol, metoprolol, and bisoprolol) reduce the frequency of death by about 35% in patients with systolic heart failure already on angiotensin-converting enzyme (ACE) inhibitors. Moreover, first-line $β_1$-blockade (bisoprolol) was at least as effective as first-line ACE inhibitors in reducing death and was superior in preventing sudden death.

The other major event relates to the role of β-blockers in hypertension. In 2006, the U.K. NICE (National Institute for Clinical Excellence) Committee, supported by the British Hypertension Society, announced that (1) β-blockers should no longer be regarded as preferred first-line agents in the treatment of hypertension, (2) the combination of β-blockers and diuretics should be discouraged owing to the increased risk of developing diabetes, (3) in patients younger than 55 years old, the first-line therapy should be ACE inhibitors or angiotensin-receptor blockers (ARBs) if ACE inhibitors were poorly tolerated. The author of this book strongly disagrees with these recommendations, not least because in the one and only comparison of first-line β-blocker and ACE inhibitor (second-line diuretics) in younger/middle-aged, high-risk hypertensive patients

(UKPDS [U.K. Prospective Diabetes Study]), the trends in reducing all seven primary end-points favored the β-blocker (atenolol) after 10 years' follow-up, with a significant 23% reduction in all-cause death after 20 years follow-up favoring those originally randomized to atenolol. That ARBs should also be considered a first-line therapy option in younger hypertensive patients is particularly worrying because the most common cause of death in younger hypertensive patients is myocardial infarction (two to three times more common than stroke) and there is a genuine worry that ARBs not only do not reduce the risk of myocardial infarction but also might even increase it. The warning against the β-blocker/diuretic combination is equally baffling because this combination was used in the UKPDS in younger patients with great success over 10 years and in the vast ALLHAT (Antihypertensive and Lipid-Lowering Treatment to Prevent Heart Attack Trial) (the largest prospective, randomized, controlled study ever performed) in the elderly, the favored treatment was diuretic (second-line β-blocker mostly)-based therapy compared with calcium antagonist or ACE inhibitor-based therapy. The diuretic-/β-blocker-based therapy was particularly effective in those with the metabolic syndrome (considered by NICE to be a virtual contraindication!).

The previous topics are discussed further in the book. Being only about 250 pages in length, great detail cannot be addressed. Only cardiovascular areas (coronary artery disease, hypertension, arrhythmias, and heart failure), being the overwhelmingly main indications for β-blockers, are covered. Hopefully, all important cardiovascular issues have been adequately covered and dealt with fairly. However, the "flavor" of the book, particularly the Summary and Conclusion sections at the end of each chapter, inevitably reflect the author's personal views.

JMC
May 2010

Contents

Chapter 1—Pharmacology   1

Introduction   1
1. Nature of the adrenoceptors   1
2. Pharmacodynamics   5
3. Pharmacokinetics   29

Summary and Conclusions   37

References   40

Chapter 2—β-Blockers and Their Effects upon Ischemic Heart Disease, Peripheral Vascular Disease (Including Aortic Aneurysms), Noncardiac Surgery (in High-Risk Cases), and the Atheromatous Process   49

Introduction   49
1. Post myocardial infarction   49
2. Angina pectoris and chronic ischemia   53
3. Peripheral arterial disease (including vascular aneurysms) and noncardiac surgery in high-risk cases   62
4. β-Blockers and the atheromatous plaque   68

Summary and Conclusions   73

References   74

Chapter 3—β-Blockers and Hypertension   81

Introduction   81
1. Recent anti-β-blocker sentiment   81
2. Pathophysiology of primary hypertension   82
3. Possible inflammatory mechanism linking central obesity and high sympathetic nerve activity in the younger/middle-aged diastolic hypertensive patient   84

4. First-line β-blockers and the young/middle-aged diastolic hypertensive patient; major randomized, controlled, hard-end-point studies 88
5. First-line β-blockers and the elderly systolic hypertensive—major hard-end-point studies 96
6. β-blockers given as second-line therapy to first-line diuretic or calcium antagonist therapy in elderly hypertensives 108
7. Are induced metabolic changes with diuretic/β-blocker-based therapy harmful? 112
8. Where do angiotensin receptor blockers fit in? 115
9. So how did the U.K. NICE committee get it so wrong? 118
10. Secondary hypertension 119
11. Is the choice of β-blocker important in relation to efficacy? 121

Summary and Conclusions 126

References 131

Chapter 4—β-Blockers and Cardiac Arrhythmias 141

Introduction 141
1. Clinical management of arrhythmias with β-blockers 142
2. Is the choice of β-blocker important? 162

Summary And Conclusions 164

References 165

Chapter 5—β-Blockers and Heart Failure 173

Introduction 173
1. Two main types of HF pathophysiology 173
2. β-Blockers and mortality in HFREF (systolic HF) 176
3. Mechanism of action of β-blockers in moderate/severe systolic HF (HFREF) 185
4. End-stage systolic HF and the salutary effect of specific $β_2$-stimulation plus specific $β_1$-blockade 187
5. Diastolic HF (HFNEF) 188
6. Contraindications to β-blockers in congestive cardiac failure 189
7. HF—prevention 190
8. Choice of β-blocker for the treatment of systolic HF (HFREF) 196

Summary And Conclusions 198

References 200

Chapter 6—Adverse Reactions 207

Introduction 207
1. Quality of life 208
2. Adverse reactions relating to the cardiovascular system 209
3. Adverse reactions relating to renal function 220
4. Adverse reactions relating to the respiratory system 221
5. Metabolic disturbance 227
6. Adverse reactions relating to the central nervous system 233
7. Sexual dysfunction 234
8. Weight gain 236
9. Skin and rashes 237
10. Arrhythmia induction 238

Summary and Conclusions 238

References 242

Index 251

Pharmacology

CHAPTER 1

INTRODUCTION

The pharmacology of β-blockers has already been well-reviewed.[1] The essential pharmacodynamics of all β-blockers is governed by $β_1$-blockade, a property possessed by all β-blockers. However, the effects of pure $β_1$-blockade are often modified by the presence of additional properties such as $β_2$-blockade; intrinsic sympathomimetic activity (ISA) involving one or more of the $β_1$, $β_2$, and $β_3$-adrenoceptors; α-blockade; and class III antiarrhythmic activity.

Pharmacokinetics is largely influenced by the lipophilicity (lipid-solubility) of the agent, affecting such properties as absorption, body distribution, metabolism and excretion, and duration of action.

1. Nature of the Adrenoceptors

A) Distribution

The $α_1$-, $α_2$-, $β_1$-, $β_2$-, and $β_3$-adrenoceptors are distributed throughout the body. **Table 1-1** shows the various organs where the adrenoceptors occur and the result of stimulation.[1]

B) Receptor Structure

The adrenoceptors are membrane glycoproteins and the various subtypes are similar in overall structure. Stimulatory agents (e.g., noradrenaline or pirbuterol) occupy the receptor site and effect

TABLE 1-1 Distribution of adrenoceptor subtypes and the physiological effects of stimulation

Organ	Predominant adrenoceptor	Physiological effect of stimulation
Myocardium	$\beta_1 > \beta_2$	Increases in contractility and heart rate
	β_3	Cardiodepression
Smooth muscle—bronchi	β_2	Bronchodilatation
Smooth muscle—blood vessels	α_1	Vasoconstriction
	α_2	Vasoconstriction
	β_2	Vasodilatation
	β_3	Vasodilatation
	β_1	Vasodilatation (coronary)
Smooth muscle—genitourinary	α_1	Muscle contraction
	β_2	Muscle relaxation
	β_3	Muscle relaxation
Smooth muscle—large bowel	β_2	Relaxation
	β_3	Relaxation
Fat tissue	α_2	Inhibition of lipolysis
	$\beta_2 > \beta_1$	Stimulation of lipolysis
	β_3	Stimulation of lipolysis and thermogenesis
Platelets	α_2	Aggregation
Liver	α_1	Glycogenolysis
	β_2	Glycogenolysis and gluconeogenesis
Pancreas	α_2	Inhibition of insulin release
	β_2	Stimulation of insulin release
Sympathetic terminals	α_2	Inhibition of noradrenaline release
	β_2	Stimulation of noradrenaline release
Skeletal muscle (slow-twitch fibers)	β_2	Less fatigue (aerobic) Increase in tremor
Blood lipids	β_2	Low triglycerides High HDL
Kidney	β_1	Renin release increase
Eye	β_2	Increase in intraocular pressure

From Cruickshank JM, Prichard BNC. Beta-blockers in clinical practice. 2nd ed. Edinburgh: Churchill Livingstone; 1994, pp 1–351.

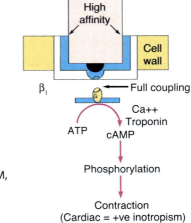

Fig. 1-1 Full agonist activity (e.g., noradrenaline [norepinephrine]) and the cardiac β_1-receptor. ATP, adenosine triphosphate; cAMP, cyclic adenosine monophosphate. (From Cruickshank JM, Prichard BNC. Beta-blockers in clinical practice. 2nd ed. Edinburgh: Churchill Livingstone; 1994, pp 1–351.)

their response via alterations in activity of intracellular effector enzymes such as adenyle cyclase or the phospholipidases and various ion channels—**Figures 1-1 and 1-2**. The coupling between the adrenergic receptors to the effector enzymes and the ion channels occurs via a process involving guanine neucleotide triphosphate—a G-protein. These G-proteins can be involved in either stimulation (Gs) or inhibition (Gi).[1]

β-Receptors can be down-regulated (internalized) or desensitized, involving phosphorylation of the receptor catalyzed by protein kinase A (PKA). The uncoupling process also involves β-adrenergic receptor kinase (β-ARK).[1]

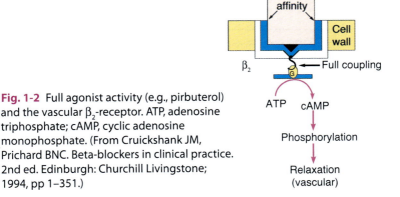

Fig. 1-2 Full agonist activity (e.g., pirbuterol) and the vascular β_2-receptor. ATP, adenosine triphosphate; cAMP, cyclic adenosine monophosphate. (From Cruickshank JM, Prichard BNC. Beta-blockers in clinical practice. 2nd ed. Edinburgh: Churchill Livingstone; 1994, pp 1–351.)

C) Nature of β-Adrenoceptor Inhibition and Stimulation, Including Intrinsic Sympathomimetic Activity

β-Blockers are competitive inhibitors of the effects of endogenous catecholamines (i.e., noradrenaline and adrenaline) at β-adrenergic sites. Noradrenaline (or norepinephrine) stimulates $β_1$-and α-receptors, and adrenaline (epinephrine) stimulates $β_1$-, $β_2$-, and α-receptors. If there is no background adrenergic tone, a β-blocker will have no effect.

Figures 1-3 and 1-4 show the effect of β-blockers with, and without, ISA under conditions of low (sleep) and high (exercise) sympathetic tone.[1]

D) Genetic Polymorphism (Pharmacogenetics)

Both the $β_1$- and the $β_2$-receptors are subject to the influence of genetic polymorphism. Certain $β_1$ variants are associated with down-regulated, insensitive $β_1$-receptors, and there is a poor or absent heart rate and blood pressure response to β-blockade;[2] in contrast, an excellent blood pressure-response occurs in the 49 Ser 389 Arg/Ser 389 Arg variant.[2] Thus, the field of pharmacogenetics will potentially enable patients, based on their phenotype, to be treated, or not treated, appropriately.

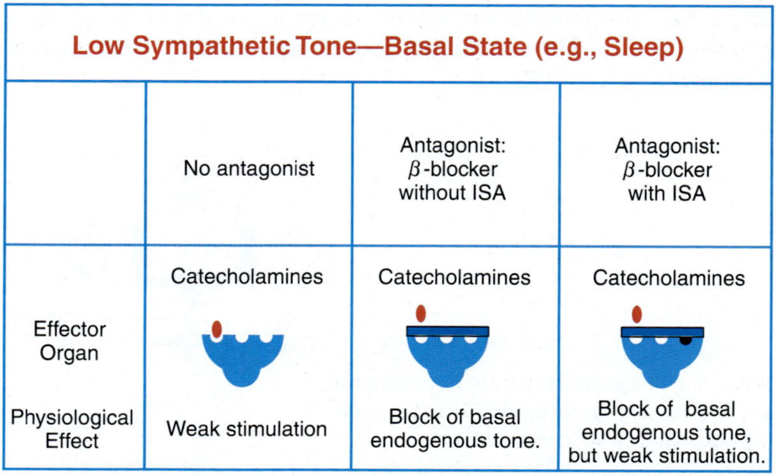

Low Sympathetic Tone—Basal State (e.g., Sleep)			
	No antagonist	Antagonist: β-blocker without ISA	Antagonist: β-blocker with ISA
Effector Organ	Catecholamines	Catecholamines	Catecholamines
Physiological Effect	Weak stimulation	Block of basal endogenous tone.	Block of basal endogenous tone, but weak stimulation.

Fig. 1-3 Nature of β-adrenoceptor inhibition; effect of intrinsic sympathomimetic activity (ISA) in the presence of low levels of catecholamines (e.g., sleep). (From Cruickshank JM, Prichard BNC. Beta-blockers in clinical practice. 2nd ed. Edinburgh: Churchill Livingstone; 1994, pp 1–351.)

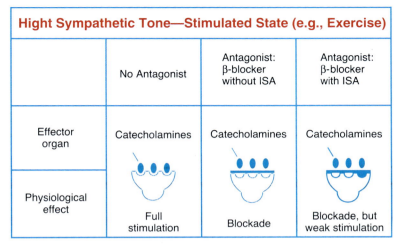

Fig. 1-4 Nature of β-adrenoceptor inhibition; effect of ISA in the presence of high levels of catecholamines (e.g., exercise). (From Cruickshank JM, Prichard BNC. Beta-blockers in clinical practice. 2nd ed. Edinburgh: Churchill Livingstone; 1994, pp 1–351.)

Certain polymorphic variants of the β_2-receptor have down-regulated, insensitive receptors, and the Gly/Gly genotype is closely linked to the development of hypertension.[3]

2. Pharmacodynamics

A) β_1-/β_2-Selectivity Ratios

Figure 1-5 illustrates the β_1-/β_2-selectivity ratios of IC118.551 (total β_2-selective antagonist); propranolol, which inhibits β_1- and β_2-receptors equally; three modestly β_1-selective agents (metoprolol, atenolol, and betaxolol); and highly β_1-selective bisoprolol.[4,5] Thus, for highly β_1-selective bisoprolol, at doses of 5-10 mg, 70%-85% of β_1-receptors are occupied compared to zero (approximate) occupancy of β_2-receptors—**Figure 1-6**.[6] Note that β_1-selectivity is diminished at higher doses (i.e., >10 mg).

There is debate as to whether nebivolol is less[7] or more[8] β_1-selective than bisoprolol; but as nebivolol contains ISA, it is addressed under the later section on ISA.

B) High β_1-Selectivity (Bisoprolol)

i) Heart Rate

Like other non-ISA β-blockers, bisoprolol 5-20 mg decreases resting and exercise heart rate by about 20%.[9]

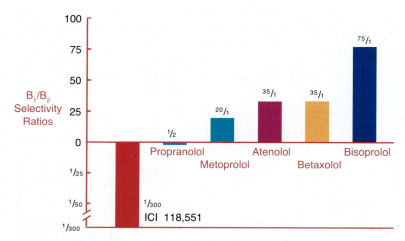

Fig. 1-5 β_1-/β_2-selectivity ratios determined in ligand-binding studies. (From Wellstein A, Palm D, Belz GG. Affinity and selectivity of beta-adrenoceptor antagonists in vitro. J Cardiovasc Pharmacol 1986;8[suppl]:S36–40.)

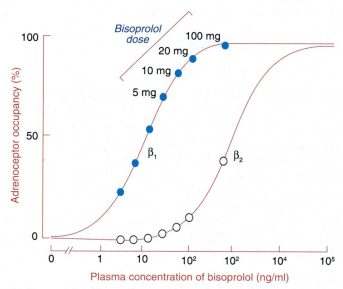

Fig. 1-6 Occupancy of β_1- and β_2-adrenoceptors after different doses of bisoprolol (rat studies). (From Brodde O. The pharmacology of bisoprolol. Rev Contemp Pharmacother 1997;8:21–33.)

ii) Cardiac Output (And Ejection Fraction and Pulmonary Capillary Pressure)

Like other non-ISA β-blockers, acutely administered bisoprolol reduces cardiac output at rest and exercise by about 20%.[7] Effects upon ejection fraction and pulmonary capillary pressure (in coronary patients) at rest and exercise were minor, indicating minimal negative inotropism.[7] However, on chronic (1-year) therapy in middle-aged hypertensive patients, bisoprolol 5 mg daily (in contrast to nonselective and moderately $β_1$-selective agents [see later]), caused no change in cardiac output, ejection fraction, or heart diameter, while at the same time effecting an antihypertensive (diastolic blood pressure [DBP]) action significantly greater than the angiotensin receptor blocker (ARB) losartan[10]—**Table 1-2a**.

iii) Muscle Blood Flow, Vascular Resistance, and Compliance

In patients with intermittent claudication, after 1 month's therapy, bisoprolol 10 mg caused no significant changes in vascular resistance or leg blood flow at rest and exercise and did not differ from the angiotensin-converting enzyme (ACE) inhibitor lisinopril in this respect; both drugs significantly improved walking distance.[11] Others have also shown that bisoprolol has no effect on vascular resistance.[12]

Vascular compliance, or elasticity, is improved by bisoprolol and pulse-wave velocity is slowed.[13]

iv) Blood Pressure

Blood pressure is positively related to both cardiac output and total peripheral resistance. Thus, because bisoprolol does not lower vascular resistance, it is clear that the initial fall in blood pressure with bisoprolol results purely from a fall in cardiac output.[7] However, if the results of the previous study comparing bisoprolol with losartan[10]—(see Table 1-2a)—are confirmed, it appears that over 1 year, there is a "hemodynamic readjustment" whereby the fall in blood pressure now stems from a fall in vascular resistance (presumably reflecting an absence of $β_2$-blockade).

Figure 1-7 illustrates the good 24-hour blood pressure control after 1 month's administration of bisoprolol 10 mg once daily.[14]

v) Airways Resistance and Alveolar Permeability

The small airways (bronchioli) are under the control of $β_2$-receptors. Thus, bisoprolol, in contrast to modestly $β_1$-selective atenolol, does not influence airways resistance (AWR) in patients with obstructive

TABLE 1-2A Effects of bisoprolol 5 mg vs losartan in hypertensives, dosed for 1 year, upon cardiac hemodynamics and blood pressure

	LOSARTAN			BISOPROLOL		
Parameter	Baseline	1-year follow-up	P value	Baseline	1-year follow-up	P value
Ejection fraction (%)	58.6±31	59.1±32	NS	60.8±33	60.3±32	NS
End-diastolic diameter	50.3±8.3	49.4±8.1	NS	49.5±7.5	50.1±8.9	NS
End-systolic diameter	31.7±2.3	32.4±2.1	NS	30.6±2.2	32.1±2.1	NS
Cardiac output (L/min)	5.63±2.13	5.67±2.7	NS	5.46±2.3	5.39±2.3	NS
Blood pressure (mm Hg)	154/92.1± 16.5/11.6	128/79.3± 12/8.4	Significant	156/94.7± 15.5/10.6	127/75.3± 12/8.8	Significant (vs. baseline for SBP and DBP and vs. losartan for DBP)

DBP, diastolic blood pressure; NS, not significant; SBP, systolic blood pressure.
From Parrinello G, Paterna S, Torres D, et al. One-year renal and cardiac effects of bisoprolol versus losartan in recently diagnosed hypertensive patients. Clin Drug Invest 2009;29:591–600.

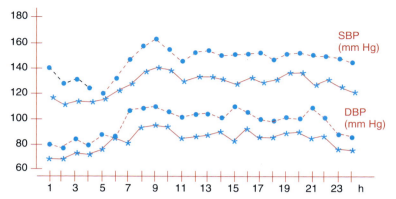

Fig. 1-7 24-hour control of blood pressure after 4-week dosing of bisoprolol 10 mg (* - - - *) compared with placebo (• - - - - •). DBP, diasystolic blood pressure; SBP, systolic blood pressure. (From Keim HJ, et al. Behandlung der leichten bis mittelschweren essentiallen hypertonic mit bisoprolol. Therapiewoche 1988;38:3507.)

airways disease[15]—**Figure 1-8**. Bisoprolol, dosed up to 10 mg daily, permits the full bronchodilator action of a β_2-stimulant such as salbutamol.[16] Thus, the avoidance of β_2-blockade offers a substantial safety factor for patients with reversible obstructive airways disease.

β-Receptors also occur on the alveolar membrane and are overwhelmingly of the β_2 variety,[17] being responsible (via regulation of

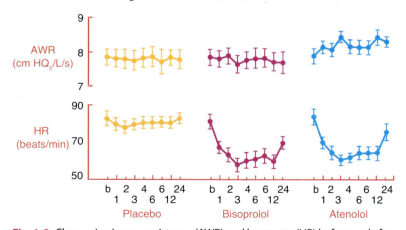

Fig. 1-8 Change in airways resistance (AWR) and heart rate (HR) before and after a single oral dose of placebo, bisoprolol 20 mg, and atenolol 100 mg (cross-over design) in 12 ischemic patients with chronic obstructive airways disease. (From Dorrow P, Bethge M, Tonnesmann V. Effects of single oral doses of bisoprolol and atenolol on airways function in non-asthmatic chronic obstructive lung disease and angina pectoris. Eur J Clin Pharmacol 1986;31:143–7.)

TABLE 1-2B Lung function with carvedilol and bisoprolol in 53 heart failure cases: randomized, Double-blind, Cross-over, 2 Months per Treatment

Double-blind, Cross-over, 2 Months per Treatment	Carbon monoxide lung diffusion (%)	Peak VO$_2$ (ml/mm/kg)
Bisoprolol	90	17.8
Carvedilol	82	17.0
P value	<.01	<.05

VO$_2$, volume of oxygen.
From Agostoni P, Contini M, Cattadori G, et al. Lung function with carvedilol and bisoprolol in chronic heart failure: is beta selectivity relevant? Eur J Heart Fail 2007;9:827–33.

sodium transport) for clearance of excess fluid in the alveolar airspace,[18] that is, β$_2$-stimulation is beneficial in pulmonary edema. Thus heat failure patients have significantly reduced carbon monoxide diffusion and exercise peak oxygen volume (VO$_2$) on nonselective carvedilol compared with bisoprolol[19]—**Table 1-2b**—exacerbated at altitude.[20]

vi) Metabolic Disturbance

As shown in (see **Table 1-1**), metabolic changes involving blood sugar and lipid disturbance are under the influence of β$_2$-receptors. Thus, bisoprolol 5-10 mg will have little, or no, effect on metabolic parameters such as lipids[21,22]—**Figure 1-9**, blood sugar/haemoglobin A1c (Hb$_{A1c}$),[23] and post-insulin blood sugar and lactate changes.[24]

vii) Neurohumoral Effects

a) Plasma Renin Activity/Angiotensin/Aldosterone Axis

In hypertensive patients, bisoprolol significantly reduced PRA,[25] the magnitude of the effect being similar to that produced by atenolol.[26] The greatest falls in PRA and blood pressure occur in those whose baseline PRA levels are high.[27]

In patients with systolic heart failure, 90% of patients respond to bisoprolol with marked falls in PRA,[28] as well as falls in angiotensin II and aldosterone levels.[29] **Table 1-2c**.

b) Plasma Catecholamine Levels

In hypertensive patients, bisoprolol has no effect upon plasma noradrenaline[25,30] concentration; and upon adrenaline levels, it has either no[30] or a depressant effect.[25]

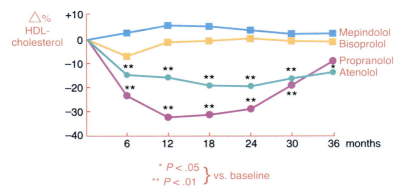

Fig. 1-9 Change in plasma triglyceride and high-density lipoprotein (HDL) levels in normocholesterolemic hypertensive patients after long-term therapy with propranolol (nonselective), atenolol (moderately β_1-selective), mepindolol (nonselective with ISA), and bisoprolol (highly β_1-selective). (From Fogari R, Zoppi A. The clinical benefits of beta-1 selectivity. Rev Contemp Pharmacother 1997;8:45–54.)

In systolic heart failure patients, bisoprolol significantly reduces plasma noradrenaline levels[29,31]— (see **Table 1-2c**). Over a 6-month period, plasma noradrenaline levels fell significantly from 533 to 402 pg/ml, compared with the significant increase in the control group from 369 to 474 pg/ml.

c) Atrial and Brain Naturetic Peptides

Atrial natriuretic peptide (ANP) and brain natriuretic peptide (BNP) are produced in cardiac myocytes in response to increased

TABLE 1-2C Effects of Bisoprolol (vs. Randomised Control) over 6 Months upon Neurohumoral Parameters in 54 Patients with Moderate/Severe Heart Failure

	BISOPROLOL		
Parameters	Baseline	6 Months	Stastistical Significance
Noradrenaline conc (pg/ml)	533	402	$P < .05$
Plasma, renin activity (ng/ml/hr)	1.2	0.42	$P < .05$
Plasma angiotensin II (pg/ml)	17.1	13.1	$P < .05$
Plasma aldosterone (pg/ml)	173	148	$P < .05$

From Belenkov IN, Skvortsov AA, Mareev V, et al. Clinical, haemodynamic and neurohumoral effects of long-term therapy of patients with heart failure with the beta-blocker bisoprolol. Kardiologia 2003;43:10-21.

myocardial wall stress. High levels of ANP and BNP in heart failure are linked to a poor prognosis.

In middle-aged hypertensive patients, bisoprolol was the best antihypertensive agent compared with the α-blockade, calcium blockers, ACE inhibitors, and diuretic therapy.[31] In that study, bisoprolol increased BNP levels threefold, in contrast to the other agents.[31]

In systolic heart failure patients, bisoprolol significantly lowered both ANP and BNP concentrations.[32] The greatest falls in BNP occurred in the β_1-receptor genotypes CC and CB (comprising 90% of all cases), in which the fall was some 35%-37%.[33]

viii) Adrenaline Interaction

Adrenaline (epinephrine) is a stimulant of the β_1-, β_2-, and α-receptors and is markedly raised during cigarette smoking[34] and insulin-induced hypoglycemia.[35] In the presence of β_1- and β_2-blockade, unopposed α-constriction occurs, leading to marked hypertensive responses and reflex marked brachycardia.[35] These changes are absent when β_2-blockade is avoided (i.e., bisoprolol 5-10 mg)[36]—Figure 1-10.

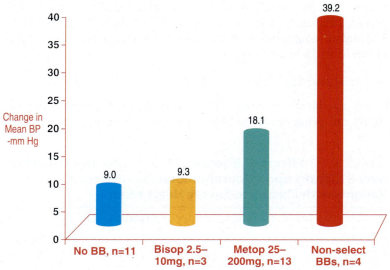

Fig. 1-10 Interaction between adrenaline (epinephrine) and β-blockers (BB); compared with control, nonselective and moderately β_1-selective (metoprolol) agents cause a significant increase in mean blood pressure (BP), in contrast to highly β_1-selective bisoprolol with which no BP change occurs. (From Tarnow J, Muller RK. Cardiovascular effect of low-dose epinephrine infusions in relation to the extent of preoperative beta-blockade. Anaesthesiology 1991;74:1035–43.)

C) Nonselectivity with No ISA (Propranolol, Timolol) and Modest β_1-Selectivity with No ISA (Atenolol, Metoprolol)

i) Heart Rate

As with highly β_1-selective bisoprolol, nonselective propranolol and timolol and modestly β_1-selective atenolol and metoprolol lower heart rates by about 20%[37]—**Figure 1-11**.

ii) Cardiac output

As with acute β_1-selective bisoprolol,[7] propranolol, timolol, atenolol, and metoprolol all decrease cardiac output by about 20%[37] (see **Figure 1-11**); but unlike chronically dosed bisoprolol,[8] with propranolol, timolol, atenolol, and metoprolol, the cardiac output remains reduced on chronic therapy (see **Figure 1-11**).

iii) Vascular Resistance, Compliance, and Muscle Blood Flow

Modestly β-selective atenolol and metoprolol increase vascular resistance on chronic oral therapy, by about 10%, and nonselective propranolol and timolol increase it by about 15%[37] (see **Figure 1-11**). This is in contrast with acute therapy in which vascular resistance is increased by 20%-30% by all four agents[37] (see **Figure 1-11**). The fall in vascular resistance over the next few days is responsible for the fall in blood pressure noted in responders on chronic therapy.

In patients with intermittent claudication, leg blood flow at rest is unaffected by propranolol.[40,41] During/after exercise, blood flow either falls[40] or remains the same[41] and walking distance (vs. placebo) is not impaired.[41]

Like propranolol, neither atenolol nor metoprolol decrease resting muscle blood flow,[40,42] but a decrease in exercise blood flows has been reported in claudicants with atenolol[40] but not metoprolol.[41] Walking distance was not shortened by metoprolol in claudicants.[41,43]

Propranolol may worsen vascular compliance,[44] whereas atenolol appears neutral.[45]

iv) Blood Pressure (Including Effects of Age and Race)

In hypertensive patients, pure β_2-blockade (e.g. ICI 118.551) was associated with a 7-to-5-mm Hg increase in blood pressure compared with placebo.[46] It would thus be predicted that nonselective and partially β_1-selective β-blockers might be less effective in

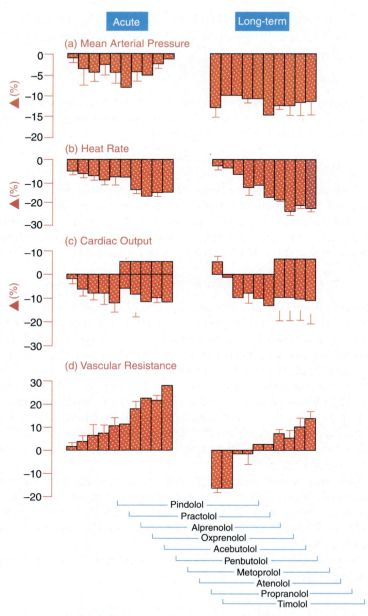

Fig. 1-11 Hemodynamic consequences of acute and chronic dosing with β-blockers with different degrees of ISA—pindolol, practolol, alprenolol, oxprenolol, acebutolol, and penbutolol—compared with those without ISA. (From Man in't Veld AJ, Schalekamp AD. Effects of ten different beta-blockers on hemodynamics, plasma rennin activity and plasma norepinephrine in hypertension. J Cardiovasc Pharmacol 1983;5:S30–45.)

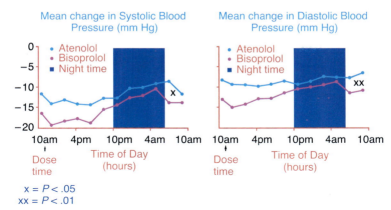

Fig. 1-12 The effects of atenolol (50-100 mg od) and bisoprolol (10-20 mg od) upon 24-hour blood pressure control in 659 hypertensive patients. (From Neutel JM, Smith DH, Ram CV, et al. Application of ambulatory blood pressure monitoring in differentiating between antihypertensive agents. Am J Med 1993;94:181–7.)

lowering blood pressure compared with an agent that blocked no β_2-receptors (i.e., bisoprolol 5-10 mg[7] (see **Figure 1-6**).

Certainly, in the numerous comparisons between nonselective propranolol and modest β_1-selective atenolol in hypertensive patients, on average, atenolol lowered DBP about 4 mm Hg more than propranolol.[47] In turn, atenolol was inferior to highly β_1-selective bisoprolol by about 4 mm Hg[48] as assessed by 24-hour ambulatory monitoring. The advantage of bisoprolol over atenolol was particularly notable during the early morning "vulnerable period" **Figure 1-12**.

Blood pressure control by β-blockade is, to a degree, age-dependent. The elderly, generally, respond less well than young/middle-aged hypertensive patients[49]—**Figure 1-13**. This is likely to be due, at least partly, to the low renin levels that predominate in the elderly. Thus, the fall in blood pressure is good in young patients[49] (see **Figure 1-13**)—in whom renin levels tend to be high but poor in the elderly. The renin/blood pressure relationship and the response to propranolol[50] are shown in **Figure 1-14**. However, another factor in the poor response to β-blockade in the elderly is decreased β_1-sensitivity.[51]

Race is important. Black patients, mostly, respond poorly to propranolol[52]—**Figure 1-15**—and this is likely to be due to low (usually) renin levels that predominate in black hypertensive patients.[53] The same applies to atenolol[54] and metoprolol.[55] However, β_1-blockers can be effective antihypertensive agents in some black subjects—again, probably renin-related.[56]

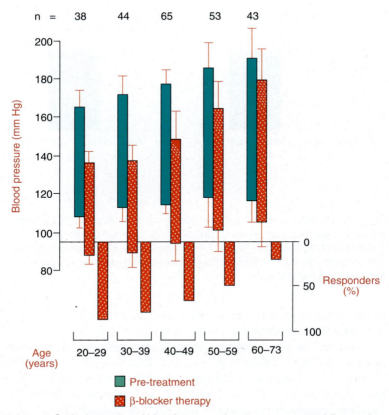

Fig. 1-13 β-Blockers control blood pressure best in younger/middle-aged hypertensives; responders are classified on the basis of achieving diastolic blood pressure of 95 mm Hg. (From Buhler FR. Age and cardiovascular response adaptation. Determination of an antihypertensive treatment concept primary based on beta-blockers and calcium entry blockers. Hypertension 1983;5:III94–100.)

By contrast, southern Asian,[57] Chinese,[58] and Japanese[59] hypertensive patients respond to β-blockers in a way similar to that of Caucasians.

Effects on central (aortic) blood pressure are covered in the Hypertension chapter.

v) Airways Resistance

Patients with labile reversible airways disease are potentially vulnerable to β-blockade. **Figure 1-16a**[60] shows the effects of various

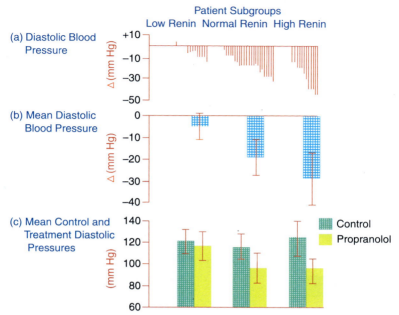

Fig. 1-14 Control of blood pressure, in relation to plasma renin status, with β-blocker (propranolol). Best control occurs in those with high renin status. (From Buhler FR, Laragh JH, Baer L, et al. Propranolol inhibition of renin secretion. N Engl J Med 1972;287:1209–14.)

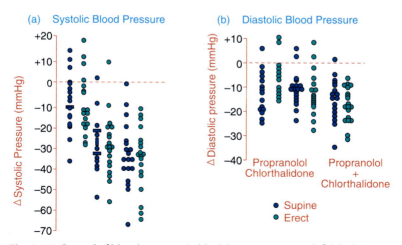

Fig. 1-15 Control of blood pressure in black hypertensives with β-blocker (propranolol), diuretic, and the combination of the two. Poor control occurs with propranolol alone. (From Richardson DW, Freund J, Gear AS, et al. Effect of propranolol on elevated arterial blood pressure. Circulation 1968;37:534–42.)

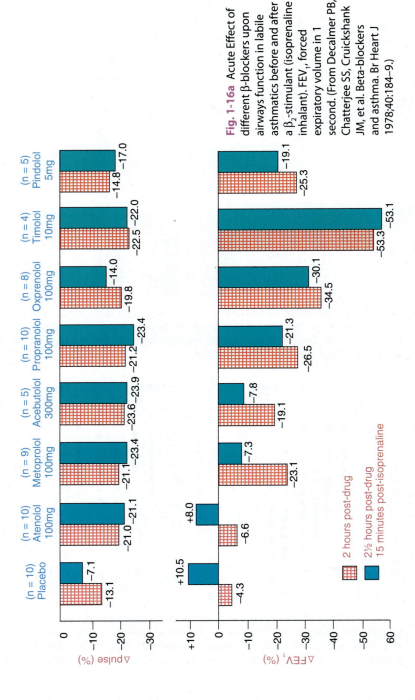

Fig. 1-16a Acute Effect of different β-blockers upon airways function in labile asthmatics before and after a β_2-stimulant (isoprenaline inhalant). FEV_1, forced expiratory volume in 1 second. (From Decalmer PB, Chatterjee SS, Cruickshank JM, et al. Beta-blockers and asthma. Br Heart J 1978;40:184–9.)

β-blockers upon forced expiratory volume in 1 second (FEV$_1$) before and after the β$_2$-stimulant isoprenaline. It is clear that modestly β$_1$-selective atenolol was the least likely to induce a fall in FEV$_1$ and largely permitted isoprenaline-induced bronchodilatation. Partially β$_1$-selective metoprolol and accebutalol caused a 20% fall in FEV$_1$ and only partly permitted the beneficial isoprenaline-induced bronchodilatation. The remaining nonselective β-blockers (including those with ISA—i.e., oxprenolol and pindolol) induced a marked fall in FEV$_1$, which was nonresponsive to β$_2$-stimulation.

The advantage of bisoprolol over atenolol under such circumstances has already been described[15]—(see **Figure 1-8**).

vi) Metabolic Disturbance

As already mentioned, potentially harmful metabolic changes are under the influence of the β$_2$-blockade—(see **Table 1-1**). Thus, metabolic disturbance involving blood sugar, Hb$_{A1c}$, insulin resistance, and lipids will be particularly apparent with nonselective β-blockers like propranolol, less so with modestly β$_1$-selective agents like atenolol and metoprolol, and essentially absent at lower doses (5-10 mg) of highly β$_1$-selective bisoprolol[21–23,61]—(see **Figure 1-9**). The clinical importance of such changes is debatable.[61]

vii) Neurohumoral Effects

a) Plasma Renin/Angiotensin/Aldosterone Axis

In hypertension, nonselective β-blockers like propranolol, timolol, and nadolol all markedly lower PRA (1). In the case of propranolol, the greatest falls in PRA and aldosterone levels occur in those patients with the highest PRA baseline levels[62]—(see **Figure 1-14**).

Moderately β$_1$-selective agents like atenolol and metoprolol lower PRA levels in hypertensive patients to a similar degree as nonselective β-blockers.[63]

In systolic heart failure patients on ACE inhibitors, metoprolol initially causes a marked fall in PRA levels, but after 1 year, this effect had worn off.[64] In that same study, there was a strong trend to lower aldosterone levels at 1 year.

b) Plasma Catecholamine Concentrations

In hypertensive patients, nonselective nadolol[65] and propranolol[63] markedly increase plasma noradrenaline levels, as do moderately β$_1$-selective atenolol and metoprolol[63]—**Figure 1-16b**.

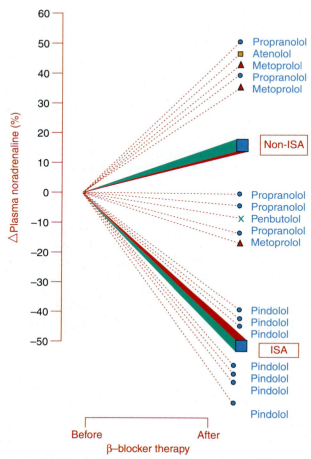

Fig. 1-16b Effect of various β-blockers upon plasma noradrenaline levels in resting hypertensive patients; ISA (pindolol) results in a fall in noradrenaline concentration. (From Man in't Veld AJ, Schalekamp AD. Effects of ten different beta-blockers on hemodynamics, plasma renin activity and plasma norepinephrine in hypertension. J Cardiovasc Pharmacol 1983;5:S30–45.)

c) Atrial and Brain Natriuretic Peptides

In patients with coronary heart disease, β-blockers increase the exercise-induced increases in ANP and BNP.[66]

In systolic heart failure, early dosing with metoprolol was associated with a rise in BNP[67] levels, which later fell significantly on chronic dosing, the degree of fall being a good prognostic marker.[68]

viii) Adrenaline Interaction

When propranolol is administered intravenously in the presence of intravenous adrenaline, the increase in mean blood pressure can be marked (60 mm Hg), but less so with modestly β_1-selective atenolol and metoprolol[69]—**Figure 1-17**). With oral β-blockade, the increase in mean blood pressure is still substantial (~30 mm Hg) with nonselective agents and 9-10 mm Hg with modestly selective metoprolol[36]—(see **Figure 1-10**). This hypertensive response is undoubtedly responsible for the absence of benefit (no reduction in the frequency of myocardial infarction) in smokers who receive nonselective β-blockers (propranolol and oxprenolol) and poorly selective metoprolol and atenolol (see later, in the Hypertension chapter), and is potentially dangerous for insulin-dependent diabetics receiving nonselective or modestly selective β-blockers.

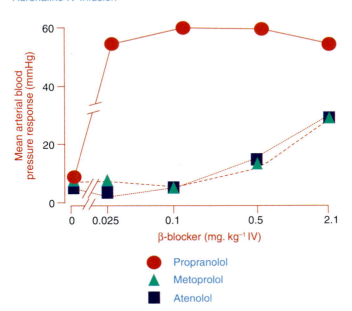

Fig. 1-17 Effect of propranolol, atenolol, and metoprolol upon blood pressure in the presence of high adrenaline levels. Marked hypertensive response occurs with nonselective propranolol. (From Ablad B, Carlsson E, Johnsson G, Regardh CG. Metoprolol. In Scrabine A [ed]. Pharmacology of antihypertensive drugs. New York: Raven Press, 1980; pp 247–62.)

D) β-Blockers with ISA (Pindolol, Oxprenolol, and Nebivolol)

The ISA of both pindolol and oxprenolol acts through the β_1-and β_2-receptors.[1] Though some claim that nebivolol contains no ISA,[70,71] others disagree.[74,75] The ISA of nebivolol may act through either (or both) the β_2- or the β_3-receptor.[61] Both β_2-[72] and β_3-[73] stimulation results in nitric oxide (NO) release. In human coronary artery[74] and ventricle,[75] the ISA of nebivolol appears to act through the β_3-receptor. There is much debate concerning the β_3-adrenoceptor as a therapeutic target.[76]

i) Heart Rate

Heart rate reduction is less with agents containing ISA[37]—(see **Figure 1-11**)—and at night (when background sympathetic nerve activity is low—(see **Figure 1-3**)), the heart rate may even be increased by pindolol[77]—**Figure 1-18**.

ii) Cardiac Output

Suppression of cardiac output is less with β-blockers with β_1 or β_2 ISA and may even be increased[37]—(see **Figure 1-11**). However, β_3-stimulation, as occurs with nebivolol, and β_2-stimulation with bopindolol and celiprolol,[61] results in NO release. β_3-Stimulation, or NO, can have a cardiac-depressant effect,[78] which may not be beneficial for heart failure subjects.[79]

iii) Muscle Blood Flow and Vascular Resistance

In contrast to non-ISA β-blockers, vascular resistance may actually fall with β-blockers containing ISA, such as pindolol and practolol[37]—(see **Figure 1-11**)—and nebivolol.[38] This may be accompanied by an increase in resting muscle blood flow.[1] However, in claudicants, calf blood flow decreases and pain-free walking distance decreases (even more so than with atenolol)[80]—**Figure 1-19**. It is possible that some form of "vascular steal" may be responsible.

It is possible that the vasodilating action of nebivolol involves, in part, estrogen-receptor stimulation, because the estrogen-antagonist tamoxifen diminishes nebivolol's vasodilator action.[39]

iv) Blood Pressure

The fall in daytime blood pressure with pindolol and oxprenolol was similar to that with other β-blockers[37]—(see **Figure 1-11**).

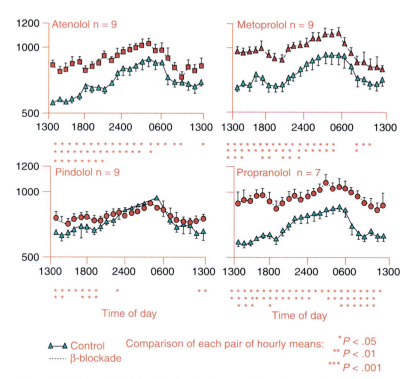

Fig. 1-18 Effect of ISA (pindolol) and absence of ISA (atenolol, metoprolol, and propranolol) upon pulse interval (long interval = slower heart rate [HR]) in hypertensive patients. Pindolol increases HR at night. (From Floras JS, Jones JV, Hassan MO, Slight P. Ambulatory blood pressure during once daily randomised double-blind administration of atenolol, metoprolol, pindolol and slow release propranolol. Br Med J 1982;285:1387–92.)

However, nocturnal blood pressure (a powerful predictor of future cardiovascular events), which is well controlled by β-blockers like bisoprolol[48]—(see **Figure 1-12**), is not lowered by pindolol[81]— **Figure 1-20**.

Effects on central blood pressure are covered in the Hypertension chapter.

v) Airways Resistance

Nonselective β-blockers with ISA, such as pindolol, act like pure β-blockers in patients with reversible airways disease, inducing a fall in FEV_1 and inhibiting the effects of $β_2$-stimulants[60] —(see **Figure 1-16a**).

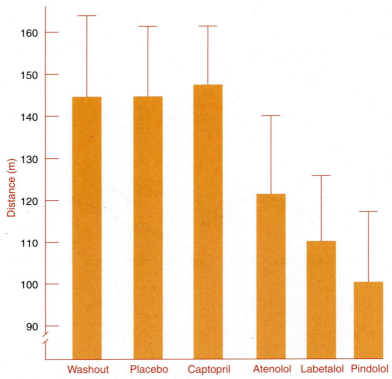

Fig. 1-19 Effect of antihypertensive drugs on walking distance in hypertensive patients with intermittent claudication. Vasodilating β-blockers (labetalol with additional α-blocking action and pindolol with high ISA) significantly shorten pain-free walking distance. (From Roberts DH, Tsao Y, McLoughlin GA, Breckeridge A. Placebo-controlled comparison of captopril, atenolol and pindolol in hypertension complicated by intermittent claudication. Lancet 1987;2:650–3.)

vi) Metabolic Disturbance

β-Blockers containing ISA cause little or no metabolic disturbance[21] —(see **Figure 1-9**). Nebivolol has no effect on insulin sensitivity.[82] The clinical significance of these findings is debatable.[61]

vii) Neurohumoral Effects

a) Plasma Renin/Angiotensin/Aldosterone Axis

In patients with hypertension, β-blockers with ISA, such as pindolol and oxprenolol, lower PRA considerably less than β-blockers without ISA[63]—**Figure 1-21**. These changes, plus the fall in aldosterone levels, do not correlate with the fall in blood pressure.[83]

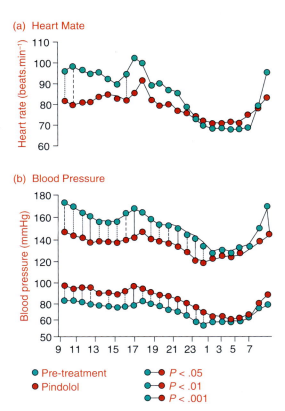

Fig. 1-20 Effects of chronic pindolol (high ISA) therapy upon 24-hour blood pressure and heart rate. No antihypertensive efficacy at night. (From Mann S, Millar-Craig M, Balasubrananian V, Raftery EB. Once daily beta-blockade in hypertension: an ambulatory assessment. Br J Clin Pharmacol 1981;12:223–8.)

b) Plasma Catecholamine Levels

In hypertension, unlike nonselective and modestly β_1-selective β-blockers (atenolol and metoprolol), pindolol (with high ISA) markedly lowers plasma noradrenaline levels[63]—(see **Figure 1-16b**). As for the decrease in PRA, the fall in blood pressure did not relate to the decrease in plasma noradrenaline.[83]

viii) Adrenaline Interaction

Nonselective β-blockers with ISA interact with adrenaline in a fashion similar to that of nonselective β-blockers without ISA (i.e., a marked increase in blood pressure can occur)[36]—(see **Figure 1-10**).

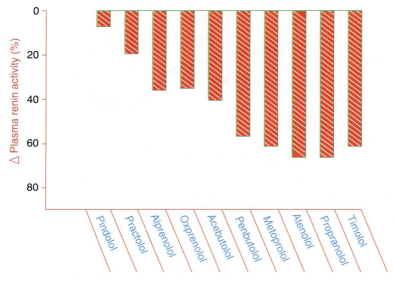

Fig. 1-21 β-Blockers with ISA (e.g., pindolol) have less effect on suppressing plasma renin activity (PRA) than β-blockers without ISA (e.g., propranolol). (From Man in't Veld AJ, Schalekamp AD. Effects of ten different beta-blockers on hemodynamics, plasma rennin activity and plasma norepinephrine in hypertension. J Cardiovasc Pharmacol 1983;5:S30–45.)

E) Nonselective β/α-Blockers (Labetalol and Carvedilol)

i) Heart Rate

Owing to α-blocking-induced vasodilatation, the effects of labetalol and carvedilol upon heart rate are somewhat less that with a classic β-blocker like propranolol.[84] With intravenous labetalol, there is little bradycardic effect[84]—**Figure 1-22**. Given orally, both labetalol and carvedilol lower heart rate at rest and exercise but to a lesser extent than a straight β-blocker.[85]

ii) Cardiac Output

Intravenous labetalol has little effect on cardiac output[84]—(**see Figure 1-22**)—and the same applies to oral labetalol and carvedilol.[85]

iii) Muscle Blood Flow and Vascular Resistance

Intravenous labetalol lowers peripheral resistance[84]—(**see Figure 1-22**)—but has little effect on muscle blood flow. In patients with

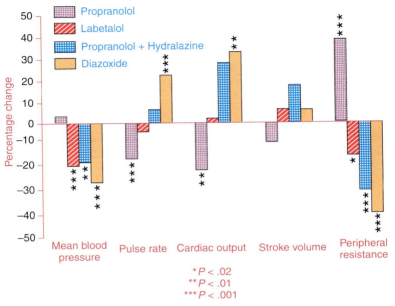

Fig. 1-22 Hemodynamic changes in hypertensive patients following intravenous labetalol, propranolol, diazoxide, and the combination of propranolol and hydralazine. (From Prichard 1975.)

intermittent claudication, oral labetalol tended to lower limb blood flow and, compared with placebo, significantly decreased pain-free walking distance[80]—(see **Figure 1-19**). The combination of β_1-blockade plus vasodilatation appears to cause a "vascular steal" effect, noted also with pindolol[80]—(see **Figure 1-19**)—and the combination of atenolol and nifedipine[86] in which not only was walking distance reduced but also the temperature in the affected foot was decreased.

iv) Blood Pressure

Unlike intravenous propranolol, intravenous labetalol effects a marked fall in blood pressure[84]—(see **Figure 1-22**). Intravenous labetalol may thus be a useful agent for the treatment of hypertensive crises.

Oral labetalol lowers both resting and exercise blood pressure,[85] though resting blood pressure may be less well controlled than with other β-blockers,[87] and at higher levels of exercise, the postexercise period can be linked to dizziness and near-syncope. The first dose of oral carvedilol can induce syncope in elderly hypertensive patients.[88]

v) Airways Resistance and Alveolar Permeability

As with other nonselective β-blockers, severe bronchospasm has been reported with labetalol[85] and carvedilol.[89] Carvedilol is inferior to bisoprolol regarding alveolar permeability, resulting in lower peak VO_2 levels in heart failure patients (worse at altitude).[19,20]

vi) Metabolic Disturbance

Metabolic disturbances involving blood lipids, blood glucose, and insulin resistance do not occur with carvedilol.[85]

vii) Neurohumoral Effects
a) Plasma Renin/Angiotensin/Aldosterone Axis

In hypertension, labetalol has been shown to lower PRA.[90] Carvedilol significantly lowers both PRA and aldosterone levels.[91]

In heart failure patients on ACE inhibitors, carvedilol induced an acute fall in PRA, but this was not apparent after 1 year's therapy.[64]

b) Plasma Catecholamine Levels

In hypertension, labetalol induces an increase in plasma noradrenaline levels.[90] Carvedilol causes no change in adrenaline concentration.[92]

In heart failure, carvedilol has been shown to decrease plasma noradrenaline levels.[93]

c) Atrial and Brain Natriuretic Peptides

In hypertension, carvedilol causes an increase in ANP levels.[94]

In heart failure, one study has suggested that after 6 months of therapy, carvedilol, in contrast to an ACE inhibitor, did not reduce, indeed increased, BNP levels.[95] By contrast, others have shown that chronic therapy with carvedilol decreases both BNP[64,68] and ANP[64] and that the fall in BNP is linked to a good prognosis.[68]

viii) Adrenaline Interaction

Because of the accompanying α-blockade, the hypertensive response observed with nonselective β-blockers like propranolol in the presence of high adrenaline levels[36,69]—(see Figures 1-10 and 1-17)—is not seen with labetalol.[96] Indeed, intravenous followed by oral labetalol is highly effective in lowering blood pressure and symptoms of pheochromocytoma[97]—Figure 1-23.

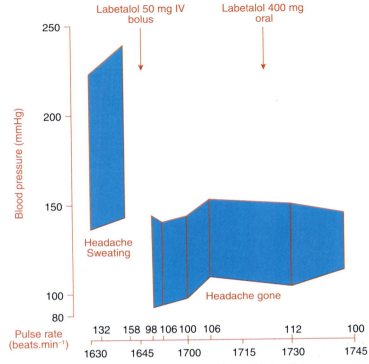

Fig. 1-23 The effect of intravenous, followed by oral, labetalol upon blood pressure and symptoms of a patient in hypertensive crisis due to a pheochromocytoma. (From Rosei EA, Brown JJ, Lever AF, et al. Treatment of phaeochromacytoma and of clonidine withdrawal hypertension with labetalol. Br J Clin Pharmacol 1976;3[suppl]:809–15.)

3. Pharmacokinetics

A major determinant of a pharmacokinetic profile of a drug, including β-blockers, is its lipid solubility (lipophilicity). As a general rule, highly lipid-soluble β-blockers, such as propranolol or metoprolol, will (a) be rapidly and completely absorbed from the gastrointestinal tract, (b) be heavily metabolized in the liver, (c) be highly bound to plasma proteins, (d) be widely distributed to all body tissues and compartments, and (e) have short plasma (and pharmacological) half-lives (which can be lengthened by slow-release formulations).

The reverse holds true for highly water-soluble, renally excreted agents such as atenolol, nadolol, and sotalol.

Table 1-3 illustrates the essential pharmacokinetic profiles of the most commonly used β-blockers.

TABLE 1-3 Pharmacokinetic profiles of some commonly used β-blockers

β-Blocker	Lipid solubility X = water-soluble xxxx = lipid soluble	Extent Absorbed (% dose)	Time to peak blood level (hr)	Plasma half-life (hr)	First-pass (liver) elimination (%)	Systemic bioavailability (%)	Metabolized (hepatic)	Active Metabolite
Atenolol	x	40-60	2-4	6-10	0	50	No	No
Bisoprolol	xx	>90%	2-3	10-12	<10	90	Yes (50%)	No
Carvedilol	xxx	85	1.5	6-7	60-75	25	Yes	No
Labetalol	xxxx	>90	1-2	3-6	60-70	30-40	Yes	No
Metoprolol tartrate	xxx	>90	1-3	3-4	25-50	50-75	Yes	Yes (weak)
slow release-succinate				12-24				
Nebivolol	xxxx	90	1-4	13	70	12-96	Yes	yes
Oxprenolol	xxx	90	1-1.5	1-2	25-80	20-75	Yes	No
Pindolol	xx	>90	0.5-1	2-5	20	80	Yes	No
Propranolol	xxxx	>90	1-3	3-4	70	30	Yes	Yes
slow release				10-12				
Sotalol	x	>90	2-3	7-15	0	>90	No	No
Timolol	xxx	>90	1-4	2-5	50-60	40-50	Yes	No

From Cruickshank JM, Prichard BNC. Beta-blockers in clinical practice. 2nd ed. Edinburgh: Churchill Livingstone; 1994, pp 1-351.

A) Absorption and Bioavailability

i) Effects of Food

The absorption of water-soluble, nonmetabolized β-blockers like sotalol and atenolol is decreased by about 20% by food.[98] By contrast, the bioavailability of lipophilic, well-absorbed agents like metoprolol and propranolol is increased by food[99] (possibly due to the increase in portal blood flow creating a functional shunt resulting in decreased clearance).

Food has no effect on the absorption/bioavailability of a β-blocker like bisoprolol with balanced (renal/hepatic) excretion/metabolism.[100]

ii) Effects of Other Drugs

Both calcium and aluminium hydroxide decrease the absorption of atenolol by about 25%. Frusimide has no effect on the absorption of atenolol but alters the clearance of propranolol, resulting in a 50% increase in blood levels with increased β-blockade.[101] Ampicillin reduces the absorption of atenolol by about 50%, with loss of β-blockade.[102] The H_2-blocker cimetidene increased the blood levels of propranolol by about 50% but had no effect on atenolol.[103]

Chronic doses of metoprolol and propranolol, but not atenolol, increase blood levels of diazepam by about 25%.[104] Propranolol can cause a significant, clinically relevant increase in serum warfarin and prothrombin time[105]—**Figure 1-24**. Both quinidine[106] and propafenone[107] markedly increase (threefold) blood levels of metoprolol—**Figure 1-25**.

B) Distribution

High lipid solubility is associated with large volumes of distribution, particular in the obese in whom propranolol's half-life is extended.[108]

Particularly important is the ability of β-blockers to cross the blood-brain banner. In humans, in contrast to water-soluble atenolol, lipophilic agents propranolol, oxprenolol, and metoprolol appeared in high concentration in brain tissue[109]—**Figure 1-26**.

C) Elimination and Metabolism

i) Renal

Water-soluble agents like atenolol and sotalol, which are solely renally excreted, accumulate in the presence of renal dysfunction resulting in a marked extension of elimination half-lives[110]—

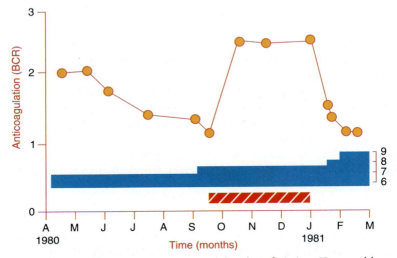

Fig. 1-24 Drug interaction with propranolol and warfarin in a 63-year-old man with deep vein thrombosis. Propranolol administration resulted in a marked increase in prothrombin time. BCR, British Corrected Ratio. (From Bax ND, Lennard MS, Al-Asady S, et al. Inhibition of drug metabolism by beta-blockers. Drugs 1983;25:121–6.)

Figure 1-27: dosage adjustment is necessary or, preferably, use a β-blocker that is removed by heptic metabolism (see later) or has a balanced mode of excretion between kidney and liver, like bisoprolol.[111] Water-soluble agents like atenolol can be removed with ease via hemodialysis,[112] as can bisoprolol.[113]

ii) Hepatic Metabolism

In patients with hepatic dysfunction, lipophilic agents like propranolol, oxprenolol, and metoprolol, which are eliminated via hepatic metabolism, will accumulate[114,115]—**Figure 1-28**—and require dosage-adjustment, unlike water-soluble sotalol and atenolol, which do not.[115]

As for renal failure, an agent with balanced excretion like bisoprolol[111] could also be considered. **Figures 1-29a and 1-29b** illustrate this point well,[116] where accumulation of the drug occurs only in the severest forms of liver and renal failure.

iii) Elderly

Renal clearance is impaired in the elderly, with glomerular filtration rate falling 35%-40% in those aged 60-80 years.[117] Likewise,

(Text continues on page 36)

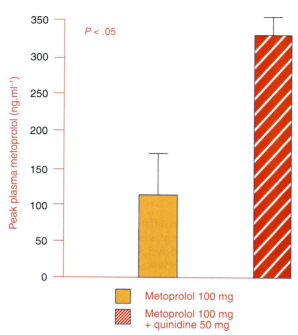

Fig. 1-25 In five extensive metabolizers of metoprolol, oral quinidine caused a threefold increase in peak metoprolol plasma concentration. (From Leeman T, Dayer P, Meyer UA. Single dose quinidine treatment inhibits metoprolol oxidation in extensive metabolisers. Eur J Clin Pharmacol 1986;29:739–41.)

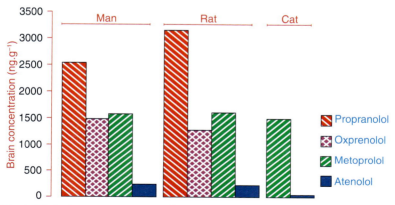

Fig. 1-26 Brain concentrations of β-blockers in man, rat, and cat. Note very low concentrations of hydrophilic atenolol compared with the high concentrations of the three lipophilic agents propranolol, metoprolol, and oxprenolol. (From Neil-Dwyer G, Bartlett J, McAinsh J, Cruickshank JM. Beta-blockers and the blood brain barrier. Br J Clin Pharmacol 1981;11:549–53.)

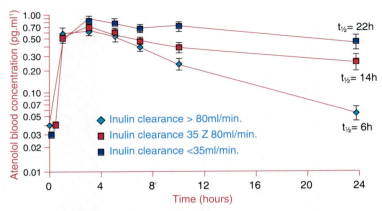

Fig. 1-27 Elimination of atenolol at different degrees of renal dysfunction. Note the mean elimination half-life of atenolol was approximately threefold longer in patients with severe renal dysfunction compared with those with normal function. (From McAinsh J. Clinical pharmacokinetics of atenolol. Postgrad Med J 1977;53(suppl 3):74–8.)

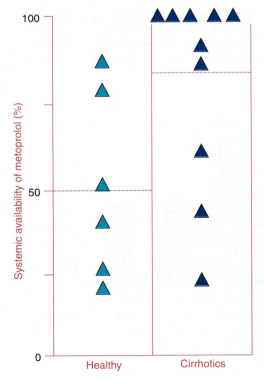

Fig. 1-28 In 10 subjects with hepatic cirrhosis, the systemic bioavailability of metoprolol is increased to 84% compared with 50% in 6 healthy subjects. (From Regardh C-G, Jordo L, Ervic M, et al. Pharmacokinetics of metoprolol in patients with hepatic cirrhosis. Clin Pharmacokinet 1981;6:375–88.).

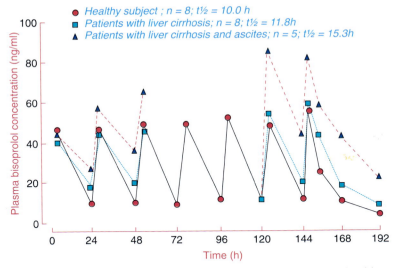

Fig. 1-29a Mean plasma levels of chronic oral (10 mg) bisoprolol in healthy and cirrhotic subjects. Only in severe cases with ascites does the half-life of bisoprolol increase by about 50%. (From Leopold G, Kutz K. Bisoprolol: pharmacokinetic profile. Rev Contemp Pharmacother 1997;8:35–43.)

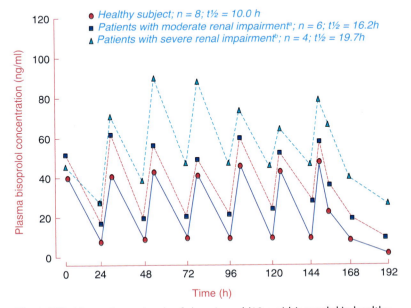

Fig. 1-29b Mean plasma levels of chronic oral (10 mg) bisoprolol in healthy and renally impaired subjects. Only in severe impairment does the half-life of bisoprolol markedly increase. (From Leopold G, Kutz K. Bisoprolol: pharmacokinetic profile. Rev Contemp Pharmacother 1997;8:35–43.)

hepatic blood-flow is reduced 40%-45% in the elderly[118] with impairment of liver enzyme action.[119]

Thus, blood levels of both renally excreted atenolol[120] and hepatically metabolized propranolol[121]—**Figure 1-30**—and metoprolol[122] are raised, possibly necessitating dosage adjustment. A β-blocker with balanced excretion (between kidney and liver; i.e. bisoprolol) has the same elimination half-life in both young and old, thus requiring no dosage adjustment.[111]

iv) Slow Metabolizers (Genetic Polymorphism)

Genetic polymorphism results in two distinct phenotypes—extensive and poor metabolizers—relevant particularly to the hepatic cytochrome P450 system. Thus, a metabolized β-blocker such as metoprolol exhibits a 17-fold variation in plasma concentration in patients taking the same dose.[123] Poor metabolizers of metoprolol can exhibit a 3-fold increase in peak blood levels plus an extended plasma half-life[124]—**Figure 1-31**—potentially resulting in an unexpected increased pharmacologic response[125] and side effects. The same applies to nebivolol.[71]

Such poor metabolizers account for about 8%-10% of the U.K. white population[126] and possibly 30% of Chinese[127].

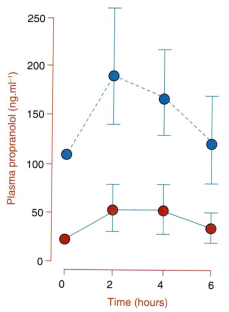

Fig. 1-30 The effect of age on propranolol (40 mg qd) blood levels in five elderly (*blue circles*) and four young (*Red circles*) hypertensive patients. Note almost a fourfold increase in peak blood levels in the elderly. (From Regardh C-G. Pharmacokinetic aspects of some beta-blockers. Acta Med Scand 1982;665[suppl]:49–60.)

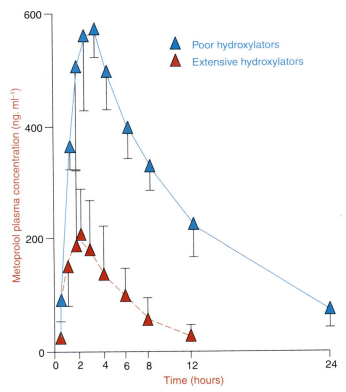

Fig. 1-31 Effect of the oxidation phenotype on the metabolism of metoprolol (200 mg). Note a threefold increase in the peak blood levels in the six poor versus the six extensive metabolizers. (From Lennard MS, Silas JH, Freestone S, et al. Oxidation phenotype—a major determinant of metoprolol metabolism and response. N Engl J Med 1982;307:1558–60.)

SUMMARY AND CONCLUSIONS

1. The adrenoceptors α_1, α_2, β_1, β_2, and β_3 are distributed throughout the body. β_1-Receptors occur mainly in the heart and kidney (stimulation resulting in renin release from the juxtaglomerular apparatus).
2. The endogenous catecholamines noradrenaline and adrenaline stimulate the adrenoceptors: β_1 and α in the case of noradrenaline and β_1, β_2, and α in the case of adrenaline.
3. β-Blockers occupy the β-receptors (and sometimes also the α-receptors, e.g., labetalol and carvediolol) and competitively inhibit the effects of adrenaline and noradrenaline (the

degree of inhibition/response will depend on the patient's β-receptor genotype—pharmacogenetics); some β-blockers not only inhibit the effects of adrenaline and noradrenaline but also partially stimulate the receptor—ISA.
4. β-Blockers occupy the $β_1$- and $β_2$-receptors to different degrees, as reflected in the $β_1$-/$β_2$-selectivity ratios; ICI 118.551 is highly $β_2$-selective, bisoprolol is highly $β_1$-selective, with intermediary positions held by propranolol and oxprenolol (both nonselective) and atenolol and metoprolol (both moderately $β_1$-selective).
5. Resting and exercise heart rate are decreased by about 20%, but less so by β-blockers with ISA or accompanying α-blockade.
6. Cardiac output is reduced acutely by β-blockers by about 20%, but less so if ISA is present (and may even be increased with high levels of ISA, e.g., pindolol). With chronic therapy, the cardiac output remains low with nonselective and moderately $β_1$-selective agents but returns to baseline levels with highly $β_1$-selective bisoprolol (1 year's therapy), presumably reflecting an absence of $β_2$-blockade.
7. Vascular resistance is increased by about 15% with chronically dosed nonselective agents, 10% by modestly $β_1$-selective (atenolol, metoprolol), and decreased by β-blockers with high levels of $β_2$ ISA (pindolol) or α-blockade (carvedilol), and after long-term, low-dose highly $β_1$-selective bisoprolol in hypertensive patients; muscle blood flow and walking distance (intermittent claudication) are little affected by β-blockers.
8. Blood pressure is increased by $β_2$-blockade via vasoconstriction. Thus, an absence of $β_2$-blockade (bisoprolol) is associated with better blood pressure control (in young/middle-aged diastolic hypertensive patients, probably overweight, with high renin/sympathetic nerve activity) than with nonselective (e.g., propranolol) or modestly selective (e.g., atenolol, metoprolol) β-blockers. α-Blockade (e.g., carvedilol) is associated with postural falls in blood pressure (particularly on first dose). $β_2$ (e.g. pindolol) and $β_3$ (e.g. nebivolol) ISA lowers blood pressure mainly via a fall in peripheral resistance. Classic β-blockers are less effective in lowering the blood pressure associated with a low-renin status (i.e., elderly systolic hypertension and hypertension in black subjects).
9. AWR and alveolar permeability are largely under the control of the $β_2$-receptor. Nonselective (e.g., propranolol and carvedilol) and modestly $β_1$ selective agents (e.g., atenolol and metoprolol) can increase AWR, inducing bronchoconstriction, and inhibit

the salutary bronchodilatory benefits of β_2-stimulants; they also decrease clearance of excess fluid from the alveolar airspace, clearly inappropriate for patients with pulmonary edema. Such potential problems can be largely avoided by low-dose, high β_1-selectivity (i.e., bisoprolol).

10. Metabolic changes affecting blood sugar, Hb_{A1c}, and lipids are largely under the influence of β_2-blockade (e.g., propranolol and to a lesser extent atenolol and metoprolol) and can be avoided by high β_1-selectivity (e.g., bisoprolol), ISA (e.g., pindolol, nebivolol), or α-blockade (e.g., carvedilol).

11. β-Blockers modify the neurohumoral system: (a) β_1-blockade is responsible for the decrease in plasma renin/angiotensin/aldosterone axis activity in both hypertension and systolic heart failure, with this effect being diminished by ISA; (b) in hypertension, nonselective and moderately β_1-selective agents cause an increase, high β_1-selectivity (bisoprolol) produces no change, and ISA agents (e.g., pindolol), a decrease, in plasma noradrenaline levels (not linked to fall in blood pressure); in systolic heart-failure, β_1-blockade is responsible for the fall in plasma noradrenaline levels; (c) in hypertension, β-blockers cause an increase in the natriuretic peptides ANP and BNP; in systolic heart failure, β_1-blockade is responsible for the fall in ANP and BNP (linked to an improved prognosis).

12. Adrenaline/β-blocker interactions occur with nonselective or modestly selective β-blockers and comprise a marked (e.g., propranolol) or moderate (e.g., metoprolol and atenolol) hypertensive response, avoided by the use of low-dose, highly β_1-selective bisoprolol. Clinically relevant situations are insulin-induced hypoglycemia and cigarette smoking.

13. Lipophilicity (fat-solubility) is a most important determinant of a β-blocker's pharmacokinetic profile.

14. In general, highly lipophilic agents such as propranolol are rapidly and completely absorbed from the gastrointestinal tract; heavily metabolized in the liver; highly bound to plasma proteins; widely distributed to all body tissues and compartments (and cross the blood-brain barrier); and have short plasma (and pharmacological) half-lives.

15. In general, hydrophilic (water-soluble) agents like atenolol, nadolol, and sotalol are poorly absorbed in the gut; are renally excreted unchanged; are lowly-bound to plasma proteins; are not widely distributed about the body (do not cross the blood-brain barrier); and have long plasma (and pharmacological) half-lives.

16. In patients with renal failure, a β-blocker that is metabolized in the liver (e.g., propranolol or metoprolol) or has a balanced excretion/metabolism between kidney and liver (i.e., bisoprolol) should be used.
17. In patients with hepatic failure, a β-blocker that is renally excreted (e.g., atenolol, sotalol, nadolol) or has a balanced excretion/metabolism between kidney and liver (i.e., bisoprolol) should be used.
18. In the elderly, hepatic and renal function tend to be impaired, thus dosing of both lipophilic (hepatically metabolized, e.g., metoprolol) and hydrophilic (renally excreted, e.g., atenolol) should be reduced; balanced hepatic and renal excretion (e.g., bisoprolol) requires no dosing adjustment.
19. β-Blockers that are metabolized via the hepatic cytochrome P450 system (e.g., metoprolol, nebivolol) are influenced by genetic polymorphism. Thus, slow metabolizers (possibly 10% of Caucasian and 30% of Chinese subjects) exhibit a threefold increase in peak blood levels plus extended half-life, potentially resulting in an unexpected increased pharmacological response plus side effects.

REFERENCES

1. Cruickshank JM, Prichard BNC. Beta-blockers in clinical practice. 2nd ed. Edinburgh: Churchill Livingstone; 1994, pp 1–351.
2. Liu J, Lui ZQ, Yu BN, et al. Beta-1 adrenergic polymorphisms influence the response to metoprolol monotherapy in hypertensive patients. Clin Pharmacol Ther 2006;80:23–32.
3. Misono M, Maeda S, Motoyuki I, et al. Combination of polymorphisms in the beta-2 adrenergic receptor and nitric oxide synthase 3 genes increases the risk for hypertension. J Hypertens 2009;27:1377–83.
4. Wellstein A, Palm D, Belz GG. Affinity and selectivity of beta-adrenoceptor antagonists in vitro. J Cardiovasc Pharmacol 1986; 8(suppl):S36–40.
5. Smith C, Teitler M. Beta-blocker selectivity at cloned human beta-1 and beta-2 adrenergic receptors. Cardiovasc Drugs Ther 1999;13:123–6.
6. Brodde O. The pharmacology of bisoprolol. Rev Contemp Pharmacother 1997;8:21–33.
7. Maack C, Tyroller S, Schnabel P, et al. Characterisation of beta-1 selectivity, adrenoceptor-Gs-protein interaction and inverse agonism of nebivolol in human myocardium. Br J Pharmacol 2001; 132:1817–26.
8. Bundkirchen A, Brixius K, Bolck B, et al. Beta-1 adrenoceptor selectivity of nebivolol and bisoprolol. Eur J Pharmacol 2003;460:119–26.

9. Steinmann E, Pfisterer M, Burkart F, et al. Acute hemodynamic effects of bisoprolol in patients with coronary artery disease. J Cardiovasc Pharmacol 1986;8:1044–50.
10. Parrinello G, Paterna S, Torres D, et al. One-year renal and cardiac effects of bisoprolol versus losartan in recently diagnosed hypertensive patients. Clin Drug Invest 2009;29:591–600.
11. Van de Ven LL, Van Leeuwen JT, Smit AJ. The influence of chronic treatment with beta-blockade on ACE inhibition on the peripheral blood flow in hypertensive patients with and without concomitant intermittent claudication. Vasa 1994;23:357–62.
12. Bailliart O, Kedra AW, Bonnin P, et al. Effects of bisoprolol on local vascular resistance. Eur Heart J 1987;8:87–93.
13. Asmar RG, Kerihuel JC, Girerd XJ, Safar ME. Effect of bisoprolol in blood pressure and arterial hemodynamic in systemic blood pressure. Am J Cardiol 1991;68:61–4.
14. Keim HJ, et al. Behandlung der leichten bis mittelschweren essentiallen hypertonic mit bisoprolol. Therapiewoche 1988;38:3507.
15. Dorrow P, Bethge M, Tonnesmann V. Effects of single oral doses of bisoprolol and atenolol on airways function in non-asthmatic chronic obstructive lung disease and angina pectoris. Eur J Clin Pharmacol 1986;31:143–7.
16. Macquin-Mavier I, Roudot-Thoraval F, Clerici C, et al. Comparative effects of bisoprolol and acebutolol in smokers with airways obstruction. Br J Clin Pharmacol 1988;26:279–84.
17. Henry PJ, Rigby PJ, Goldie RG. Distribution of beta-1 and beta-2 adrenoceptors in mouse trachea and lung. Br J Pharmacol 1990;99:136–44.
18. Mutiu GM, Factor P. Alveolar epithelial beta-2 adrenoceptors. Am J Respir Cell Mol Biol 2008;38:127–34.
19. Agostoni P, Contini M, Cattadori G, et al. Lung function with carvedilol and bisoprolol in chronic heart failure: is beta selectivity relevant? Eur J Heart Fail 2007;9:827–33.
20. Agostoni P, Palermo P, Contini M. Respiratory effects of beta-blocker therapy in heart failure. Cardiovasc Drugs Ther 2009;Sep 30 Epub ahead of print.
21. Fogari R, Zoppi A. The clinical benefits of beta-1 selectivity. Rev Contemp Pharmacother 1997;8:45–54.
22. Frithz G, Weiner L. Long-term effects of bisoprolol on blood pressure, serum lipids, and HDL-cholesterol in patients with essential hypertension. J Cardiovasc Pharmacol 1986;8(suppl 11):S134–8.
23. Janka HU, Ziegler AG, Disselhof G, Mehnhert H. Influence of bisoprolol on blood glucose, glucosuria and haemoglobin A-1 in non-insulin-dependent diabetes. J Cardiovasc Pharmacol 1986;8 (suppl 11):S96–9.
24. Leopold G, Ungethum, Pabst J, et al. Pharmacodynamic profile of bisoprolol. Br J Clin Pharmacol 1986;22:293–300.

25. Sun N, Hong T, Zhang R, Yang X. The effects of verapamil SR and bisoprolol on reducing the sympathetic nervous system's avtivity. Hypertens Res 2000;23:537–40.
26. Bolli P, Maller FB, Linder L, et al. Cardiac and vascular beta-adrenoceptor-mediated responses before and during treatment with bisoprolol and atenolol. J Cardiovasc Pharmacol 1986;8(suppl 11):S1–4.
27. Suonsyrga T, Hannila-Handeberg T, Paavonen KJ, et al. Laboratory tests as predictors of the anti-hypertensive effects of amlodipine, bisoprolol, hydrochlorthiazide and losartan in men (GENRES Study). J Hypertens 2008;26:1250–6.
28. Bruck H, Leineweber K, Temme T, et al. The Arg389Gly beta-1 adrenoceptor polymorphism and catecholamine-effects on plasma renin activity. J Am Coll Cardiol 2005;46:2111–5.
29. Belenkov IN, Skvortsov AA, Mareev V, et al. Clinical, haemodynamic and neurohumoral effects of long-term therapy of patients with heart failure with the beta-blocker bisoprolol. Kardiologia 2003;43:10–21.
30. Kirsten R, Neff J, Heintz B, et al. Influence of different bisoprolol doses on haemodynamics, plasma catecholamine, in hypertensive patients. J Cardiovasc Pharmacol 1986;8(suppl 11):S113–21.
31. Deary AJ, Schulmann AL, Murfet H, et al. Influence of drugs and gender on the arterial pulse-wave and naturetic peptide secretion in untreated patients with essential hypertension. Clin Sci 2002; 103:493–9.
32. de Groote P, Delour P, Lamblin N, et al. Effects of bisoprolol in patients with stable congestive heart failure. Ann Cardiol Angeiol 2004;53:167–70.
33. Yu WP, Lou M, Deng B, et al. Beta-1 adrenergic receptor polymorphism and response to bisoprolol in patients with chronic heart failure. Zhong Xin Xue Guan Bing Za Zin 2006;34:776–80.
34. Cryer PE, Haymond MW, Santiago JV, Shak SD. Norepinephrine and epinephrine release and adrenergic mediation of smoking-associated hemodynamic and metabolic events. N Engl J Med 1976; 295:573–7.
35. Lloyd-Mostyn RH, Oram S. Modification by propranolol of cardiovascular effects of induced hypoglycaemia. Lancet 1975;1: 1213–5.
36. Tarnow J, Muller RK. Cardiovascular effect of low-dose epinephrine infusions in relation to the extent of preoperative beta-blockade. Anaesthesiology 1991;74:1035–43.
37. Man in't Veld AJ, Schalekamp AD. Effects of ten different beta-blockers on hemodynamics, plasma rennin activity and plasma norepinephrine in hypertension. J Cardiovasc Pharmacol 1983;5:S30–45.
38. Cockcroft JR, Chowienczyk PJ, Brett SE, et al. Nebivolol vasodilates human forearm vasculature: evidence for l-arginine/NO-dependent mechanism. J Pharmacol Exp Ther 1995;274:1067–71.

39. Hillebrand U, Lang D, Telgmann RG, et al. Nebivolol decreases endothelial cell stiffness via the oestrogen receptor beta: a nano-imaging study. J Hypertens 2009;27:517–26.
40. Smith RS, Warren DJ. Effect of beta-blocking drugs on peripheral blood flow in intermittent claudication. J Cardiovasc Pharmacol 1982;4:2–4.
41. Hiatt WR, Stoll S, Niess AS. Effect of beta-blockers on the peripheral circulation in patients with peripheral vascular disease. Circulation 1985;72:1226–31.
42. Hiatt WR, Fradl DC, Zerbe GO, et al. Selective and non-selective beta-blockade of the peripheral circulation. Clin Pharmacol Ther 1984;35:12–8.
43. Lepantalo M. Beta-blockade and intermittent claudication. Acta Med Scand 1985;700(suppl):3–48.
44. Ting CT, Chen CH, Chang MS, Yin FC. Short and long-term effects of antihypertensive drugs on arterial reflections, compliance and impedance. Hypertension 1995;26:524–30.
45. De Cesaris R, Ranieri G, Filitti V, Andriani A. Large artery compliance in essential hypertension. Effects of calcium antagonism and beta-blocking. Am J Hypertens 1992;5:624–8.
46. Robb OJ, Petrie JC, Webster J, Harry J. ICI 118,551 does not reduce blood pressure in hypertensive patients responsive to atenolol and propranolol. Br J Clin Pharmacol 1985;19:541P-2P.
47. Cruickshank JM, Prichard BN. Beta-blockers in clinical practice. 2nd ed. Edinburgh Churchill Livingstone; 1994, pp 391–427.
48. Neutel JM, Smith DH, Ram CV, et al. Application of ambulatory blood pressure monitoring in differentiating between antihypertensive agents. Am J Med 1993;94:181–7.
49. Buhler FR. Age and cardiovascular response adaptation. Determination of an antihypertensive treatment concept primary based on beta-blockers and calcium entry blockers. Hypertension 1983;5:III94–100.
50. Buhler FR, Laragh JH, Baer L, et al. Propranolol inhibition of renin secretion. N Engl J Med 1972;287:1209–14.
51. Wilkins MR, Kendall MJ. Beta-blockers and the elderly. J R Coll Physicians Lond 1984;18:42–5.
52. Richardson DW, Freund J, Gear AS, et al. Effect of propranolol on elevated arterial blood pressure. Circulation 1968;37:534–42.
53. Banks RA, Markandu ND, Roulston JE, MacGreggor GA. Differing effects of sodium restriction, spironolactone, propranolol and captopril in black and white patients with hypertension. 8th Scientific Meeting of the International Society of Hypertension, Milan, May-June 1981, 35 (abstr).
54. Poulter N, Sanderson JE, Sever PS, Obel A. Comparative efficacy of first-line drugs in the treatment of hypertension in the Black African. 10th Scientific Meeting of the International Society of Hypertension, Interlaken, June 1984 (abstr).

55. Hollifield JW, Moore LC. How beta-blockers lower blood pressure. Drug Ther 1983;13:91–9.
56. Prichard BN, Cruickshank JC, Graham BR. Beta-adrenergic blocking drugs in the treatment of hypertension. Blood Press 2001;10: 366–86.
57. Seedat YK, Stewart-Wynne EG, Reddy J, Randeree M. Experiences with beta-blockers in hypertension. S Afr Med J 1973;47:259–62.
58. Cheah JS, Shia BL. Propranolol in the treatment of Asians. J Trop Med Hyg 1974;77: 150–4.
59. Tsukiyama H, Otsuka K, Higuma K. Effect of beta-blockers on central haemodynamics in essential hypertension. Br J Clin Pharmacol 1982;24:218–27.
60. Decalmer PB, Chatterjee SS, Cruickshank JM, et al. Beta-blockers and asthma. Br Heart J 1978;40:184–9.
61. Cruickshank JM. Are we misunderstanding beta-blocker? Int J Cardiol 2007;120:10–27.
62. Buhler FR, Laragh JH, Baer L, et al. Propranolol inhibition of renin secretion. N Engl J Med 1972;287:1209–14.
63. Man in't Veld AJ, Schalekamp AD. Effect of ten different beta-blockers on haemodynamics, plasma renin activity and plasma norepinephrine in hypertension. J Cardiovasc Pharmacol 1983;5(suppl):S30–45.
64. Fung JW, Yu CM, Chan S, et al. Effect of beta-blockade (carvedilol and metoprolol) on activation of the renin-angiotensin-aldosterone system and naturetic peptides in chronic heart failure. Am J Cardiol 2003;92:406–10.
65. Mitenko PA, McKenzie JK, Sitar DS, et al. Nadolol antihypertensive effect and disposition in young and elderly adults with mild to moderate hypertension. Clin Pharmacol Ther 1989;46:56–62.
66. Marie PY, Mertes PM, Hassan-Sebbag N, et al. Exercise release of cardiac naturetic peptides is markedly enhanced when patients with coronary heart disease are treated chronically with beta-blockers. J Am Coll Cardiol 2004;43:353–9.
67. Davis ME, Richards AM, Nicholls MG, et al. Introduction of metoprolol increases BNP in mild, stable heart failure. Circulation 2006;113:977–85.
68. Ollson LG, Swedberg K, Cleland JG, et al. Prognostic importance of plasma NT-pro BNP in chronic heart failure in patients treated with a beta-blocker (COMET trial). Eur J Heart Fail 2007;9:795–801.
69. Ablad B, Carlsson E, Johnsson G, Regardh CG. Metoprolol. In Scrabine A (ed). Pharmacology of antihypertensive drugs. New York: Raven Press, 1980; pp 247–62.
70. Brixius K, Bundkirchen A, Bolck B, et al. Nebivolol, bucindolol, metoprolol and carvedilol are devoid of ISA activity in human myocardium. Br J Pharmacol 2001;133:1330–8.
71. Prisant LM. Nebivolol: pharmacologic profile of an ultraselective, vasodilatory beta-1 blocker. J Clin Pharmacol 2008;48:225–39.

72. Broeders MA, Doevendans PA, Bekkers BC, et al. Nebivolol a third generation beta-blocker that augments vascular nitric oxide release. Circulation 2000;102:677–84.
73. Ignaro LJ. Experimental evidences of nitric oxide-dependent vasodilatory activity of nebivolol, a third generation beta-blocker. Blood Press 2004;13(suppl):2–16.
74. Dessy C, Saliez J, Ghisdal P, et al. Endothelial beta-3 adrenoceptors mediate nitric oxide-dependent vasorelaxation of coronary microvessels in response to nebivolol. Circulation 2005;112:1198–205.
75. Rozec B, Erfanian M, Laurant K, et al. Nevivolol, a vasodilating selective beta-1 blocker and beta-3 adrenergic agonist in the non-failing transplanted human heart. J Am Coll Cardiol 2009;53;1539–42.
76. Ursino MG, Vasiva V, Raschi E, et al. The beta-3 adrenoceptor as a therapeutic target: current perspectives. Pharmacol Res 2009;59:221–34.
77. Floras JS, Jones JV, Hassan MO, Slight P. Ambulatory blood pressure during once daily randomised double-blind administration of atenolol, metoprolol, pindolol and slow release propranolol. Br Med J 1982;285:1387–92.
78. Moniotte S, Balligaid J-L. Potential use of beta-3 antagonists in heart failure therapy. Cardiovasc Drug Rev 2002;20:19–26.
79. Flather MD, Shibata MC, Coats J, et al. Randomised trial to determine the effect of nebivolol on mortality and cardiovascular hospital admissions in elderly patients with heart failure (SENIORS). Eur Heart J 2005;26:215–25.
80. Roberts DH, Tsao Y, McLoughlin GA, Breckeridge A. Placebo-controlled comparison of captopril, atenolol and pindolol in hypertension complicated by intermittent claudication. Lancet 1987;2:650–3.
81. Mann S, Millar-Craig M, Balasubrananian V, Raftery EB. Once daily beta-blockade in hypertension: an ambulatory assessment. Br J Clin Pharmacol 1981;12:223–8.
82. Kaiser T, Heise T, Nosek L, et al. Influence of nebivolol and enalapril on metabolic parameters and arterial stiffness in hypertensive type 2 diabetic patients. J Hypertens 2006;24:1397–403.
83. Wilcox CS, Lewis PS, Peart WS, et al. Renal function, body fluid volume, renin, aldosterone and noradrenaline during treatment of hypertension with pindolol. J Cardiovasc Pharmacol 1981;3: 598–611.
84. Prichard BN, Thompson FO, Boakes AJ, Joekes AM. Some haemodynamic effects of compound AH 5158 compared with propranolol, propranolol plus hydralazine and diazoxide. Clin Sci Mol Med 1975;48:97S-100S.
85. Cruickshank JM, Prichard BN. Beta-blockers in clinical practice. 2nd ed. Edinburgh: Churchill Livingstone; 1994, pp 206–15, 1119–26.
86. Solomon SA, Ramsey LE, Yeo WW, et al. Beta-blockade and intermittent claudication. BMJ 1991;303:1100–4.

87. Wright JT, DiPette DJ, Goodman RP, et al. Renin, race and antihypertensive efficacy with atenolol and labetalol. J Hum Hypertens 1991;5:193–8.
88. Krum H, Conway EL, Broadbear JH, et al. Postural hypotension in elderly patients given carvedilol. BMJ 1994;309:775–6.
89. McTavish D, Campoli-Richards D, Sorkin EM. Carvedilol. A review of its pharmacology and therapeutic efficacy. Drugs 1993;45:232–58.
90. Kock G, Fronsson L. Acute effects of combined alpha/beta-adrenoceptor blockade in ischemic heart disease complicated by hypertension. Am J Hypertens 1991;4:709–13.
91. Dupont AG. Effects of carvedilol on renal function. Eur J Clin Pharmacol 1990;38(suppl 2):S96–100.
92. Leonetti G, Sampieri L, Cuspidi C, et al. Resting and post exercise haemodynamic effects of carvedilol. J Cardiovasc Pharmacol 1987;10(suppl 11):S94–6.
93. Yanagi M, Tsutamoto T, Tanaka T, et al. Effect of carvedilol on plasma adiponectine concentration in patients with chronic heart failure. Circ J 2009;73:1067–73.
94. Higaki J, Ogihara T, Nakamuru M, et al. Effect of carvedilol on plasma hormonal and biochemical factors in Japanese patients with hypertension. Drugs 1988;36(suppl 6):64–8.
95. Rosenberg J, Gustafsson F, Remme WJ, et al. Effect of beta-blockade and ACE-inhibition on B-type naturetic peptides in stable patients with systolic heart failure. Cardiovasc Drugs Ther 2008;22:305–11.
96. Struthers AD, Whitesmith R, Reid JL. Metabolic and haemodynamic effects of increased circulating adrenalin in man. Br Heart J 1983;50:277–81.
97. Rosei EA, Brown JJ, Lever AF, et al. Treatment of phaeochromacytoma and of clonidine withdrawal hypertension with labetalol. Br J Clin Pharmacol 1976;3(suppl):809–15.
98. Kahela P, Antilla M, Tikkanen R, Sundquist H. Effect of food on the bioavailability of sotalol. Acta Pharmacol Toxicol 1979;44:7.
99. Melander A, Stenbury P, Liedholm H, et al. Food-induced reduction in bioavailability of atenolol. Eur J Clin Pharmacol 1979;16:327–30.
100. Leopold G, Pabst J, Ungethum W, Buhring KU. Basic pharmokinetics of bisoprolol. J Clin Pharmacol 1986;26:616–21.
101. Chiariello M, Volpe M, Rengo F, et al. Effects of furosemide on plasma concentration and beta-blockade by propranolol. Clin Pharmacol Ther 1979;26:433.
102. Schafer-Korting M, Kirch W, Axthelm T, et al. Atenolol interaction with aspirin, allopurinol, and ampicillin. Clin Pharmacol Ther 1983;33:283–8.
103. Kirch W, Kohler H, Spahn H, Mutschler E. Interaction of cimetidene with metoprolol, propranolol or atenolol. Lancet 1981;2:521–2.
104. Hawksworth G, Betts T, Crowe A, et al. Diazepam/beta-blocker interactions. Br J Clin Pharmacol 1984;17(suppl):69S-76S.

105. Bax ND, Lennard MS, Al-Asady S, et al. Inhibition of drug metabolism by beta-blockers. Drugs 1983;25:121–6.
106. Leeman T, Dayer P, Meyer UA. Single dose quinidine treatment inhibits metoprolol oxidation in extensive metabolisers. Eur J Clin Pharmacol 1986;29:739–41.
107. Wagner F, Kalusche D, Trenk D, et al. Drug interaction between propafenone and metoprolol. Br J Clin Pharmacol 1987;24: 213–20.
108. Bowman SL, Hudson SL, Hudson SA, et al. A comparison of the pharmacokinetics of propranolol in obese and normal volunteers. Br J Clin Pharmacol 1986;21:529–32.
109. Neil-Dwyer G, Bartlett J, McAinsh J, Cruickshank JM. Beta-blockers and the blood brain barrier. Br J Clin Pharmacol 1981;11: 549–53.
110. McAinsh J. Clinical pharmacokinetics of atenolol. Postgrad Med J 1977;53(suppl 3):74–8.
111. Leopold G. Balanced pharmacokinetics and metabolism of bisoprolol. J Cardiovasc Pharmacol 1986;8 (suppl 11):S16.
112. Seiler K-U, Albrecht H-U, Niedermayer W, Wassermann O. Pharmacokinetics of atenolol in dialysis patients. Royal Society Medicine, International Congress and Symposium Series 1980;19:25–31.
113. Kanegae K, Hiroshige K, Suda T, et al. Pharmacokinetics of bisoprolol and its effect on dialysis refractory hypertension. Int J Artif Organs 1999;22:798–804.
114. Regardh C-G, Jordo L, Ervic M, et al. Pharmacokinetics of metoprolol in patients with hepatic cirrhosis. Clin Pharmacokinet 1981; 6:375–88.
115. Sotaniemi EA, Pelkoven RO, Arranto AJ, et al. Effects of liver function on beta-blocker kinetics. Drugs 1983;25(suppl 2):113–20.
116. Leopold G, Kutz K. Bisoprolol: pharmacokinetic profile. Rev Contemp Pharmacother 1997;8:35–43
117. Rowe JW, Andres R, Tobin JD, et al. The effects of age on creatinine clearance in man. J Gerontol 1976;31:155–63.
118. Geokas MC, Haverback BJ. The aging gastrointestinal tract. Am J Surg 1969;117:881–92.
119. Greenblatt DJ, Sellers EM, Shader RI. Drug disposition in old age. N Engl J Med 1982;306:1081–8.
120. Petrie JC (personal communication).
121. Regardh C-G. Pharmacokinetic aspects of some beta-blockers. Acta Med Scand 1982;665(suppl):49–60.
122. Rigby JW, Scott AK, Hawksworth GM, Petrie JC. A comparison of the pharmacokinetics of atenolol, metoprolol, oxprenolol and propranolol in elderly hypertensive and young healthy subjects. Br J Clin Pharmacol 1985;20:327–31.
123. Von Bahr C, Collste P, Frisk-Holmberg M, et al. Plasma levels and effects of metoprolol on blood pressure, adrenergic beta-blockade and plasma renin activity in essential hypertension. Clin Pharmacol Ther 1976;20:130–7.

124. Lennard MS, Silas JH, Freestone S, et al. Oxidation phenotype—a major determinant of metoprolol metabolism and response. N Engl J Med 1982;307:1558–60.
125. Bijl MJ, Visser LE, van Schaik RH, et al. Genetic variation in the CYP2 D6 gene is associated with a lower heart rate and blood pressure in beta-blocker users. Clin Pharmacol Ther 2009;85:45–50.
126. Evans DA, Mahgoub A, Sloan TP, et al. A family and population study of the genetic polymorphism of debrisoquine oxidation in a white British population. J Med Genet 1980;17:102–5.
127. Kalow W. The metabolism of xenobiotics in different populations. Can J Physiol Pharmacol 1982;60:1–12.

CHAPTER 2

β-Blockers and Their Effects upon Ischemic Heart Disease, Peripheral Vascular Disease (Including Aortic Aneurysms), Noncardiac Surgery (in High-Risk Cases), and the Atheromatous Process

INTRODUCTION

It was James Black's original idea that a molecule that was able to inhibit the action of the stress hormones adrenaline and noradrenaline should, in theory, be able to modify their effects upon the ischemic myocardium—that is, reduce or abolish angina pectoris and diminish the risk of infarction. β-Blockers were the result of this thinking, for which he was awarded the Nobel Prize for Medicine and a Knighthood.

1. Post myocardial infarction

This topic has been extensively reviewed.[1]

A) Early intervention (intravenous followed by oral within 12-24 hours after onset of pain)

i) Pain Relief

Several studies have demonstrated that intravenous β-blockade results in marked pain relief.[1] This benefit was particularly well illustrated with atenolol (vs. saline) in which both subjective and objective pain scores were significantly reduced—**Figure 2-1**.[2] Pain relief was closely linked to a reduction of blood pressure-heart rate product and reduced diamorphine requirement.[2]

ii) Infarct size and reinfarction

Infarct size reduction (CK-MB [MB isoenzyme of creatine kinase] enzyme-release) is closely linked to heart rate reduction in those receiving β-blockers—**Figure 2-2a**.[3] β-Blockers reduce infarct size as assessed by enzyme release by about 30%,[4] but the benefit is present only when the intravenous β-blocker is given within 4 hours or so from the onset of symptoms—**Figure 2-2b**.[5] When infarct size is assessed by electrocardiogram (ECG) R-wave loss, the process is almost complete by 12 hours,[6] and R-wave recovery in those randomized to β-blockade (atenolol) continues to increase up to 1 year post infarction—**Figure 2-3**.[7]

Reinfarction rate, like infarct size, is also linked to heart rate reduction.[3] In the large (n = 45,852) COMMIT (Clopidogrel and Metoprolol in Myocardial Infarction) trial,[8] the reinfarction rate was reduced by metoprolol (intravenous followed by oral) by a significant 18% vs. placebo.

iii) Mortality

The MIAMI (Metoprolol in Acute Myocardial Infarction) study[9] in 5778 patients comparing placebo vs. intravenous (within 24 hr of onset) followed by oral (200 mg/day) metoprolol for 2 weeks resulted in a nonsignificant 13% reduction in mortality. The larger ISIS-1 (First International Study of Infarct Survival) study in 16,105 patients involving intravenous followed by oral atenolol/100mg/day) for 1 week vs. randomized control resulted in a significant 15% reduction in in-hospital cardiovascular death (mainly due to prevention of cardiac rupture)[10]—**Figure 2-4**. At 1-year follow-up, vascular deaths were still significantly reduced. The more recent large COMMIT trial,[8] involving placebo vs. intravenous (unlike MIAMI and ISIS-1 was proceeded by the thrombolysis) followed by

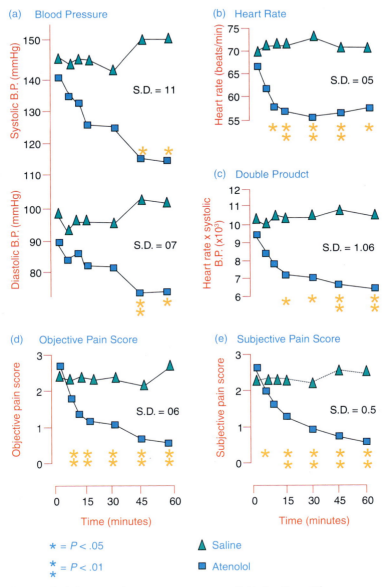

Fig. 2-1 Early intervention post acute myocardial infarction with randomized saline or intravenous atenolol. A significant reduction of objective and subjective pain scores occurred with atenolol. (From Ramsdale DR, Faragher EB, Bennett DH, et al. Ischemic pain relief in patients with acute myocardial infarction by intravenous atenolol. Am Heart J 1982;103:459–67.)

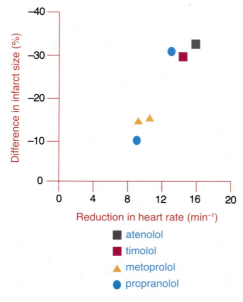

Fig. 2-2a Effect of β-blockers on infarct size (assessed by CK-MB [MB isoenzyme of creatine kinase] release) in relation to reduction of heart rate. β-blockers were started IV within 12 hours of pain onset and continued orally. (From Kjekshus JK. Importance of heart rate in determining beta-blocker efficacy in acute and long-term acute myocardial infarction intervention trials. Am J Cardiol 1986;57: 43F–49F.)

oral metoprolol for 1 month, resulted in no reduction in mortality but a significant 18% reduction in reinfarction and a significant 17% reduction in ventricular fibrillation. However, this benefit was counterbalanced by a 30% increase in cardiogenic shock.

Thus, intravenous followed by oral β-blockade should be given only to those who are hemodynamically stable.

B) Late intervention with oral β-blockade (2-28 days post myocardial infarction)— mortality and reinfarction rates

An overview of these studies[4] revealed a marked difference of effect of β-blockers with and without intrinsic sympathomimetic activity (ISA). Those without ISA (mainly metoprolol, propranolol, and timolol) effected an approximate 30% reduction in mortality, in contrast to agents with ISA (alprenolol, oxprenolol, and pindolol) that effected only a nonsignificant 10% reduction in mortality— **Figure 2-5**. β-Blockers with ISA are less effective in lowering heart rate, which undoubtedly accounts for their poor efficacy in reducing mortality—**Figure 2-6**.[11] Metoprolol was at least as effective as nonselective propranolol and timolol, indicating that $β_1$-blockade is the active ingredient. Post-infarct patients with heart failure who received β-blockers at admission and discharge from hospital

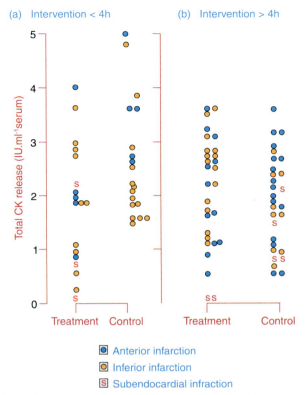

Fig. 2-2b The importance of early (<4 hr from onset of pain) intervention with IV plus oral β-blocker upon infarct size. (From Peter T, Norris R, Clarke ED, et al. Reduction of enzyme levels by propranolol after acute myocardial infarction. Circulation 1978;57:1091–5.)

experienced an approximate 50% reduction in 3-year mortality rate compared with patients who received no β-blockade.[12]

Nonfatal reinfarction rate was reduced by a significant 25%[4] and, like mortality, was closely related to heart rate reduction—Figure 2-7.[3]

2. Angina pectoris and chronic ischemia

This topic has been extensively reviewed.[13]

Angina pectoris is usually accompanied by ECG ST segment depression. However, the vast majority (~85%) of ECG ischemic episodes are "silent"[14] and their numbers peak between 06:00 a.m. and 12:00 noon[15] —the so-called vulnerable period.

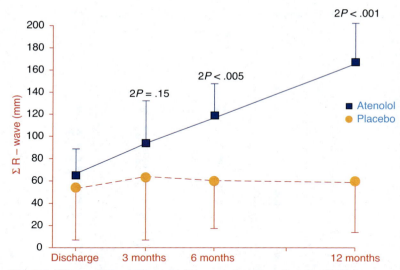

Fig. 2-3 Effects of long-term atenolol upon electrocardiogram (ECG) R-wave scores. Return of R-wave amplitude reflects initial limitation of infarct size. (From Yusuf S, Lopez R, Sleight P. Effect of atenolol on recovery of the electrocardiographic signs of myocardial infarction. Lancet 1979;2:868–9.)

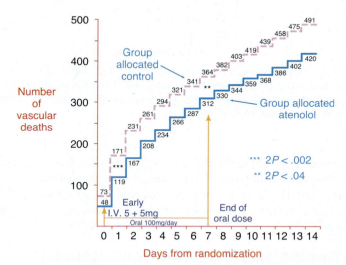

Fig. 2-4 ISIS-1 Study: In 16,027 cases of acute myocardial infarction, administration of early intravenous (followed by oral) atenolol significantly reduced in-hospital vascular mortality. (From ISIS-1 [First International Study of Infarct Survival] Collaborative Group. Randomised trial of intravenous atenolol among 16,027 cases of suspected acute myocardial infarction. Lancet 1986;2:57–66.)

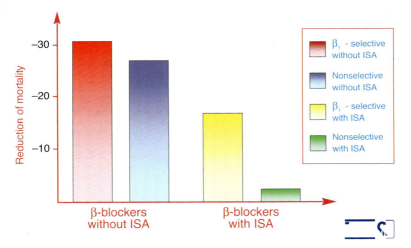

Fig. 2-5 Secondary prevention of post myocardial death by oral β-blockade. The possession of intrinsic sympathomimetic activity (ISA) reduces efficacy of β-blockers. (From Yusuf S, Peto R, Lewis J, et al. Beta-blockade during and after myocardial infarction: an overview of the randomised trials. Prog Cardiovasc Dis 1985;27;335–71.)

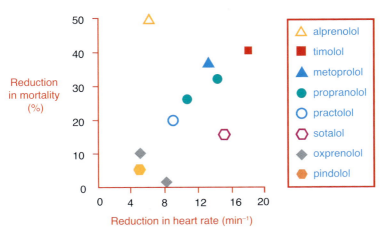

Fig. 2-6 Relationship between reduction in heart rate and mortality after late-intervention post myocardial infarction (MI) with oral β-blockers. The greater the heart rate reduction, the greater the reduction in mortality. (From Kjekshus J. Comments—beta-blockers: heart rate reduction a mechanism of benefit. Eur Heart J 1985;6[suppl A]:9–30.)

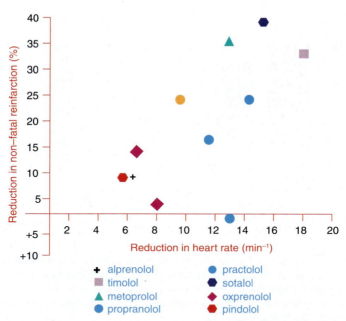

Fig. 2-7 Relation between reduction in heart rate and nonfatal infarction with oral β-blocker. The greater the heart rate reduction, the greater the reduction in reinfarction frequency. (From Kjekshus JK. Importance of heart rate in determining beta-blocker efficacy in acute and long-term acute myocardial infarction intervention trials. Am J Cardiol 1986;57: 43F–49F.)

A) Pain relief and effort tolerance

i) Non-ISA β-blockers

Such agents, for example, nadolol,[16] reduce episodes of pain and glyceryl trinitrate (GTN) tablets taken per week by about 30% (vs. placebo) and increase exercise time and total work by 25%-30%—**Figure 2-8**.

Non-ISA β-blockers for example, propranolol,[17] are more effective than the dihydropyridine calcium blocker nifedipine in reducing anginal episodes—**Figure 2-9**—and GTN consumption. The combination of propranolol and nifedipine was the most effective in reducing anginal episodes and reducing GTN consumption. Highly $β_1$-selective bisoprolol was equivalent to verapamil in improving effort tolerance in ischemic patients,[18] indicating that $β_1$-blockade is the active antianginal ingredient.

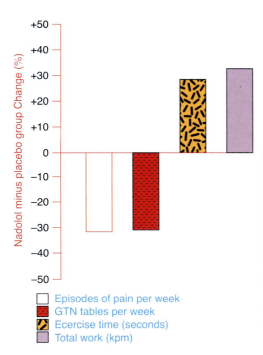

Fig. 2-8 Chronic nadolol oral therapy (vs. placebo) significantly improves symptoms and effort tolerance of patients with chronic angina pectoris. GTN, glyceryl trinitrate. (From Shapiro W, Park J, DiBianco R, et al. Comparison of nadolol and placebo in the treatment of stable angina pectoris. Chest 1981;80:425–30.)

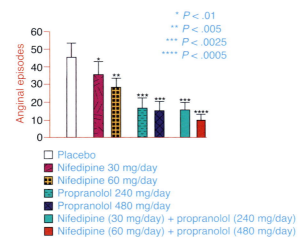

Fig. 2-9 In patients with severe angina pectoris, oral propranolol was superior to nifedepine in reducing the number of angina episodes. The combination of the highest doses of propranolol and nifedepine was the most effective therapy. (From Lynch P, Dargie H, Krikler S, Krickler D. Objective assessment of anti-anginal treatment: a double-blind comparison of propranolol, nifedipine and their combination. Br Med J 1980;281:184–7.)

ii) β-Blockers with ISA

In a blind, randomized, cross-over study comparing atenolol and pindolol (high ISA) in patients with chronic angina[19] atenolol was significantly superior in decreasing the number of anginal attacks and increasing the duration of exercise. These benefits were related to greater fall in heart rate with atenolol over a 24-hour period.

iii) Syndrome X

This syndrome, more common in women, mimics classic angina pectoris but has apparently clear coronary arteries. However, abnormalities in the microvascular bed have been detected, leading to impaired vasodilatory reserve.

One placebo-controlled study showed propranolol to be inferior to diltiazem in controlling symptoms;[20] whereas other studies showed atenolol to be superior to both nitrates and amlodipine as regards symptom relief[21] and propranolol to be superior to verapamil.[22,23]

B) Reduction in the number of silent and painful ECG ST segment depression episodes (total ischemic burden) by β-blockade

Silent ischemia has a prognosis as poor as that of painful ischemia[24] and is closely linked to ventricular fibrillation and sudden death.[25] Thus, the suppression of these episodes is important.

Both silent and painful ischemia (total ischemic burden) are linked to higher heart rates. One would thus predict that β-blockers with ISA would be less effective in suppressing these ischemic episodes; this is indeed the case. A double-blind, randomized, cross-over study comparing atenolol and pindolol[19] showed that pindolol was less effective in lowering heart rate, and even slightly raised it at night—**Figure 2-10**. Accordingly, pindolol, unlike atenolol, was unable to reduce nocturnal episodes of ischemia and was less effective than atenolol in reducing daytime painful and painless episodes.

In the large TIBBS (Total Ischemic Burden Bisoprolol) study involving 330 patients with stable angina with ST segment depression, the number of ischemic episodes related directly to later cardiac events; randomized bisoprolol was more effective than randomized nifedipine in suppressing ischemic episodes over a 24-hour period[26,27]—**Figure 2-11**. The advantage of bisoprolol was particularly apparent between 6:00 a.m. and noon, which is the "vulnerable"

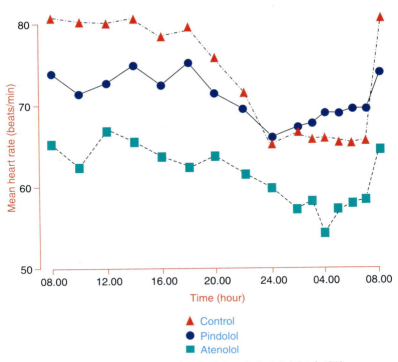

Fig. 2-10 The effect of chronic oral atenolol and pindolol (high ISA) upon 24-hour heart rate in patients with effort-induced or nocturnal angina. Note that pindolol increases nocturnal heart rate. (From Quyyumi AA, Wright C, Mockus L, Fox KM. Effect of partial agonist activity in beta-blockers in severe angina pectoris: a double-blind comparison of pindolol and atenolol. Br Med J 1984;289:951–3.)

period in which ischemic episodes peak. Similar results have been noted with metoprolol.[27] The "vulnerable" period is associated with a peaking of sympathetic nerve activity (the "waking" or "alarm" response) and is linked to an increased risk of myocardial infarction (MI) and sudden death, which is abolished by β-blockade.[28]

C) Smoking and silent ischemia

In patients with coronary artery disease, smoking increases myocardial oxygen demand by increasing heart rate and blood pressure and decreasing coronary blood flow,[29] resulting in diminished myocardial perfusion.[30]

Cigarette smoking accordingly increased the degree of ST segment depression and exacerbated angina symptoms in both the absence and the presence of propranolol[31]—**Figure 2-12**. The efficacy of

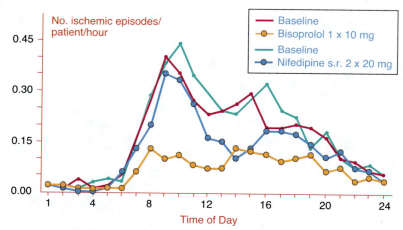

Fig. 2-11 Circadian profile of ischemic episodes in patients (*n* = 330) with stable angina at baseline and during bisoprolol 10-20 mg od or slow-release (s.r.) nifedipine 20-40 mg bid. Bisoprolol was markedly superior, particularly at the "vulnerable period" between 6:00 a.m. and noon. (TIBBS trial; von Arnim T. Medical treatment to reduce total ischaemic burden: Total Ischemic Burden Bisoprolol Study (TIBBS), a multicentric trial comparing bisoprolol and nifedipine. J Am Coll Cardiol 1995;25:231–8.)

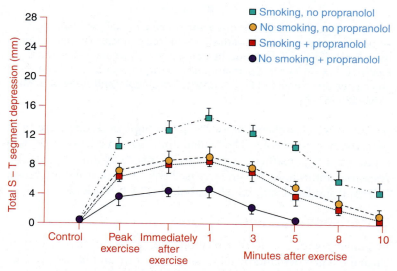

Fig. 2-12 Cigarette smoking worsens exercised-induced ischemic episodes (on ECG) and abolishes the anti-ischemic effect of chronic oral propranolol in patients with angina. (From Fox K, Johnathon A, Williams H, Selwyn A. Interaction between cigarettes and propranolol in treatment of angina pectoris. Br Med J 1980;281:191–3.)

nifedipine is also reduced by smoking, even more so than is the case with propranolol and atenolol.[32]

D) Reduction in the risk of cardiovascular events by β-blockade in patients with chronic, stable myocardial ischemia

In preinfarction angina, as in the HINT (Holland Interuniversity Nifedipine Trial) study,[33] metoprolol was superior to nifedipine in preventing cardiac events. In the more common "stable" situation, both atenolol and bisoprolol have shown benefit. In the ASIST (Atenolol Silent Ischaemia Study)[34] involving 306 patients with daily ischemia, randomized atenolol was superior to placebo in increasing event-free survival at 1 year and also increased the time to the first cardiovascular event. The TIBBS study[35] in 307 patients with stable myocardial ischemia showed that randomized bisoprolol was superior to nifedipine in achieving event-free survival at 1 year—**Figure 2-13**.

E) Likely mechanism of β-blocker benefits in ischemic heart disease

These have been extensively discussed[36] and stem from the effects of $β_1$-blockade.

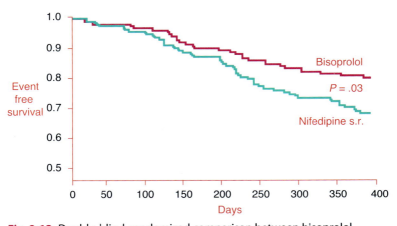

Fig. 2-13 Double-blind, randomized comparison between bisoprolol 10-20 mg od and slow-release (s.r.) nifedepine 20-40 mg bid over 1 year in 307 patients with stable angina. Event-free survival was superior ($P < .02$) with bisoprolol. (From von Armin T, for the TIBBS Investigators. Prognostic significance of transient ischemic episodes: response to treatment shows improved prognosis. J Am Coll Cardiol 1996;28:20–4.)

1. Reduction in myocardial oxygen requirements via a decrease in heart rate, blood pressure and ventricular contractility.
2. Slowing of the heart rate prolongs coronary diastolic filling period.
3. Redistribution of coronary flow toward vulnerable subendocardial regions.
4. Increase in the threshold to ventricular fibrillation.
5. Reduction in infarct size and reduction in the risk of cardiac rupture.
6. Reduction in the rate of reinfarction.
7. Regression of the atheromatous process.
8. Atheromatous plaque stabilisation (rupture less likely).

3) Peripheral arterial disease (including vascular aneurysms) and noncardiac surgery in high-risk cases

A) Pain-free walking distance

In the chapter on pharmodynamics, it was shown that β-blockers had little or no effect on resting and exercise-related leg muscle blood flow (p. 13) and did not diminish pain-free walking distance. However, interestingly and counterintuitively, β-blockers with vasodilatory properties (e.g., pindolol with ISA, labetalol with a-blocking properties) significantly decreased pain-free walking distance (pp. 22, 24, and 27) possibly due to a vascular steal phenomenon. The same detrimental effect was noted when a nonvasodilating β-blocker (atenolol) was combined with a vasodilator (nifedipine) (p. 27).

B) High-risk cases coming to noncardiac surgery

A classic example of high-risk (coronary artery disease and peripheral arterial disease) patients coming to vascular surgery was the DECREASE (Dutch Echocardiographic Cardiac Risk Evaluation Applying Stress Echo) I study.[37] One hundred and twelve patients were randomized to either placebo or bisoprolol 5-10 mg starting about 1 month presurgery and continuing for 1 month postsurgery.[37] There was a highly significant reduction in cardiac deaths and nonfatal MI (primary end-point) in the bisoprolol group—**Figure 2-14**. After 2 years follow-up, there was a threefold reduction in the primary end-point in the bisoprolol group.[38]

To the surprise of many, a similar very large trial involving metoprolol did not confirm the previous findings. The POISE

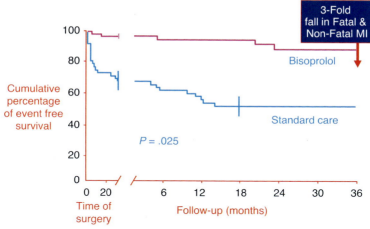

Fig. 2-14 The DECREASE 1 study showed that in high-risk patients undergoing noncardiac surgery, perioperative β_1-blockade with bisoprolol significantly reduced the combined primary end-point of cardiac death and myocardial infarction. (Poldermans D, Boersma, Bax JJ, et al. Bisoprolol reduces cardiac death and myocardial infarction in high-risk patients as long as 2 years after vascular surgery. Eur Heart J 2001;22:1353–8.)

(Peri-Operative Ischaemic Evaluation) trial[39] randomized a high-risk (atherosclerotic disease, mainly coronary artery disease and peripheral arterial disease) group of 8351 to either placebo or metoprolol 100 mg extended-release 2-4 hours presurgery and continued on 200 mg daily for 30 days postoperation. There was a significant reduction in the primary end-point and MI, but stroke, and death rates were significantly increased by metoprolol—**Figure 2-15**. The authors explained the results as due to intra- and postoperative hypotension. The fact that this did not happen in the bisoprolol DECREASE 1 trial was explained by the fact that bisoprolol was started 1 month before the surgery and at a low-modest dose. β-Blockers given immediately presurgery can increase stroke rate,[40] though perioperative β-blockade is not, in general, associated with stroke.[41]

A meta-analysis[42] of perioperative β-blockers in noncardiac surgery concluded that the evidence did not support the use of β-blockers. However, the accompanying editorial[43] pointed out that the previously discussed conclusion was based almost entirely on the negative POISE result, as illustrated in the current European guidelines[44]—**Figure 2-16**.

Confirmation of the benefits of β_1-blockade (bisoprolol) in noncardiac surgery was soon forthcoming. The DECREASE IV study[45]

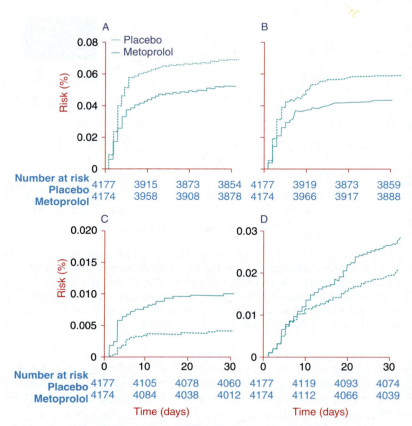

Fig. 2-15 POISE trial. In 8351 patients at risk of atherosclerotic disease, metoprolol (vs. placebo) significantly reduced the rate of myocardial infarction (B), but there was a significant increase in the rates of all deaths (D) and stroke (C). (From Effects of extended-release metoprolol succinate in patients undergoing non-cardiac surgery [POISE trial]: a randomised controlled trial. Lancet 2008;371:1839–47.)

involved 1066 moderately high-risk patients coming to noncardiac surgery, randomized to control therapy, fluvastin, bisoprolol, and the combination of fluvastatin and bisoprolol. The treatment was started about 1 month presurgery, the starting dose of bisoprolol was 2.5 mg, and continued for 1 month postsurgery. The composite end-point of cardiac death and MI was reduced by a significant 66% with bisoprolol, and the effect of the combination with fluvastin was even more marked—**Figure 2-17**. Importantly, when the results of DECREASE IV were combined with those of DECREASE I and III,[46] it was apparent that bisoprolol did not increase the

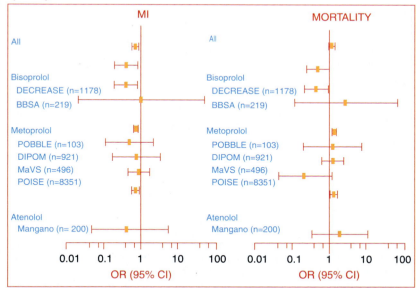

Fig. 2-16 "Only bisoprolol (vs. metoprolol and atenolol), given perioperatively to high-risk, noncardiac surgical cases, had significant beneficial effects on the frequency of myocardial infarction and all-cause death, probably due to a low-moderate dose given a few weeks prior to surgery." (From The Task Force for Preoperative Cardiac Risk Assessment and Perioperative Cardiac Management in Non-cardiac Surgery of the European Society of Cardiology (ESC) and endorsed by the European Society of Anaesthesiology (ESA). Guidelines for pre-operative cardiac risk assessment and perioperative cardiac management in non-cardiac surgery. Eur Heart J 2009;30:2769-812.)

frequency of stroke in contrast to metoprolol (in POISE), which did—**Table 2-1**.

An editorial seeking clarity on the subject concluded that the evidence supports the use of perioperative β-blockers in patients already on this therapy or those with cardiac ischemia, with careful titration of dose in the days and weeks prior to surgery.[47]

C) Dangers of sudden perioperative β-blocker withdrawal

In 140 cases of vascular surgery patients who were on preoperative β-blockers, 8 patients had β-blocker withdrawn suddenly in the postoperative period, resulting in an increased mortality some 50% greater than those who remained on β-blockers.[48]

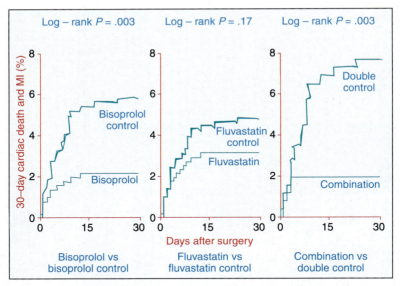

Fig. 2-17 In intermediate-risk surgical patients, bisoprolol or bisoprolol-plus-fluvastatin significantly reduced 30-day cardiac death and myocardial infarction (MI). (From Poldermans D, Schouten O, Bax J, et al. Reducing cardiac risk in non-cardiac surgery: evidence from the DECREASE studies. Eur Heart J Suppl 2009;11:A9–A14.)

D) Cardiac surgery and β-blockers

The benefits of β_1-blockade in noncardiac surgery probably occur also in patients undergoing coronary artery bypass graft (CABG) surgery.[49]

Certainly, bisoprolol 2.5-5.0 mg given within 6 hours post CABG ($n = 200$) and continued for 1 month was at least as effective

TABLE 2-1 Prophylactic β-blocker therapy and the effect upon stroke frequency after noncardiac surgery in high-moderate risk patients; POISE (metoprolol) vs. DECREASE I + II + IV (bisoprolol)

Studies	n	Odds ratio for stroke (CI)	Statistical significance
POISE (metoprolol)	8351	2.2 (1.3–3.8)	Significant
DECREASE I, II, IV (bisoprolol)	3884	1.16 (0.4–3.4)	Nonsignificant

CI, confidence interval.
From Van Lier F, Schouten O, Hoeks SE, et al. Impact of beta-blocker therapy to prevent stroke after non-cardiac surgery. Am J Cardiol 2010;105:43–7.

as amiodarone in reducing the frequency of atrial fibrillation.[50] This contrasts strongly with preoperative angiotensin-converting enzyme (ACE) inhibition, which not only increases the risk of atrial fibrillation but also doubles the perioperative mortality rate.[51]

E) Aneurysms

i) Abdominal aortic aneurysms

Certainly, patients with aortic aneurysms coming to surgery benefit significantly from perioperative β-blockade (particularly if coprescribed with a statin) in terms of reduced perioperative mortality and nonfatal MI.[52]

In terms of abdominal aortic aneurysm growth, early evidence suggested that β-blockers slowed the expansion rate.[53,54] Even in current times, β-blockers are recommended[55] in contrast to calcium blockers, which may increase the chance of an abdominal aortic aneurysm appearing.[56] However, the results of a large placebo-controlled study[57] and a systematic meta-analysis of the data[58] indicate that β-blockers do not slow the growth rate of abdominal aortic aneurysms.

ii) Dissecting aneurysms

Most dissecting aneurysms arise from cystic medial necrosis, usually associated with atherosclerosis. A small percentage (~4%) result from Marfan's syndrome, but most are linked to hypertension (82%) and smoking (62%).[59] The condition has a fearsome mortality level; untreated cases have a 22% mortality at 6 hours, 50% at 48 hours, 70% at 1 week, and 90% at 3 months.[60] Thus, urgent treatment is mandatory.

Type A aneurysms affect the proximal or ascending aorta, and most of these cases go straight to surgery.[61] Type B, or distal, descending dissections may often be treated with chronic medical therapy.[61]

Acute therapy (on admission to hospital) requires immediate lowering of blood pressure and reduction of ejection velocity. Thus, patients require intravenous nitroprusside plus β-blocker,[61] aiming for heart rates between 50 and 60 beats/min and a systolic blood pressure of 90 to 120 mm Hg.[61] Twenty percent to 30% of type B patients require surgery.[59,62] For those who are managed on chronic medical therapies, β-blockers are the cornerstone of treatment,[63] reducing the need for surgery, time in hospital, and cost compared with other antihypertensive therapies[62]—**Table 2-1a**.

β-Blockers are clearly acting via $β_1$-blockade and have been shown to diminish the underlying inflammatory response as

TABLE 2-1a Effect of β-blockade upon the management of type b (distal) dissecting aneurysms

Antihypertensive treatment	Need for surgery (%)	Mean days in hospital	Cost (euros) per patient
BB therapy	20	2	644
Non-BB therapy	53	16	12,748

BB, β-blocker.
From Genoni M, Paul M, Jenni R, et al. Chronic beta-blocker therapy improves outcome and reduces treatment costs in chronic type B aortic dissection. Eur J Cardiothorac Surg 2001;19:606–10.

evidenced by a fall in C-reactive protein (CRP) and white blood cell (WBC) levels.[64] However, in Marfan's syndrome, β-blockers appear to be not as effective in preventing dissection as inhibitors of matrix metalloproteinase–2 and -9.[65]

4. β-Blockers and the atheromatous plaque

A) Animal models

This topic has been reviewed.[66] It is apparent that animals fed atherogenic diets are prone to atherosclerotic changes on the aorta and coronary vessels and these lesions are retarded by β-blockade. Propranolol induced blood lipid changes in cocks and monkeys but reduced coronary atheroma lesions by about 60%. Of particular interest was the ability of propranolol to be antiatherogenic under hyperadrenergic states.

B) Humans and the atheromatous process

The human atheromatous process clearly has an underlying inflammatory process[67,68] as evidenced by high CRP and interleukin-6 (IL-6) levels. The siting of atheromatous plaque appears to be under the control of pulsatile blood flow patterns.[69] Low and oscillatory shear stress patterns encourage plaque formation in contrast to high shear force (laminar flow) areas, which are free of atheromatous plaque[70]—**Figure 2-18**—probably due to nitric oxide (NO) release.[71] The frequency of flow pulsation is under the control of heart rate and desirable high shear force (laminar)—flow patterns are encouraged by low heart rates.[69]

Most cases (75%) of MI result from fissuring of a vulnerable plaque resulting in intravascular thrombus formation[71]—**Figure 2-19**. Thus, plaque stabilization is an important concept concerning the prevention of plaque fissuring and infarction.

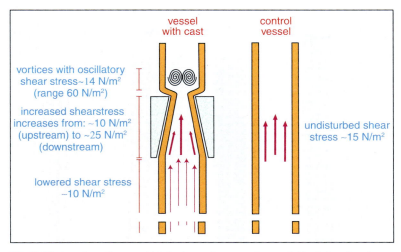

Fig. 2-18 Laminar-flow and high shear stress on the endothelial wall reduce the risk of atheromatous plaque formation. (From Cheng C, Tempel D, van Haperen R, et al. Atherosclerotic lesion size and vulnerability are determined by patterns of fluid shear stress. Circulation 2006;113:2744–53.)

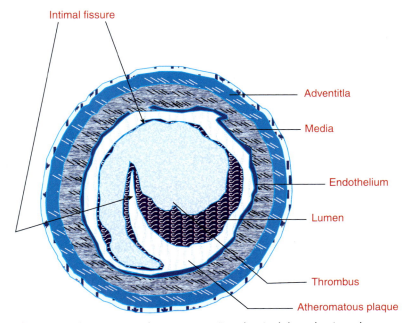

Fig. 2-19 Atheromatous plaque rupture/intraluminal thrombosis and myocardial infarction. Thrombus is also present beneath the intima.

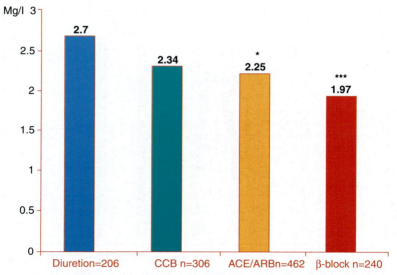

Fig. 2-20 The effect of monotherapy antihypertensive treatments upon plasma C-reactive protein levels. ACE/ARB, angiotensin-converting enzyme/ACE receptor blocker; CCB, calcium channel blocker. (From Palmas W, Ma S, Psaty B, et al. Antihypertensive medications and C-reactive protein in the multi-ethnic study of atherosclerosis. Am J Hypertens 2007;20:233–41.)

i) β-Blockers and the inflammatory process

Many factors underlie the inflammatory process, a major component being high sympathetic nerve (β_1) activity/noradrenaline levels.[72] Thus, in patients with ischemic heart disease[73] and hypertensives, β-blockers were more effective than diuretics, calcium blockers, ACE inhibitors, and angiotensin receptor I blockers in reducing CRP levels[74]—**Figure 2-20**.

ii) β-Blockers and blood velocity patterns

As already noted, low and oscillatory blood flow patterns encourage, and laminar blood flow discourages, atheromatous plaque formation. Thus, the effect of various antihypertensive agents upon this process is important.

Most of the relevant work has been done by Spence and colleagues utilizing Doppler echo flow techniques in patients with carotid stenosis[75-77]—**Table 2-2**. Hydralazine and nifedipine were associated with an increased frequency of disturbed flow patterns, ACE inhibition was neutral, and β-blockade was associated with a laminar flow

TABLE 2-2 Effect of antihypertensive agents on arterial flow patterns in human

	Neutral	Turbulent flow	Laminar flow
Placebo	Yes	No effect	No effect
Hydralazine	No	Worse	No (discouraged)
Nifedipine	No	Worse	No (discouraged)
Captopril	Yes	No effect	No effect
Metoprolol	No	Diminished	Yes (encouraged)

From Spence JD. Effects of hydralazine versus propranolol on blood velocity patterns in patients with carotid stenosis. Clin Sci (Lond) 1983;65:91–3; Spence JD. Quantitative spectral analysis of carotid Doppler signal: evaluation of a method for measurement of drug effects. Clin Invest Med 1989;12:82–9; and Spence JD. Effects of antihypertensive drugs on flow-disturbance: nifedipine, captopril and metoprolol evaluated by quantitative spectral analysis of Doppler flow patterns in patients with carotid stenosis. Clin Invest Med 1994;17:319–25.

pattern. Thus, it might be predicted that β-blockade would be effective in beneficially modifying the atheromatous process in humans.

iii) β-Blockers and atheromatous plaque regression/progression/vulnerability stability

Coronary plaque disruption was closely related to a high heart rate, which was reversed by the presence of β-blockade;[78] β-blockade also reduces coronary artery wall stress.[79] Thus, β-blockers appear to stabilize the vulnerable plaque.

β-Blockers can also decrease the coronary artery atheromatous plaque volume as assessed directly by intravascular ultra sonography.[80] In patients with known coronary artery disease (80% of whom had hypertension) followed up for 1 year, those on β-blockers (n = 1154, nonrandomized) experienced a significant regression of plaque volume compared with those who were not on β-blockers (n = 361)—**Figure 2-21**; the effect of statins is included for comparison.

In contrast, a prospective placebo-controlled study with nifedipine showed that after 2 years follow-up, although there was improvement in endothelial function, there was no effect on coronary plaque volume.[81] Also, in a substudy of the CAMELOT Study,[82] involving middle-aged subjects with coronary heart disease and raised blood pressure, over a 2-year period, plaque volume showed progression in the placebo group, a trend toward progression in the enalaptil group, and a mild trend toward progression in the amloipine group—**Figure 2-22**.

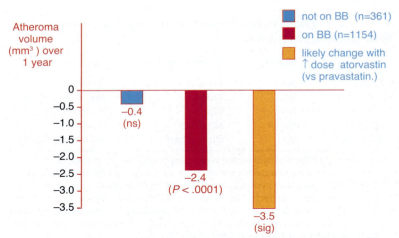

Fig. 2-21 Decrease in coronary atheromatous plaque volume (as assessed by intracoronary ultrasound) by β-blockers (BB) over 1 year (independent of statins, ACE inhibitors, other drugs, low-density lipoprotein concentration, and heart rate). ns, not significant; sig, significant. (From Sipahi I, Tuzcu EM, Woski KE, et al. Beta-blockers and progression of coronary atherosclerosis: pooled analysis of 4 intravascular ultrasonography trials. Ann Intern Med 2007;147:10–18.)

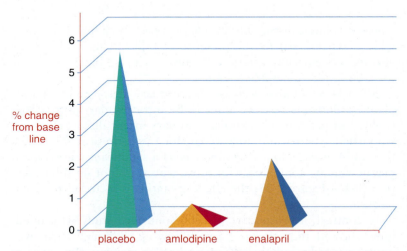

Fig. 2-22 Camelot Study. In middle-aged patients with mild hypertension plus coronary disease, over a 2-year period, atheromatous plaque volume (intravascular ultrasound) progressed significantly in the randomized placebo group. In the randomized calcium antagonist and ACE inhibitor groups, there was only a trend toward progression. (From Nissen SE, Tuzcu LM, Libby P et al. Effect of antihypertensive agents on cardiovascular events in patients with coronary disease and normal blood pressure. The CAMELOT Study: randomised controlled trial. JAMA 2004;292:2217–26.)

SUMMARY AND CONCLUSIONS

1. Early post-MI intervention (12-24 hr post event), comprising intravenous followed by oral therapy (mainly atenolol and metoprolol) results in (a) significant pain relief and reduction in opiate requirement; (b) reduction in infarct size and reinfarction rates; (c) significant (15%) reduction in in-hospital mortality (but only in absence of preceding thrombolysis); (d) if preceded by thrombolysis, no mortality reduction was noted, but significant falls in reinfarction and ventricular fibrillation rates were present; (e) however, there is a 30% increase in cardiogenic shock; (f) thus, early β-blockade should be administered only under stable hemodynamic conditions; (g) $β_1$-blockade is the active ingredient.
2. Late-intervention post-MI with oral β-blockade (non-ISA) results in (a) a 30% reduction in mortality rate; (b) reinfarction rate is reduced by a significant 25%; (c) these benefits are directly related to heart rate reduction (i.e., $β_1$-blockade); (d) β-blockers with ISA (e.g., oxprenolol, pindolol) lower heart rate less and do not significantly reduce mortality.
3. In patients with chronic myocardial ischemia, non-ISA β-blockers (a) significantly reduce the number of both silent (85% of total) and painful ST segment depression episodes, particularly in the early morning "vulnerable" period (when sympathetic nerve activity is maximal); (b) reduce the number of painful episodes and GTN requirement and increase exercise time by 25%-30%; (c) are more effective than dihydropyridine calcium blockers in these respects, and the combination of these two agents is more effective than each individual component separately; (d) these benefits result from $β_1$-blockade; (e) β-blockers with ISA are less effective owing to a lesser action on heart rate (pindolol even increases heart rate at night).
4. $β_1$-blockade is (a) superior to placebo in prolonging event-free survival (atenolol) and (b) superior to nifedipine (bisoprolol) in prolonging event-free survival.
5. Smoking impairs the antianginal effects of propranolol and atenolol (and even more so nifedipine).
6. β-Blockade is at least as effective as nitrates and calcium blockers in reducing the pain of syndrome X (no demonstrable coronary artery obstruction).
7. In patients with peripheral arterial disease (a) β-blockers without ISA do not decrease muscle blood flow at rest and exercise and do not reduce pain-free walking distance; (b) β-blockers with vasodilatory properties (e.g., ISA/pindolol or α-blockade/

labetalol) diminish pain-free walking distance, possibly via a "vascular steal" effect; combining a nonvasodilating β-blocker (e.g., atenolol) with a vasodilator (e.g., nifedipine) also results in a decrease in pain-free walking distance.
8. High-risk patients (with peripheral arterial disease/aortic aneurysm) coming to noncardiac surgery who receive a low dose of highly $β_1$-selective bisoprolol 1 month pre- and postsurgery experience a highly significant reduction in cardiac deaths and nonfatal MI with no change in the frequency of stroke, still apparent after 2 years' follow-up; these benefits were not seen with metoprolol (significant increase in stroke and death rate) possibly owing to starting the β-blocker on the day before surgery, at too high a dose (inducing intra- and perisurgical hypotension).
9. The death rate of abdominal aneurysm cases coming to surgery is reduced by β-blockade; the growth rate of abdominal aneurysms is not slowed by β-blockade; early mortality of dissecting aneurysms of the thoracic aorta is exceedingly high and the type A proximal variety should receive intravenous β-blockade and go straight to surgery; the type B distal variety (non-Marfan's) are closely linked to hypertension and cigarette smoking and are often treated medically—the cornerstone of treatment is β-blockade ($β_1$-blockade), reducing the need for surgery and hospital admission.
10. In humans, the development of atheromatous plaque is linked to an inflammatory process and disturbed blood flow patterns (nonlaminar); $β_1$-blockade has been shown to (a) reduce the inflammatory response (decrease CRP levels); (b) encourage optimal (laminar) blood flow patterns (probably via lowering heart rate); (c) regress atheromatous plaque volume (assessed by intravascular ultrasonography) over 1 year; (d) stabilize the "vulnerable" plaque (prone to fissure, intravascular thrombosis, and MI). In contrast, dihydropyridine calcium antgonists and ACE inhibitors do not regress plaque volume in humans and show only trends in slowing progression.

REFERENCES

1. Cruickshank JM, Prichard BNC. Beta-Blockers in Clinical Practice. 2nd ed. Edinburgh: Churchill Livingstone; 1994, pp 559–629.
2. Ramsdale DR, Faragher EB, Bennett DH, et al. Ischemic pain relief in patients with acute myocardial infarction by intravenous atenolol. Am Heart J 1982;103:459–67.

3. Kjekshus JK. Importance of heart rate in determining beta-blocker efficacy in acute and long-term acute myocardial infarction intervention trials. Am J Cardiol 1986;57:43F–49F.
4. Yusuf S, Peto R, Lewis J, et al. Beta-blockade during and after myocardial infarction: an overview of the randomised trials. Prog Cardiovasc Dis 1985;27;335–71.
5. Peter T, Norris R, Clarke ED, et al. Reduction of enzyme levels by propranolol after acute myocardial infarction. Circulation 1978;57: 1091–5.
6. Yusuf S, Lopez R, Maddison A, Sleight P. Variability of ECG and enzyme evolution of myocardial infarction in man. BMJ 1981;45:271–80.
7. Yusuf S, Lopez R, Sleight P. Effect of atenolol on recovery of the electrocardiographic signs of myocardial infarction. Lancet 1979;2:868–9.
8. COMMIT (Clopidogrel and Metoprolol in Myocardial Infarction Trial). Early intravenous and oral metoprolol in 45,852 patients with acute myocardial infarction; randomised, placebo-controlled trial. Lancet 2005;366:1622–32.
9. MIAMI Trial Research Group. Metoprolol in Acute Myocardial Infarction (MIAMI). A randomised, placebo-controlled international trial. Eur Heart J 1985;6:199–226.
10. ISIS-1 (First International Study of Infarct Survival) Collaborative Group. Randomised trial of intravenous atenolol among 16,027 cases of suspected acute myocardial infarction. Lancet 1986;2:57–66.
11. Kjekshus J. Comments—beta-blockers: heart rate reduction a mechanism of benefit. Eur Heart J 1985;6(suppl A):9–30.
12. Califf RM, Lokhaygina Y, Velazquez EJ, et al. Usefulness of beta-blockers in high-risk patients after myocardial infarction in conjunction with captopril and/or valsartan (VALIANT). Am J Cardiol 2009;104:151–7.
13. Cruickshank JM, Prichard BNC. Beta-Blockers in Clinical Practice. 2nd ed. Edinburgh: Churchill Livingstone; 1994, pp 631–704.
14. Selwyn AP, Fox K, Eves M, et al. Myocardial ischaemia in patients with frequent angina pectoris. Br Med J 1978;2:1594–6.
15. Campbell S, Barry J, Rebecca JS, et al. Active transient myocardial ischemia during daily life in asymptomatic patients with positive exercise tests and coronary artery disease. Am J Cardiol 1986;57: 1010–16.
16. Shapiro W, Park J, DiBianco R, et al. Comparison of nadolol and placebo in the treatment of stable angina pectoris. Chest 1981;80:425–30.
17. Lynch P, Dargie H, Krikler S, Krickler D. Objective assessment of antianginal treatment: a double-blind comparison of propranolol, nifedipine and their combination. Br Med J 1980;281:184–7.
18. Di Divitiis O, et al. Bisoprolol in the treatment of angina pectoris: a double-blind comparison with verapamil. Eur Heart J 1987;8(suppl): 43–54.
19. Quyyumi AA, Wright C, Mockus L, Fox KM. Effect of partial agonist activity in beta-blockers in severe angina pectoris: a double-blind comparison of pindolol and atenolol. Br Med J 1984;289:951–3.

20. Ferrini D, Bugiardini F, Galvani M, et al. Opposing effects of propranolol and diltiazem on angina threshold during exercise in patients with syndrome X. Ital Cardiol 1986;16:224–31.
21. Lanza GA, Colonna G, Pasieri V, Maseri A. Atenolol versus amlodipine versus isosorbide-5 mononitrate on angina symptoms in syndrome X. Am J Cardiol 1999;85:854–6.
22. Bugiardini R, Borghi A, Biagetti L, Puddu P. Comparison of verapamil versus propranolol therapy in syndrome X. Am J Cardiol 1989;63:286–90.
23. Borghi A, Sassone B, Trevasi M, et al. Long-term efficacy of beta-blockers in syndrome X. Eur Heart J 1991;238:abstract 1254.
24. Theroux DD, Halpen C, Debaissieux JC, et al. Prognostic value of exercise testing soon after myocardial infarction. N Engl J Med 1979;301:341–5.
25. Pepine CJ, Morganroth J, McDonald JT, Gottlieb SO. Sudden death during ambulatory monitoring. Am J Cardiol 1991;68:785–9.
26. von Arnim T. Medical treatment to reduce total ischaemic burden: Total Ischemic Burden Bisoprolol Study (TIBBS), a multicentric trial comparing bisoprolol and nifedipine. J Am Coll Cardiol 1995;25:231–8.
27. von Arnim T. Prognostic significance of transient ischemic episodes: response to treatment shows improved prognosis results of the TIBBS follow-up. J Am Coll Cardiol 1995;25(suppl):88A.
28. Muller JE, Stone PH, Turi ZG, et al, and the MILIS Study Group. Circadian variation in the frequency of onset of acute myocardial infarction. N Engl J Med 1985;313:1315–22.
29. Martin JL, Wilson JR, Ferraro N, et al. Acute coronary vasoconstrictive effects of cigarette smoking on coronary heart disease. Am J Cardiol 1984;54:56–60.
30. Deanfield JE, Shea MJ, Wilson RA, et al. Direct effects of smoking on the heart: silent ischemic disturbances of coronary flow. Am J Cardiol 1986;57:1005–9.
31. Fox K, Johnathon A, Williams H, Selwyn A. Interaction between cigarettes and propranolol in treatment of angina pectoris. Br Med J 1980;281:191–3.
32. Deanfield JE, Wright C, Krikler S, et al. Cigarette smoking and the treatment of angina with propranolol, atenolol and nifedipine. N Eng J Med 1984;310:951–4.
33. Lubsen J, Tijssen JG. Efficacy of nifedipine and metoprolol in the early treatment of unstable angina in the coronary care unit (HINT). Am J Cardiol 1987;60:18A–25A.
34. Pepine CJ, Cohn PF, Deedwania PC, et al. Effect of treatment outcome in mildly symptomatic patients with ischaemia during daily life. The Atenolol Silent Ischaemia Study (ASIST). Circulation 1994;90:762–8.
35. von Armin T, for the TIBBS Investigators. Prognostic significance of transient ischemic episodes: response to treatment shows improved prognosis. J Am Coll Cardiol 1996;28:20–4.
36. Cruickshank JM, Prichard BNC. Beta-Blockers in Clinical Practice. 2nd ed. Edinburgh: Churchill Livingstone; 1994, pp 559–81.

37. Poldermans D, Boersma E, Bax JJ, et al. The effect of bisoprolol on perioperative mortality and myocardial infarction in high risk patients undergoing vascular surgery. N Engl J Med 1999;341: 1789–94.
38. Poldermans D, Boersma, Bax JJ, et al. Bisoprolol reduces cardiac death and myocardial infarction in high-risk patients as long as 2 years after vascular surgery. Eur Heart J 2001;22:1353–8.
39. Effects of extended-release metoprolol succinate in patients undergoing non-cardiac surgery (POISE trial): a randomised controlled trial. Lancet 2008;371:1839–47.
40. Fleisher LA, Poldermans D. Peri-operative beta-blockade: where do we go from here? Lancet 2008;371:1813–4.
41. Von Lier F, Schouten O, van Domberg RT, et al. Effect of chronic beta-blocker use on stroke after non-cardiac surgery. Am J Cardiol 2009;104:429–33.
42. Bangalore S, Wetterslev J, Pranesh S, et al. Perioperative beta-blockers in patients having non-cardiac surgery: a meta-analysis. Lancet 2008; 372:1962–76.
43. Boersma E, Poldermans D. Beta-blockers in non-cardiac surgery: haemodynamic data needed. Lancet 2008;372:1930–2.
44. The Task Force for Preoperative Cardiac Risk Assessment and Perioperative Cardiac Management in Non-cardiac Surgery of the European Society of Cardiology (ESC) and endorsed by the European Society of Anaesthesiology (ESA). Guidelines for pre-operative cardiac risk assessment and perioperative cardiac management in non-cardiac surgery. Eur Heart J 2009;30:2769-812.
45. Poldermans D, Schouten O, Bax J, et al. Reducing cardiac risk in non-cardiac surgery: evidence from the DECREASE studies. Eur Heart J Suppl 2009;11:A9–A14.
46. Van Lier F, Schouten O, Hoeks SE, et al. Impact of beta-blocker therapy to prevent stroke after non-cardiac surgery. Am J Cardiol 2010;105:43–7.
47. Chopra V, Eagle KA. Perioperative beta-blockers for cardiac risk reduction. JAMA 2010;303:551–2.
48. Shammash JB, Trost JC, Gold JM, et al. Perioperative beta-blockers withdrawal and mortality in vascular surgical patients. Am Heart J 2001;141:148–53.
49. Ferguson TB, Coombs LP, Peterson ED. Pre-operative beta-blocker use and mortality and morbidity following CABG surgery in North America. JAMA 2002;287:2221–7.
50. Sleilaty G, Madi-Jebara S, Yazigi A, et al. Post-operative oral amiodarone versus oral bisoprolol as prophylaxis again atrial fibrillation after CABG: a prospective randomised trial. Int J Cardiol 2009;137:116–22.
51. Miceli A, Capoun R, Fino C, et al. Effects of angiotensin-converting enzyme inhibitor therapy on clinical outcome in patients undergoing coronary artery bypass surgery. J Am Coll Card 2009;54:1778–84.

52. Kertai MD, Boersma E, Westerhout CM, et al. A combination of statins and beta-blockers is independently associated with a reduction in the incidence of perioperative mortality and non-fatal MI in patients undergoing abdominal aortic aneurysm surgery. Eur J Vasc Endovasc Surg 2004;28:343–52.
53. Leach SD, Toole AL, Stern H, et al. Effect of beta-adrenergic blockade on the growth rate of abdominal aortic aneurysms. Arch Surg 1988;123:606–9.
54. Englund R, Hudson P, Hanel K, Stanton A. Expansion rates of small abdominal aortic aneurysms. Aust N Z J Surg 1998;68:21–4.
55. Sule S, Aronow WS. Management of abdominal aortic aneurysms. Compr Ther 2009;35:3–8.
56. Wilmink AB, Vardulaki KA, Hubbard CS, et al. Are antihypertensive drugs associated with abdominal aortic aneurysms? J Vasc Surg 2002;36:751–7.
57. Propranolol Aneurysm Trial Investigators. Propranolol for small abdominal aortic aneurysms: results of a randomised trial. J Vasc Surg 2002;35:72–9.
58. Guessous I, Periard D, Lorenzetti D, et al. The efficacy of pharmacotherapy for decreasing the expansion rate of abdominal aortic aneurysms: a systematic review and meta-analysis. PLoS One 2008;3:e 1895.
59. Tefera G, Acher CW, Hoch JR, et al. Effectiveness of intensive medical therapy in type B aortic dissection. J Vasc Surg 2007;45:1114–8.
60. Wheat MW. Treatment of dissecting aneurysms of the aorta. Prog Cardiovasc Dis 1973;XV1:87–101.
61. Doroghazi R, Slater EE, DeSanctis RW. Medical therapy for aortic dissections. J Cardiovasc Med 1981;6:187–97.
62. Genoni M, Paul M, Jenni R, et al. Chronic beta-blocker therapy improves outcome and reduces treatment costs in chronic type B aortic dissection. Eur J Cardiothorac Surg 2001;19:606–10.
63. Mukherjee D, Eagle KA. Aortic dissection- an update. Curr Probl Cardiol 2005;30:287–325.
64. Jo Y, Anzai T, Sugano Y, et al. Early use of beta-blockers attenuates systemic inflammatory response after distil type aortic dissection. Heart Vessels 2008;23:334–40.
65. Chung AW, Yang HH, Radomski MW, van Breeman C. Long-term doxycycline is more effective than atenolol to prevent thoracic aortic aneurysm in Marfan's syndrome through the inhibition of matrix metalloproteinase-2 and -9. Circ Res 2008;102:e73–85.
66. Cruickshank JM, Smith JC. The beta-receptor, atheroma and cardiovascular damage. Pharm Ther 1989;42:385–404.
67. Ross R. Atherosclerosis—an inflammatory disease. N Engl J Med 1999; 340:115–26.
68. Pande RL, Perlstein TS, Beckman JA, Creager MA. Association of insulin resistance and inflammation with peripheral arterial disease. Circulation 2008;118:33–41.

69. Chatzizisis YS, Giannoglou GD. Pulsatile flow: a critical modulator of the natural history of atherosclerosis. Med Hypothesis 2006;67: 338–40.
70. Cheng C, Tempel D, van Haperen R, et al. Atherosclerotic lesion size and vulnerability are determined by patterns of fluid shear stress. Circulation 2006;113:2744–53.
71. Dimmeler S, Zeiher AM. Exercise and cardiovascular health: get active to AKTivate your endothelial nitric oxide synthase. Circulation 2003;107:3118–20.
72. Banfi C, Cavalia-V, Veglia F, et al. Neuro-hormonal activation is associated with increased level of plasma matrix metalloproteinase-2 in human heart failure. Eur Heart J 2005;26:481–8.
73. Doo Y-C, Kim D-M, Oh D-J, et al. Effect of beta-blockers on expression of interleukin-6 and C-reactive protein in patients with unstable angina pectoris. Am J Cardiol 2001;88:422–4.
74. Palmas W, Ma S, Psaty B, et al. Antihypertensive medications and C-reactive protein in the multi-ethnic study of atherosclerosis. Am J Hypertens 2007;20:233–41.
75. Spence JD. Effects of hydralazine versus propranolol on blood velocity patterns in patients with carotid stenosis. Clin Sci (Lond) 1983;65:91–3.
76. Spence JD. Quantitative spectral analysis of carotid Doppler signal: evaluation of a method for measurement of drug effects. Clin Invest Med 1989;12:82–9.
77. Spence JD. Effects of antihypertensive drugs on flow-disturbance: nifedipine, captopril and metoprolol evaluated by quantitative spectral analysis of Doppler flow patterns in patients with carotid stenosis. Clin Invest Med 1994;17:319–25.
78. Heidland VE, Stauer BE. Left ventricular muscle mass and elevated heart rate are associated with coronary plaque disruption. Circulation 2001;104:1477–82.
79. Williams MJ, Low CJ, Wilkins GT, Stewart RA. Randomised comparison of the effects of nicardipine and esmolol on coronary artery wall stress implications for the risk of plaque rupture. Heart 2000;84: 377–82.
80. Sipahi I, Tuzcu EM, Woski KE, et al. Beta-blockers and progression of coronary atherosclerosis: pooled analysis of 4 intravascular ultrasonography trials. Ann Intern Med 2007;147:10–18.
81. Luscher TF, Pieper M, Tendera M, et al. A randomised, placebo-controlled study on the effect of nifedipine on coronary endothelial function and plaque formation in patients with coronary artery disease: the ENCORE II study. Eur Heart J 2009;30:1590–7.
82. Nissen SE, Tuzcu LM, Libby P, et al. Effect of antihypertensive agents on cardiovascular events in patients with coronary disease and normal blood pressure. The CAMELOT Study: randomised controlled trial. JAMA 2004;292:2217–26.

β-Blockers and Hypertension

CHAPTER 3

INTRODUCTION

It was not initially envisaged that β-blockers would lower high blood pressure (BP). In 1964, Brian Prichard[1] first noted their (propranolol) antihypertensive action, and there was much lively debate as to the veracity of that claim. Of course, β-blockers were later to become a cornerstone in the treatment of hypertension.

Essential hypertension (BP ≥ 140/90 mm Hg) is extremely common. In developed and developing countries alike, it occurs in 25%-35% of the adult population and up to 60%-70% of those older than 60 years,[2] being a particular problem in China.[3] Hypertension may affect more than 90% of individuals over their lifetimes.[4] Hypertension is a potentially dangerous condition, accounting for up to 50% of heart disease risk and 75% of stroke risk.[5] This risk is continuous down to pressures as low as 115/75 mm Hg,[4] and for each 10 mm Hg decrease in systolic blood pressure (SBP), the average risk of heart disease mortality and cerebrovascular disease mortality decreases by 30% and 40%, respectively.[5] With increasing age, the adverse cardiovascular consequences of elevated BP shift in importance from diastolic to systolic and finally to pulse pressure.[6]

1. Recent anti-β-blocker sentiment

In the last few years, several publications by eminent experts have expressed strong anti-β-blocker sentiments as regards their use in the treatment of hypertension.[7-11]

Until June 2006, the recommendations of the British Hypertension Society[12] were according to the AB/CD rule—for younger/middle-aged hypertensive patients, first-line therapy was a choice between angiotensin-converting enzyme (ACE) inhibition and β-blockade, and for older hypertensive patients, a choice between low-dose diuretic or calcium blocker.

Then came the new recommendations from the U.K. NICE (National Institute for Clinical Excellence) committee, supported by the British Hypertension Society.[13] The essence of the new recommendations was (a) β-blockers are no longer preferred as a routine initial therapy, (b) that the combination of a β-blocker and a diuretic is to be discouraged owing to the increased risk of the patient developing diabetes, (c) in patients aged 55 years or younger, the first-choice for initial therapy should be an ACE inhibitor, or an angiotensin receptor-1 antagonist (angiotensin receptor blocker [ARB]) if an ACE inhibitor is not tolerated.

Could so many experts have got it wrong? The author (JMC) of this book strongly disagrees with these guidelines.[14,15]

The 2007 ESH/ESC (European Society of Hypertension/European Society of Cardiology) Guidelines for the management of hypertension[16] and 2009 reappraisal[17] are more reasonable concerning β-blockers: (a) all five major classes of antihypertensive agent are suitable for first-line therapy, irrespective of age, and they suggest that the fall in BP and not the type of drug is the important factor, but (b) they warn against the combination of β-blockers and diuretics in patients with the metabolic syndrome or at high risk of developing type 2 diabetes (i.e., centrally obese), (c) in diabetes, they favor inhibitors of the renin-angiotensin system owing to their renoprotective actions, and (d) in moderate to severe hypertension, recommend starting with a low-dose, fixed combination of two compatible antihypertensive agents.

To understand the possible "rights and wrongs" of U.K. and European recommendations, it is necessary to consider the pathophysiology of primary hypertension.

2. Pathophysiology of primary hypertension

The Framingham Group[18] have recently shown that the development of diastolic hypertension resulted from high peripheral resistance, occurred in the young/middle-aged and was closely linked to overweight/obesity; whereas the development of isolated systolic hypertension occurred in the elderly and was a function of aging of the arteries and impaired vascular compliance—**Table 3-1** (though

TABLE 3-1 The Framingham Heart Study—different predictors of diastolic hypertension (± systolic hypertension) and isolated systolic hypertension

Predictors of DH (± systolic hypertension) = DBP > 90 mm Hg (± SBP > 140 mm Hg)	Predictors of ISH – SBP > 140 mm Hg + < 90 mm Hg
1. Young age.	1. Older age.
2. Male sex.	2. Female sex.
3. High BMI at baseline.	3. Increasing BMI during follow-up (but much weaker than in young).
4. Increasing BMI during follow-up.	4. ISH arises more commonly from normal and high-normal BP than "burned out" diastolic hypertension.
5. Main mechanism of DH is raised peripheral resistance.	5. Only 18% with new-onset ISH had a previous DBP > 95 mm Hg.
	6. Main mechanism of ISH is increased arterial stiffness (poor vascular compliance).

N = 3915 untreated normal subjects, mean age 48.5 yr, followed-up for 10 yr.
BMI, body mass index; BP, blood pressure; IDH, isolated diastolic hypertension; ISH, isolated systolic hypertension.
From Franklin SS, Pio JR, Wong ND, et al. Predictors of new-onset diastolic and systolic hypertension. The Framingham Heart Study. Circulation 2005;111:1121–7.

isolated systolic hypertension can occur in younger subjects and is linked to low socioeconomic status and lifestyle factors such as smoking[19]). Others have confirmed the link between obesity and hypertension in the young/middle-aged[20-22]—**Figure 3-1**, and the relationship between increased visceral adipose tissue and high BP is independent of BMI[21]—**Figure 3-2**. Moreover, the hypertension associated with central obesity (increased waist circumference) is also linked to a high heart rate and cardiac output[23]—**Figure 3-3**.

These previously discussed combined phenomena in the younger/middle-aged diastolic hypertensive patient suggest increased sympathetic nerve activity; and indeed, this is the case with central (as opposed to peripheral) obesity[24]—**Figure 3-4**. Not surprisingly, the two conditions that are closely associated with central obesity (i.e., the metabolic syndrome[25] and type 2 diabetes[26]) are also linked to high sympathetic nerve activity, particularly when accompanied by hypertension—**Figures 3-5 and 3-6**. The high sympathetic activity appears to affect all tissues except the skin.[27]

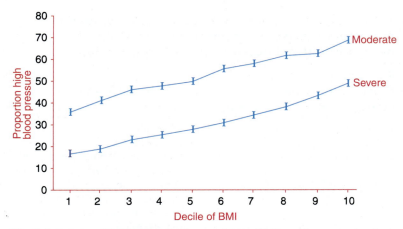

Fig. 3-1 Relationship between body mass index (BMI) and hypertension in 37,027 middle-aged subjects. (From Timpson NJ, Harbord R, Davey-Smith G, et al. Does greater adiposity increase blood pressure and hypertension risk? Hypertension 2009;54:84–90.)

The high adrenergic drive of overweight subjects results in an increase in stroke volume and cardiac output of about 20%[28] plus an increase in heart rate. High BP results from an increased peripheral resistance due to inadequate compensatory (to a high cardiac output) vasodilatation, presumably due to endothelial dysfunction.[29]

3. Possible inflammatory mechanism linking central obesity and high sympathetic nerve activity in the younger/middle-aged diastolic hypertensive patient

This important topic has been discussed.[15] The centrally located adipocytes produce several vasculotoxic adipokinins (e.g., tumor necrosis factor-α [TNF-α] and interleukin-6 [IL-6]),[30,31] which act upon the liver, which releases C-reactive protein (CRP). The adipokinins also induce an endothelial inflammatory response resulting in endothelial dysfunction and insulin resistance—**Figure 3-7**. Insulin resistance is accompanied by a compensatory increased insulin secretion that acts centrally resulting in increased sympathetic outflow[32] and renin release (via β1-stimulation of the renal juxtaglomerular apparatus).[33] Central adipocytes also produce the "thin hormone" leptin that, like insulin, also acts centrally, resulting in increased

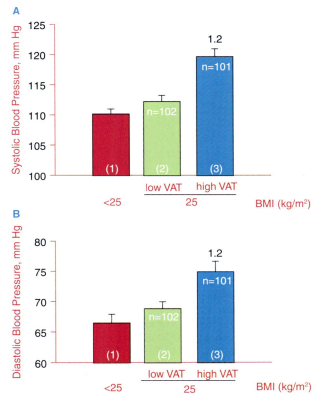

Fig. 3-2 Relationship between BMI and visceral adipose tissue (VAT) and blood pressure in middle-aged subjects. (From Rheaume C, Arsenault BJ, Belanger S, et al. Low cardiorespiratory fitness levels and elevated blood pressure. What is the contribution of visceral adiposity? Hypertension 2009;54:91–7.)

sympathetic outflow.[34] In middle-aged hypertensive patients, raised leptin levels are significantly linked to both a high body mass index (BMI) and high BP.[35] The high renin levels result in increased angiotensin II levels, which also act centrally resulting in increased sympathetic outflow.[36] There is thus a "vicious circle" that results in high noradrenaline activity leading to chronic β_1-stimulation and its concomitant injurious effects upon the periphery (e.g., cardiac necrosis and apoptosis),[37] increased risk of ventricular fibrillation and sudden death,[38] increased rate of atheroma formation[39] and left ventricular hypertrophy (LVH)[40]—**Figure 3-8**.

All of these problems in young/middle-aged, probably centrally obese, hypertensive patients are, theoretically, solved by β_1-blockade.

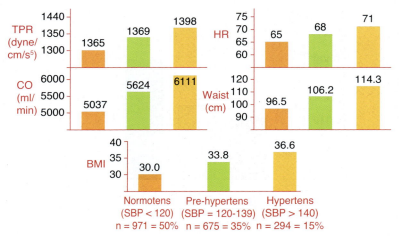

Fig. 3-3 The Strong Heart Study, comprising 1940 young (age 14-39 yr) subjects (50% normotensive, 35% prehypertensive, and 15% hypertensive), studied the relationship between hypertension/prehypertension and BMI, waist circumference, heart rate (HR), and cardiac output (CO). SBP, systolic blood pressure; TPR, total peripheral resistance. (From Drukteinis JS, Roman MJ, Fabsitz RR, et al. Cardiac and systemic haemodynamic characteristics of hypertension and prehypertension in adolescents and young adults. The Strong Heart Study. Circulation 2007;115:221–7.)

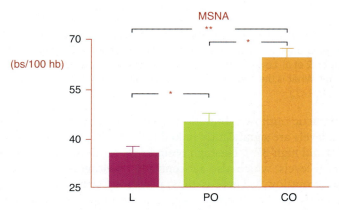

Fig. 3-4 Patients with central obesity (CO; $n = 26$) have significantly increased muscle sympathetic nerve activity (MSNA) compared with those with peripheral obesity (PO; $n = 20$) or who are lean (L; $n = 30$). bs, bursts per minute corrected for heart rate; hb, heart rate. (From Grassi G, Dell'Oro R, Facchini A, et al. Effect of central and peripheral body fat distribution on sympathetic and baroreflex function in obese hypertensive. J Hypertens 2004;22:2363–9.)

Chapter 3: β-Blockers and Hypertension   87

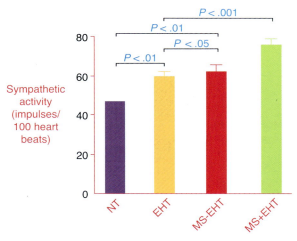

Fig. 3-5 In obese, nondiabetic subjects (*n* = 69), sympathetic nerve activity is highly significantly raised in patients with combined hypertension (EHT) and the metabolic syndrome (MS). EHT + MS n = 18; MS only *n* = 17; EHT only *n* = 16; no MS + no EHT *n* = 18. NT, normotensive. (From Huggett RJ, Burns J, Mackintosh AF, Mary DA. Sympathetic neural activation in non-diabetic metabolic syndrome and its further augmentation by hypertension. Hypertension 2004;44:847–52.)

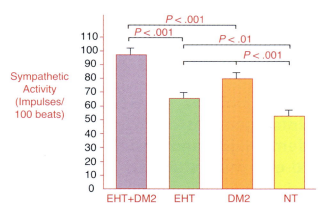

Fig. 3-6 Sympathetic nerve activity is markedly raised in those with hypertension and type 2 diabetes (EHT + DM2; *n* = 17) compared with those with hypertension (*n* = 17) or DM2 alone (*n* = 17) or who were normotensvie (NT; *n* = 17). (From Huggett RJ, Scott EM, Gilbey SG, et al. Impact of type-2 diabetes mellitus on sympathetic neural mechanisms in hypertension. Circulation 2003;108:3097–4001.)

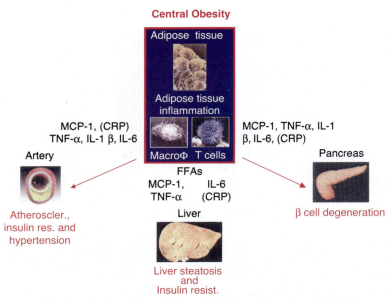

Fig. 3-7 Central obesity, inflammation (raised C-reactive protein [CRP]), adipokinins (e.g., interleukin-6 [1L-6], tumor necrosis factor-α [TNF-α]), the immune response, and the likely effect on peripheral organs (e.g., insulin resistance). FFAs, free fatty acids; MMP-1, matrix metalloproteinase-1. (From Cruickshank JM. Are we misunderstanding beta-blockers? Int J Cardiol 2007;120:10–27.)

What is the evidence that this is the case—that $β_1$-blockade is beneficial to young/middle-aged (probably overweight/obese) hypertensive patients in terms of reducing hard cardiovascular end-points?

4. First-line β-blockers and the young/middle-aged diastolic hypertensive patient; major randomized, controlled, hard-end-point studies

This issue has been addressed[14] and the conditions for selection/nonselection of studies for consideration were outlined.

The four major hard-end-point studies were the Medical Research Council (MRC) mild hypertension study,[41] IPPPSH[42] (The International Prospective Primary Prevention Study in Hypertension), MAPHY[43] (Metoprolol in Patients with Hypertension), (a substudy of HAPPHY (Heart Attack Primary Prevention in Hypertension),

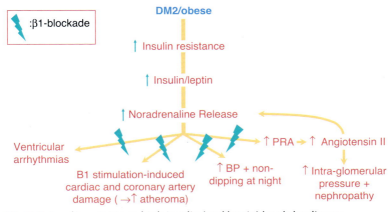

Fig. 3-8 Insulin resistance, high insulin (and leptin) levels leading to noradrenaline release, and the effects of chronic β_1-stimulation and β_1-blockade on the periphery. BP, blood pressure; DM2, type 2 diabetes mellitus; PRA, plasma renin activity. (From Cruickshank JM. Are we misunderstanding beta-blockers? Int J Cardiol 2007;120:10–27.)

chosen because it highlighted the β-blocker/smoking interaction), U.K. Prospective Diabetes Study (UKPDS) 38[44] and UKPDS 39[45]— Table 3-2.

In order to appreciate the strengths and the weaknesses of the β-blockers propranolol,[41] oxprenolol,[42] and metoprolol,[43] it is important to view the results in terms of cigarette-smoking status.

TABLE 3-2 Randomized, controlled, hard-end-point studies in younger/middle-aged diastolic hypertensives (± diabetes) involving first-line β-blocker therapy

Trial	BB (vs. comparator)	Mean age (yr)	Initial BB (mm Hg)	PP (mm Hg)
IPPPSH	Oxprenolol (vs. diuretic)	52	173/108	65
MRC Mild Hypertension	Propranolol (vs. diuretic vs. placebo)	51	161/98	63
MAPHY	Metoprolol (vs. diuretic)	52	167/108	59
UKPDS	Atenolol (vs. captopril)	56	159/94	65

BB, β-blocker; IPPPSH, The International Prospective Primary Prevention Study in Hypertension; MAPHY, Metoprolol in Patients with Hypertension; MRC, Medical Research Council; PP, pulse pressure; UKPDS, U.K. Prospective Diabetes Study.
From Cruickshank JM. Are we misunderstanding beta-blockers? Int J Cardiol 2007;120:10–27.

A) The vital β-blocker/smoking interaction

Emphasis is on myocardial infarction (MI) and men, because MI occurs mainly in men and is three times more common than stroke in the young/middle-aged diastolic hypertensive patient.[41] However, stroke (men and women) was also affected by smoking—a 54% reduction in stroke rate by propranolol vs. placebo in nonsmokers was converted to a 21% increase in smokers—**Figure 3-9** (the diuretic-induced reduction in stroke was unaffected by smoking).

In the MRC-1,[41] IPPPSH,[42] and MAPHY[43] studies, about one third of the populations were smokers. The dramatic effect of smoking on the rate of MI in men is shown in **Figure 3-10**. A 33%-49% reduction in coronary events by the β-blockers vs. placebo or diuretic therapy in nonsmokers was nullified in smokers and was even converted to a worrying 10%-35% increase in the case of nonselective oxprenolol and propranolol.

A rather startling conclusion is that as cardiovascular events in the young/middle-aged are about twice as common in smokers,[41] who comprise about one third of the whole, about 50% of all cardiovascular events occur in smokers and will be "out of reach" of nonselective (e.g., propranolol and oxprenolol) and modestly selective (e.g., metoprolol) β-blockers. In countries with much higher

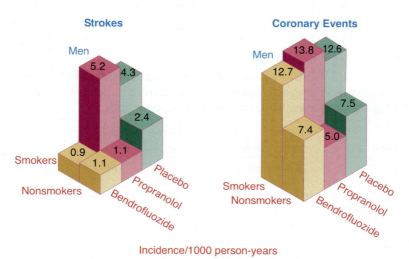

Incidence/1000 person-years

Fig. 3-9 Medical Research Council (MRC)-1 trial. The beneficial effects of propranolol in middle-aged hypertensive patients in the prevention of myocardial infarction and strokes (in nonsmokers) are negated in those who smoke cigarettes. (From Medical Research Council Working Party. MRC trial of treatment of mild hypertension principal results. Br Med J 1985;291:97–104.)

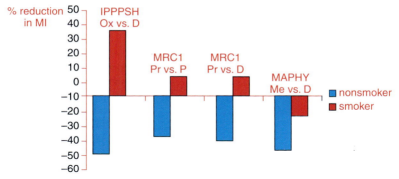

Fig. 3-10 In the MRC-1, IPPPSH, and MAPHY trials, the beneficial effects of nonselective propranolol (Pr) and oxprenolol (Ox) and moderately β-$_1$-selective metoprolol (Me) in young/middle-aged hypertensive patients upon the prevention of myocardial infarction (MI) in nonsmokers (vs. placebo [P] or diuretics [D]) are negated in smokers. (From Cruickshank JM. Are we misunderstanding beta-blockers? Int J Cardiol 2007;120:10–27.)

smoking rates (e.g., China), the cardiovascular events "out of reach" to nonselective and modestly $β_1$-selective agents would be much higher than 50%.

B) What is the likely mechanism of the β-blocker/cigarette smoking interaction?

Cigarette smoking is associated with a two- to threefold increase in adrenaline (epinephrine) secretion,[46] lasting for at least 30 minutes—**Figure 3-11**. Adrenaline stimulates $β_1$-, $β_2$-, and α-receptors, so that in the presence of nonselective (oxprenolol, propranolol) or modestly $β_1$-selective (metoprolol, atenolol) agents, there would be unopposed (total or partial) α-constriction, resulting in an increase in BP. **Figure 3-12** illustrates this point vividly[47] where, in the presence of modestly raised adrenaline concentrations, the increase in mean BP (vs. control) is marked (~30mm Hg) with nonselective agents, moderate (9-10 mg Hg) with partially $β_1$-selective metoprolol, and absent with highly $β_1$-selective bisoprolol. Such BP increases will coincide with raised adrenaline-levels (i.e., for 30-45 min during/post smoking) and may thus be missed in the clinic. However, BP-control in smokers who received propranolol in the MRC mild hypertension study[41] was somewhat inferior to that in the nonsmokers receiving propranolol.

An inevitable conclusion is that, with, say, a 20-a-day smoker taking a nonselective or poorly selective β-blocker, the BP will be

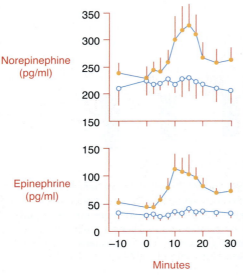

Fig. 3-11 Effect of smoking (*orange circles*) and sham-smoking (*blue circles*) upon plasma catecholamines. Note the two- to threefold increase in adrenaline (epinephrine) levels. (From Cryer PE, Haymond MW, Satiago JV, Shar SP. Norepinephrine and epinephrine release and adrenergic mediation of smoking-associated hemodynamic and metabolic events. N Engl J Med 1976;295:573–7.)

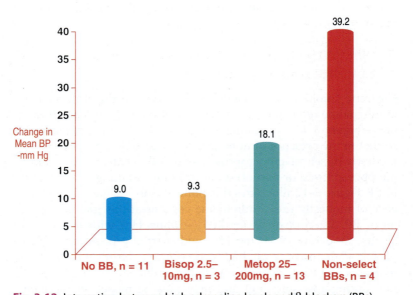

Fig. 3-12 Interaction between high adrenaline levels and β-blockers (BBs). Note the marked increase in blood pressure (vs. control) with nonselective and poorly β_1-selective (metoprolol) agents compared with no blood pressure change with highly β_1-selective bisoprolol. (From Tarnow J, Muller RK. Cardiovascular effects of low-dose epinephrine infusions in relation to the extent of pre-operative beta-blockade. Anaesthesiology 1991;74:1035–43.)

little different (or maybe considerably higher) from pretreatment levels for most of the day; hence, the "out of reach" cardiovascular events with such β-blockers. These smoking-related "out of reach" cardiovascular events could be brought "within reach" by avoidance of β_2-blockade (i.e., use of a highly β_1-selective agent).

C) β-Blockers and the overweight/obese, high-risk hypertensive patient with type 2 diabetes

UKPDS study 38[44] examined the effect of tight hypertension control (with randomized first-line captopril or atenolol, plus second-line diuretic) vs. less-tight control (acting as surrogate placebo) in obese (mean BMI = 30) hypertensive patients with type 2 diabetes. The beneficial effects, over a 9- to 10-year follow-up period, of tight control (10/5 mm Hg < less-tight control) on the seven primary end-points are shown in **Figure 3-13**; 23% were smokers (but no separate analysis is available).

UKPDS 39[45] looked at the contribution (in the tight-control group) of the randomized ACE inhibitor and β-blocker to the benefits observed over 10 years. When compared with less-tight control, the trends in benefits in all seven primary end-point, plus heart failure prevention, all favored the β-blocker—**Figure 3-14**. Notable was the approximate 50% reduction in stroke, 60% reduction in peripheral arterial disease-related end-points, 45% reduction in

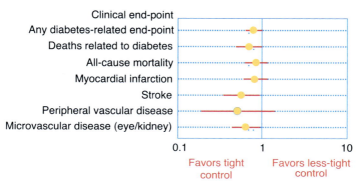

Fig. 3-13 The UKPDS (U.K. Prospective Diabetes Study) 39. The favorable effect of tight control (10/5 mm Hg < less-tight control) vs. less-tight control of blood pressure upon the seven primary end-points in middle-aged, obese hypertensive patients with type 2 diabetes. Relative risk + 95% confidence interval. (From U.K. Prospective Diabetes Study Group. Efficacy of atenolol and captopril in reducing risk of macrovascular and microvascular complications in type-2 diabetes: UKPDS 39. BMJ 1998;317:713-20.)

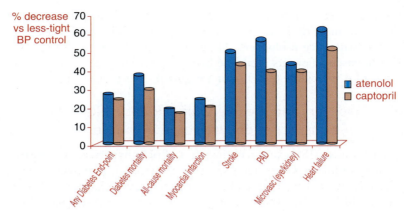

Fig. 3-14 The UKPDS 38. The trends in prevention of all seven primary end-points (plus secondary end-point of heart failure) all favor the β-blocker atenolol vs. the angiotensin-converting enzyme (ACE) inhibitor captopril (compared with less-tight control of blood pressure). PAD, peripheral artery disease. (From U.K. Prospective Diabetes Study Group. Tight blood pressure control and risk of macrovascular and microvascular complications in type-2 diabetes. UKPDS 38. BMJ 1998;317:703–13.)

microvascular (kidney and eye) end-points, and 65% reduction in heart failure by the β-blocker compared with less-tight control. There was no evidence of "special" ACE inhibitor-induced "reno-protection" as assessed by both albuminuria and serum creatinine changes. The beneficial trends of the β-blocker over the ACE inhibitor tended to increase over the 10-year observation period, and after 20 years' follow-up[48] (patients discharged to primary care after 10 years' follow-up), there was now a significant 23% reduction in all-cause death in those originally allocated to the β-blocker group— Figure 3-15; there were also strong trends favoring the β-blocker over ACE inhibition in reduction of MI and peripheral arterial disease. Relevant to these long-term benefits of β-blocker therapy may be the ability of these drugs to regress the atheromataous plaque (see Chapter 2).

Thus, first-line $β_1$-blockade has a powerful role to play in the treatment of the younger/middle-aged diastolic hypertensive patient.[49]

D) Are the benefits of antihypertensive therapy purely a function of the fall in blood pressure?

In the MRC mild hypertension study,[41] the fall in BP was somewhat greater in the diuretic than in the propranolol group and this was reflected in significantly fewer strokes. In contrast, seen also in

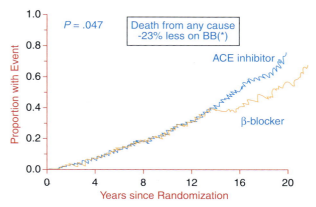

Fig. 3-15 The UKPDS at 20-year follow-up. Death from any cause was a significant 23% less in those randomized to the β-blocker (BB) group. ACE, angiotensin-converting enzyme. (From Holman RR, Paul SK, Bethel MA, et al. Long-term follow-up after tight control of blood pressure in type-2 diabetes. N Engl J Med 2008;359:1565–76.)

the IPPPSH study,[42] MI was reduced only in men randomized to β-blockade; the combined benefits of both propranolol and oxprenolol in men are shown in **Table 3-3**.[50] In particular, Q-wave MI (electrocardiogram [ECG]) and sudden death were reduced only in the propranolol group vs. placebo and diuretics—**Table 3-4**.[51] Support for these findings came from the Australian placebo-controlled study in 3427 middle-aged mild hypertensive patients[52] in whom diuretic-based therapy (albeit in doses higher than used today)

TABLE 3-3 Pooled results for young/middle-aged men (n = 7717) in the MRC mild hypertension and IPPPSH studies (rate/1000 patient-yr)

End-point	DIURETIC (N = 3827)		BETA-BLOCKER (N = 3890)		PERCENTAGE DIFFERENCE	P VALUE
	n	Rate (%)	n	Rate (%)		
Total mortality	164	9.4	137	7.7	−18	.09
Cardiovascular mortality	105	6.0	77	4.3	−28	.03
Nonfatal plus fatal chronic heart disease	186	10.7	151	8.5	−21	.04

From Wikstrand J. Beta-blockers and cardioprotection—is there any good news from the recent trials? J Clin Pharm Ther 1987;12:347–50.

TABLE 3-4 The incidence of sudden death and electrogardiogram changes compatible with transmural (Q-wave) infarction (Minnesota code 1_{1-3}) (rate/1000 person-yr of observation in over 17,000 mild hypertensives) in MRC mild hypertension study

	BENDROFLUAZIDE		PROPRANOLOL		PLACEBO	
	n	Rate (%)	n	Rate (%)	n	Rate (%)
Q-wave infarction	353	22.7†	271	16.8*	629	19.8
Sudden death	33	1.6	16	0.7	45	1.1

Rate differs significantly from control group,* $P < .05$.
Rate differs significantly from propranolol group,† $P < .001$.
From Miall W, Greenberg G (eds). Mild Hypertension: Is There Pressure to Treat? An account of the MRC trial. Cambridge, Cambridge University Press; 1987, pp 78-94 and 101–18.

resulted in a significant 45% reduction in stroke but a small increase in MI. Similar results were obtained in the Oslo Study in which diuretic therapy was compared with a randomized untreated control group over a 10-year period.[53] A mega-meta-analysis[54] claiming that all antihypertensive drug classes are equally effective in reducing cardiovascular events (combined stroke, MI, and heart failure) in both younger and older hypertensive patients persisted in lumping together β-blocker- and diuretic-based therapy as "conventional therapy" (even though they possess quite different hemodynamic profiles and modes of action), but did not (surprisingly) directly compare β-blocker and diuretic therapy in younger hypertensive patients regarding their ability to prevent the number one killer (i.e., MI) and did not relate to the powerful β-blocker/smoking interaction in this context. Had they done so they would have discovered that in young/middle-aged hypertensive patients, diuretics prevent stroke but not MI and that nonselective and moderately $β_1$-selective β-blockers prevent both stroke and MI in nonsmokers but not in smokers.

Thus, stroke prevention, unlike prevention of MI, is directly related to fall in BP and there are marked differences between drug classes in their ability to prevent MI.

5) First-line β-blockers and the elderly systolic hypertensive—major hard-end-point studies

A recent mega-meta-analysis of 147 randomized trials involving elderly (60-69 yr) hypertensive patients[55] concluded that all the classes of antihypertensive drugs have similar effects in reducing cardiovascular end-points, for a given reduction in BP (though calcium blockers may be superior in preventing stroke). Such conclusions seem to be at odds with recent studies involving first-line atenolol.

In order to better understand the complex hemodynamics of isolated systolic hypertension and the interaction with various drug therapies, the importance of pulse pressure (both peripheral and central) needs to be appreciated.

A) Arterial stiffening and pulse pressure

As arteries age and stiffen, they become less compliant and pulse pressure (PP) widens. In the elderly, a wide brachial artery PP is a somewhat better predictor of cardiovascular events than SBP and both are better than the diastolic blood pressure (DBP).[56] However, it now seems likely that central (aortic) PP is the most important predictor of cardiovascular events in the elderly.[57]

B) Central blood pressure and pulse pressure amplification; implications for β-blockers

This complex topic has recently been well described.[58,59] PP as measured at the brachial artery is higher (amplified) than the central aortic PP, and this is particularly the case in the younger/middle-aged subjects[58]—**Figure 3-16**. Hence, in the young, brachial PP is about 70% greater than central PP, but only by about 20% in the elderly. Thus, drugs that increase the amplification in the elderly (i.e., vasodilatory agents) will be associated with lower central PPs. Bradycardia (β-blockers) is associated with a decrease in the PP amplification[59]—**Figure 3-17**—and would thus be associated with wider central PPs (i.e., theoretically not good). However, a substudy of the ASCOT (Anglo-Scandinavian Cardiac Output Trial) study has shown that the higher central SBP on atenolol vs. amlodipine is not due to bradycardia but to a greater magnitude of wave reflection owing to the absence of vasodilatation.[60] This is clearly a complex area that needs further clarification.[61]

Thus, the combination of (a) the higher central SBP due to the absence of vasodilatation, (b) the age-related fall in plasma renin (particularly in hypertensive patients),[62] cardiac output,[17] β-receptor sensitivity and affinity,[63] and (c) the decreasing antihypertensive action of β-blockers in the elderly[64] suggest that classic β-blockade may not be the ideal first-line therapy for the elderly systolic hypertensive patient without coronary artery disease.

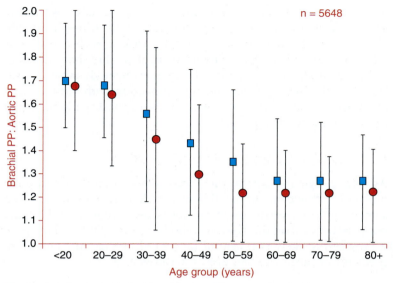

Fig. 3-16 Pulse pressure (PP) amplification lessens with increasing age in both men (*squares*) and women (*circles*). (From Avolio AP, van Bortel LM, Boutouyrie JR, et al. Role of pulse-pressure amplification in arterial hypertension. Experts opinion on review of the data. Hypertension 2009;54:3375–83.)

C) Results of first-line β-blockade in elderly hypertensives

i) No Coronary artery disease

The results of the four prospective, randomized, controlled studies involving first-line β-blockade (all atenolol) are shown in **Table 3-5**.[65-68]

In all four studies, atenolol faired poorly against placebo,[66] nontreatment,[65] diuretics,[66] losartan,[67] and amlodipine[68] in reducing the risks of cardiovascular events. In the LIFE (Losartan Intervention for Endpoint Reduction) study, the worst results for atenolol vs. losartan were in those with the widest PP.[69]

ii) With coronary artery disease (and the J-curve phenomenon)

In the large (N = 22,576) INVEST (International Verapamil/Trandolopril Study) study,[70] there was no difference in morbidity and mortality in patients randomized to either atenolol/diuretic or verapamil/ACE inhibitor therapy—**Figure 3-18a**. However, patients with poor left ventricular function at baseline fared better on atenolol/diuretic-based therapy.

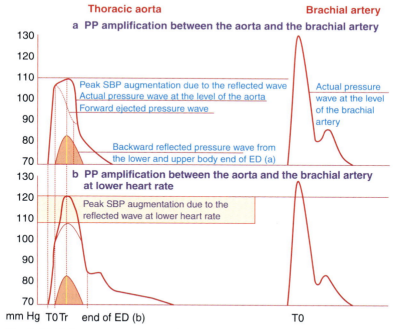

Fig. 3-17 Pulse pressure (PP) amplification between the aorta and the brachial artery. The peak central systolic blood pressure (SBP) is greater at lower heart rates. ED, end-diastole. (From Safar ME, Protogarou AD, Blacher J. Statins, central blood pressure, and blood pressure amplification. Circulation 2009;119:9–12.)

It is worth noting that in the INVEST study, a J-curve relationship was noted for treated BP and MI. This important phenomenon was first highlighted by the present author[71] who noted a J-curve relationship between treated DBP and MI in patients with myocardial ischemia (but not in nonischemic patients)—**Figure 3-18b**—but not for stroke. It was surmised that coronary diastolic filling pressure was compromised in patients whose coronary flow reserve was exhausted. This controversial topic was resolved by the large prospective Hypertension Optimal Treatment (HOT) study;[72] though the data on the 3000+ ischemic patients was not highlighted in detail in the HOT publication, the vital data finally came to light in a published J-curve debate.[73] The data are shown in **Tables 3-6 and 3-6a**, where it is apparent that in the high-risk ischemic group, for stroke prevention, the lower the BP the better; by contrast, for MI, prevention, low achieved DBP was associated an increased risk of infarction—aiming to lower DBP to less than 80 mm Hg compared

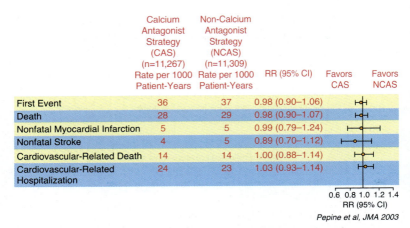

Fig. 3-18a The INVEST (International Verapamol/Trandolopril Study) studies in elderly (mean age 66 yr) hypertensive patients ($N = 22{,}576$) with coronary heart disease. The atenolol/thiazide combination was equivalent to the calcium antagonist/ACE inhibitor combination in reducing primary endpoints. CI, confidence interval; RR, relative risk. (From Pepine CJ, Handberg EM, Cooper-Dehoff RM, et al. A calcium antagonist vs non-calcium antagonist hypertension treatment strategy for patients with coronary artery disease [INVEST]. JAMA 2003;290:2805–16.)

with less than 85 mm Hg was associated with a 22% increase in the risk of MI.

D) Why was first-line atenolol so ineffective in elderly systolic hypertensive patients (without coronary heart disease)?

i) Effects on central (aortic) hemodynamics

In a double-blind, randomized, cross-over study involving elderly isolated systolic hypertensive patients, the effects of atenolol, diuretic, calcium antagonist, and ACE inhibitor upon central pressures were studied.[74] Unlike the three other drugs, atenolol had no significant effect upon central SBP or PP—**Figure 3-19**. This result was confirmed by others[75] who also showed that whereas the calcium antagonist, ACE inhibitor, and diuretic all reduced the augmentation index (ratio of augmentation pressure over the PP), atenolol increased it. The CAFE (Conduit Artery Function Evaluation) substudy of the ASCOT study[76] also showed that atenolol was inferior to calcium blocker-based therapy in its effects upon central hemodynamics (not reflected in peripheral values).

TABLE 3-5 First-line β-blockers (atenolol) perform poorly in elderly systolic hypertension (wide pulse pressure)

Trial	β-blocker	Mean age (yr)	Initial BP (mm Hg)	Pulse pressure (mm Hg)	Result
MRC Elderly	Atenolol (vs. placebo vs. diuretic)	70	185/91	94	Only diuretics differed from placebo in stroke prevention; diuretic was superior to atenolol in reducing coronary events.
HEP	Atenolol (vs. nontreatment)	69	196/99	97	Significant reduction in stroke but no effect on coronary events by atenolol.
LIFE	Atenolol (vs. losartan)	67	174/98	76	Losartan was superior to atenolol in reducing cardiovascular mortality and nonfatal and fatal stroke.
ASCOT	Atenolol ± Diuretic (vs. amlodipine ± perindopril)	63	164/94	70	Amlodipine ± perindopril was superior to atenolol ± diuretic in reducing all-cause mortality and all coronary and stroke end-points.

ASCOT, Anglo-Scandinavian Cardic Output Trial; BP, blood pressure; HEP, Hypertension in Primary Care; LIFE, Losaratan Intervention for Endpoint Reduction; MRC, Medical Research Council.
From Cruickshank JM. Are we misunderstanding beta-blockers? Int J Cardiol 2007;120:10–27.

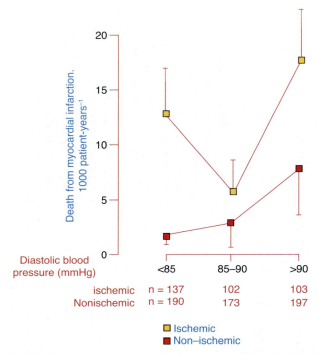

Fig. 3-18b The J-curve phenomenon. In hypertensive patients with ischemic heart disease, excessive lowering of diastolic blood pressure results in an increased frequency of death from myocardial infarction. (From Cruickshank JM, Thorp JM, Zacharias FJ. Benefits and potential harm in lowering high blood pressure. Lancet 1987;1:581–4.)

ii) Effects on left ventricular hypertrophy in elderly and younger hypertensives

Meta-analysis has indicated that β-blockers reverse LVH only modestly compared with ACE inhibitors.[77] However, the important age effect was not taken into account—an error still being made in 2009!.[78] In the younger/middle-aged hypertensive patient, LVH is related to both high BP and increased sympathetic nerve activity. So-called inadequate LVH has a high wall stress and is linked to high BP,[79] whereas inappropriate LVH (probably eccentric) has a low wall stress and is linked to neurohumoral activation.[80] Such LVH should be reversible by $β_1$-blockade. In contrast, LVH (probably concentric) in the elderly isolated systolic hypertensive results from poor vascular compliance associated with a high central augmented SBP, wide PP,[81] and low PP amplification[58] and should be reversible by agents that improve vascular compliance and lower

TABLE 3-6 J-curve phenomenon; excessive lowering of diastolic blood pressure in hypertensive patients with ischemic heart disease may increase the risk of myocardial infarction; HOT study

Group	Target DBP	N	Base SBP/DBP	Achieved SBP/DBP	ALL MI + SILENT MI		
					Events/1000 patient/yr	Comparison	RR
Non IHD	≤90	5245	169/105	143/85	4.7	90 vs. 85	1.13
	≤85	5228	169/105	141/83	4.1	85 vs. 80	1.07
	≤80	527	169/105	139/81	3.9	90 vs. 80	1.21
With IHD	≤90	1019	174/106	146/85	9.3	90 vs. 85	1.37
	≤85	1036	173/106	144/83	6.8	85 vs. 80	0.82
	≤80	1025	173/106	143/81	8.3	90 vs. 80	1.12

DBP, diastolic blood pressure; HOT, Hypertension Optimal Treatment; IHD, ischemic heart disease; MI, myocardial infarction; RR, relative risk; SBP, systolic blood pressure.

From Cruickshank JM. The J-curve in hypertension. Curr Cardiol Rep 2003;5:441–52.

TABLE 3-6a J-curve phenomenon; excessive lowering of diastolic blood pressure in hypertensive patients with ischemic heart disease does not increase the risk of stroke; HOT study

Group	Target DBP	N	Base SBP/DBP	Achieved SBP/DBP	ALL STROKE Events/1000 patient/yr	Comparison	RR
Non IHD	≤90	5245	169/105	143/85	3.0	90 vs. 85	0.73
	≤85	5228	169/105	141/83	4.1	85 vs. 80	1.17
	≤80	5237	169/105	139/81	3.5	90 vs. 80	0.85
With IHD	≤90	1019	174/106	146/85	9.3	90 vs. 85	1.18
	≤85	1036	173/106	144/83	7.9	85 vs. 80	1.48
	≤80	1025	173/106	143/81	5.3	90 vs. 80	1.75*

*P value for trend = .046.
DBP, diastolic blood pressure; HOT, Hypertension Optimal Treatment; IHD, ischemic heart disease; RR, relative risk; SBP, systolic blood pressure.
From Cruickshank JM. The J-curve in hypertension. Curr Cardiol Rep 2003;5:441–52.

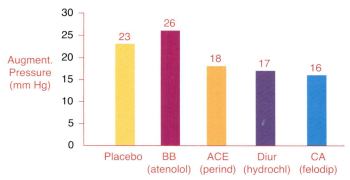

Fig. 3-19 Effect of different antihypertensive agents (vs. placebo) central/aortic systolic pressure in 52 elderly (mean age 77 yr) systolic hypertensive patients (randomized, double-blind, cross-over times 1 mo. ACE, angiotensin-converting enzyme inhibitor; BB, β-blocker; CA, calcium antagonist; Diur, diuretic. (From Morgan T, Lauri J, Bertram D, Anderson A. Effect of different antihypertensive drug classes on central aortic pressure. Am J Hypertens 2004;17:118–23.)

central SBP, decrease PP, and increase PP amplification (i.e., not classic β-blockers).

In accordance with these predictions, atenolol, in contrast to verapamil, had an absence of effect upon echocardiographic LVH reversal in elderly hypertensive patients;[82] similar poor results in the elderly for atenolol occurred in comparisons with perindopril[83] and ibesartan[84] and in the LIFE study, in which losartan was more effective than atenolol in reversing both ECG LVH[67] and echocardiographic LVH.[85]

In stark contrast, β-blockers are highly effective in reversing LVH in younger/middle-aged hypertensive patients. Atenolol is highly effective in reversing LVH whether assessed by ECG[86,87] or echocardiogram (particularly effective in reducing wall thickness vs. diuretic[88]) and is equivalent to the ACE inhibitor ramipril in this respect.[89] Metoprolol is likewise effective.[90] Highly β_1-selective bisoprolol also significantly reduces left ventricular mass and reduces wall thickness,[91,92] being at least as good as ACE inhibition in this respect[93]—**Figure 3-20**. This reversal of LVH with bisoprolol is accompanied by a 20% increase in coronary flow reserve[94]—**Figure 3-21**.

Interestingly, in a large comparative study involving 1105 middle-aged men, with almost 60% black hypertensive patients, at 1-year follow-up, only hydrochlorothiazide, captopril, and atenolol effected significant falls in left ventricular mass (atenolol

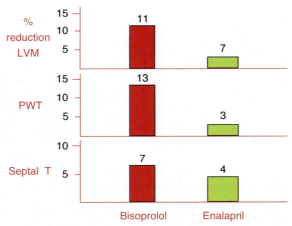

Fig. 3-20 Effect of randomized bisoprolol and enalapril on left ventricular hypertrophy (LVH) over a 6-mo period in 56 middle-aged (mean age 50 yr) hypertensive patients. The β-blocker is at least as effective as the ACE inhibitor. LVM, left ventricular mass; PWT, posterior wall thickness; Septal T, septal thickness. (From Goss P, Routaut R, Herreo G, Dallocchio M. Beta-blockers vs ACE-inhibition in hypertension: effects on left-ventricular hypertrophy. J Cardiovasc Pharmacol 1990;16:S 145–50.)

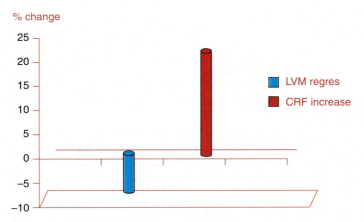

Fig. 3-21 Effect of bisoprolol dosed for over 1 year on left ventricular mass (LVM) and coronary flow reserve (CFR) in 10 hypertensive patients with ischemic heart disease. (From Motz W, Vogt M, Scheler S, et al. Improvement of coronary reserve following regression of hypertrophy resulting from blood pressure lowering with a beta-blocker. Dtsch Med Wochen 1993;118:535–40.)

particularly effective in reducing wall thickness) compared with clonidine, diltiazem, and prazosin, which did not (in spite of good BP control).[95]

iii) β-Blocker/smoking interaction in the elderly hypertensive

The powerful β-blocker (propranolol, oxprenolol, and metoprolol)/smoking interaction described earlier in young/middle-aged hypertensive patients[41-43] was also noted with atenolol in the MRC elderly study,[66] whether given first-line (second-line diuretics) or second-line (to first-line diuretics)—**Figure 3-22**. In the MRC elderly study, about 20% were smokers, and the modest 16% reduction vs. placebo in cardiovascular events with first-line atenolol in nonsmokers was converted to a worrying 38% increase in smokers. Likewise, the marked 39% decrease vs. placebo in cardiovascular events in the diuretic (second-line atenolol) group who were nonsmokers is converted to a meager 7% reduction in the smoking group.

Interestingly the adverse atenolol/smoking interaction was not apparent in the LIFE study,[96] where the advantage of losartan over atenolol was noted mainly in the nonsmokers.

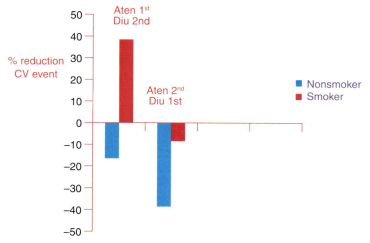

Fig. 3-22 β-blocker/smoking interaction in the MRC elderly trial. With first-line atenolol/second-line diuretic, cardiovascular (CV) events were markedly increased (vs. placebo) in smokers. In second-line atenolol/first-line diuretic, the CV benefits were abolished in smokers. (From Medical Research Council Working Party. MRC trial of treatment of hypertension in older adults: principal results. Br Med J 1992;304:405–12.)

6. β-blockers given as second-line therapy to first-line diuretic or calcium antagonist therapy in elderly hypertensives

A) Hard-end-point trials

In considering the advantages and disadvantages of a diuretic/β-blocker combination, it has become clear that results depend on which agent is given first. The MRC elderly study[66] addressed this very issue, comparing (vs. placebo) first-line diuretic/second-line β-blocker and first-line β-blocker/second-line diuretic. In spite of BP control being roughly equal with the two treatment arms, the effects upon hard cardiovascular end-points were quite different—Table 3-7. First-line atenolol/second-line diuretic (vs. placebo) produced little benefit, having no impact on coronary events and a nonsignificant reduction in stroke. In contrast, first-line diuretic/second-line atenolol effected a significant 44% reduction in coronary and 31% reduction in stroke events. A possible explanation is that a first-line diuretic[97] (or indeed calcium antagonist[98]) increases sympathetic nerve activity (and renin levels) in addition to improving vascular compliance and central hemodynamics,[74] thus pro-

TABLE 3-7 Reducing the rate of stroke and coronary events (vs. placebo) in elderly hypertensive patients with the combination of diuretic and atenolol when atenolol is first-line therapy and second-line therapy

Placebo-controlled studies involving atenolol as first- or second-line therapy		Reduction in coronary events vs. placebo (%)	Reduction in stroke events vs. placebo (%)
Atenolol as first-line (diuretic second-line)	MRC Elderly	0 (NS)	17 (NS)
Atenolol as second-line (diuretic first-line) therapy	MRC Elderly	44 (sig)	31 (sig)
Atenolol as second-line (diuretic first-line) therapy	SHEP	27 (sig)	36 (sig)

MRC, Medical Research Council; NS, not significant; SHEP, Systolic Hypertension in the Elderly Program; sig, significant.
From Cruickshank JM. Are we misunderstanding beta-blockers? Int J Cardiol 2007;120:10–27.

ducing a hemodynamic scenario suited to β_1-blockade—that is, not dissimilar to that occurring in younger, overweight diastolic hypertensive patients (in whom first-line β-blockers perform well at least in nonsmokers).

The impressive results of first-line diuretic/second-line β-blocker shown in the MRC elderly study[66] were reproduced in the SHEP[99] and ALLHAT[100] studies. In SHEP, stroke frequency was reduced by a significant 36% and fatal and nonfatal coronary events were reduced by a significant 27% by chlorthalidone/β-blocker-based therapy vs. placebo. ALLHAT (Antihypertensive and Lipid-Lowering Treatment to Prevent Heart Attack Trial) is the largest (N = 42,418) prospective, randomized study ever completed, though the numbers were reduced to 33,357 owing to the removal of the α-blocker doxazasin (owing to an excess of heart failure). The investigators concluded that after 5 years' follow-up, comparing chorthalidone- (second-line mainly β-blocker), amlodipine-, and lisinopril-based therapy, the diuretic-based therapy was the favored treatment—**Table 3-8**.

The diuretic/β-blocker combination is superior to a diuretic/calcium antagonist combination in the prevention of MI.[101]

An attractive "bonus" of the diuretic/β-blocker combination in the elderly hypertensive patient is the fact that this combination reduced the risk of bone fracture by about 30%[102]—**Figure 3-23.**

The INSIGHT (International Nifedipine GITS Study: Intervention as a Goal in Hypertension Treatment) study[103] was a double-blind

TABLE 3-8 ALLHAT (N = 33,357, mean age 67 yr)—results

a. Treated BP at 5 yr = Chorthalidone 133.9/75.4; amlodipine 134.7/74.6; lisinopril 135.9/75.4
b. Primary outcome (combined fatal & nonfatal CHD)—No difference
c. Secondary Outcome:
   Chlorthalidone vs. Amlodipine—CCF on amlodipine increased × 38%
   Chlorthalidone vs. Lisinipine—Combined CVD on lisinopril increased × 10%
   Stroke on lisinopril increased × 15%
   CCF on lisinopril increased × 19%
d. Thiazide is preferred first-line antihypertensive agent (β-blocker usually second-line)

ALLHAT, Antihypertensive and Lipid-Lowering Treatment to Prevent Heart Attack Trial; BP, blood pressure; CCF, congestive cardiac failure; CHD, coronary heart disease; CVD, cardiovascular disease.
From The ALLHAT Officers and Coordinators for the ALLHAT Collaborative Research Group. Major outcomes in high-risk hypertensive patients randomised to ACE-inhibitor or calcium channel blocker vs diuretic. JAMA 2002;288:2981–97.

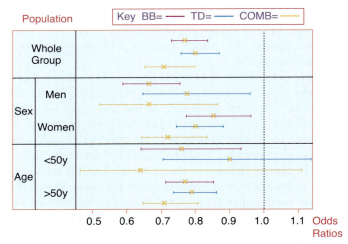

Fig. 3-23 Decline in risk of bone fracture (N = 30,6001) by β-blockers (BB), thiazide diuretics (TD), and their combination (COMB). Controls N = 120,819. (From Schlienger RG, Kraenzlin ME, Meier CR. Use of beta-blockers and risk of fractures. JAMA 2004;292:1326–32.)

comparison of slow-release nifedipine/second-line atenolol vs. hydrochlorothiazide-amiloride/second-line atenolol. The result showed no difference in the primary end-point, though fatal MI and nonfatal heart failure were increased in the calcium antagonist group.

Both men and women gain equal benefit from antihypertensive therapy.[104]

B) Fixed, low-dose β-blocker/diuretic combination therapy

Fixed, low-dose combination therapy is optimal in terms of simplicity and patient compliance, particularly in the elderly.[105]

There are no hard-end-point trials involving low fixed-dose diuretic/β-blocker combinations. However, such combinations involving high $β_1$-selectivity are highly effective in lowering BP in both old and young, with minimal or absent adverse reactions and metabolic disturbance, as shown with various bisoprolol doses (2.5-40 mg) combined with hydrochlorothiazide (6.25 mg).

Under placebo-controlled conditions, there is little value in going above the dose of 5 mg od bisoprolol in terms of controlling SBP[106]—Figure 3-24. Response rates (DBP < 90 mm Hg or a fall of ≥ 10 mm Hg SBP) are excellent compared with placebo, amlodipine, and enalapril[107]—Figure 3-25—and losartan alone or combined

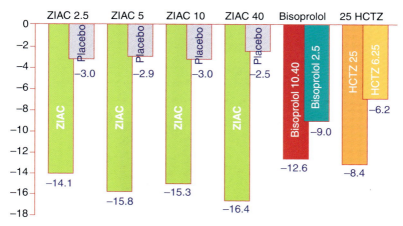

Fig. 3-24 The fixed combination of β₁-blockade (bisoprolol) at low dosage with low-dose diuretic (Ziac) is highly effective at reducing systolic blood pressure (vs. placebo). HCTZ, hydrochlorothiazide. (From Frishman WH, Burris JF, Mroczek WJ, et al. First-line therapy option with low-dose bisoprolol fumarate and low dose hydrochlorothiazide with stage I and stage II systemic hypertension. J Clin Pharmacol 1995;35:182–8.)

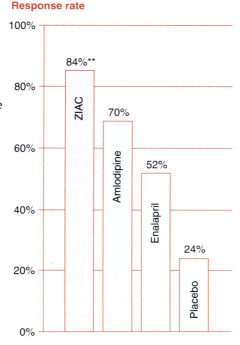

Fig. 3-25 Fixed combination of low-dose β₁-blockade (bisoprolol) and low-dose diuretic (Ziac) controls blood compared well with calcium blocker or ACE inhibitor-based therapy and placebo (response rate is the achievement of diastolic blood pressure [DBP] <90 mm Hg or fall of at least 10 mm Hg systolic blood pressure [SBP]). **, significant vs. amlodipine, enalapril, and placebo. (From Neutel JM, Rolf CN, Valentine SN, et al. Low dose combination therapy at first-line treatment of mild to moderate hypertension the efficacy and safety of bisoprolol/6.25 mg HCTH versus amlodipine, enalapril and placebo. Cardiovasc Rev Rep 1996;17:33–45.)

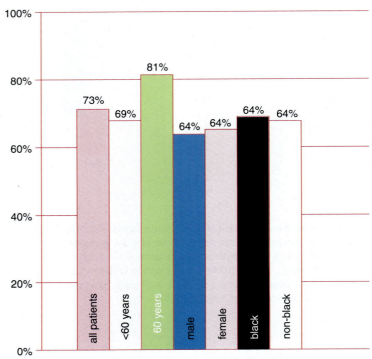

Fig. 3-26 The response rate (DBP < 90 mm Hg or fall of SBP > 10 mm Hg) to the fixed combination of low-dose β_1-blockade and diuretic (Ziac) is excellent, and similar, in elderly and younger patients and also in black and white subjects. (From Frishman WH, Burris JF, Mroczek WJ, et al. First-line therapy option with low-dose bisoprolol fumarate and low dose hydrochlorothiazide with stage I and stage II systemic hypertension. J Clin Pharmacol 1995;35:182–8.)

with diuretic.[108] Adverse reactions and metabolic disturbance were minimal or absent. Response rates were particularly good in the elderly (>60 yr) and were the same in both black and white subjects[106]—**Figure 3-26**, and BP was well controlled throughout the whole 24-hr period[109]—**Figure 3-27**.

7. Are Induced metabolic changes with diuretic/β-blocker-based therapy harmful?

β-blocker-associated metabolic disturbances involving blood sugar, hemoglobin$_{A1c}$ (Hb$_{A1c}$), insulin sensitivity, free fatty acids, plasma triglycerides, and very low density lipoprotein (VLDL) and high-density lipoprotein (HDL) cholesterol are closely linked to β_2-blockade.[110]

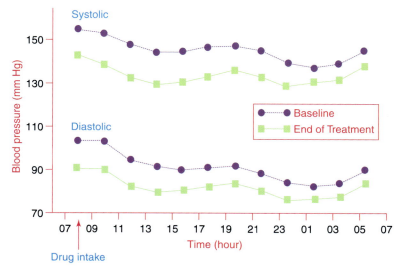

Fig. 3-27 The fixed combination of low-dose β_1-blockade and diuretic is effective in lowering blood pressure over 24 hr. (From Lewin AJ, Lueg MC, Targum S, et al. A clinical trial evaluating the 24 hour effects of bisoprolol 5/ hydrochlorothiazide 6.25 mg combination in patients with mild to moderate hypertension. Clin Cardiol 1993;16:732–6.)

Thus, nonselective agents like propranolol, timolol, and nadolol will be the worst offenders, followed by modestly β_1-selective agents like atenolol and metoprolol. Highly β_1-selective β-blockers like bisoprolol (at doses of ≤ 10 mg or less) will be essentially free of metabolic disturbances involving blood sugar, insulin sensitivity, and lipids,[111,112] as will agents containing α-blockade (e.g., carvedilol[113,114]) or β_2/β_3 intrinsic sympathomimetic activity (ISA; e.g., nebivolol[115]).

With diuretics, biochemical disturbance is minimal with low doses, particularly with hydrochlorothiazide.[116]

Do these drug-induced surrogate end-points for cardiovascular events actually predict what will happen to the patient? In the UKPDS study,[45] atenolol (diuretic second-line)-based therapy was associated with an increase in Hb_{A1c} concentration, yet after 9 years follow-up, the Kaplan-Meier plots of patients who died of cardiovascular causes related to diabetes were separating at 5-6 years in favor of atenolol, over captopril-based, therapy—**Figure 3-28**. Importantly, at 20 years' follow-up,[48] there was now a significant 23% reduction in all-cause death in the group originally allotted to the β-blocker group—(see **Figure 3-15**).

Perhaps even more revealing were the results stemming from the 14.3-year follow-up of the placebo-controlled SHEP study[126]

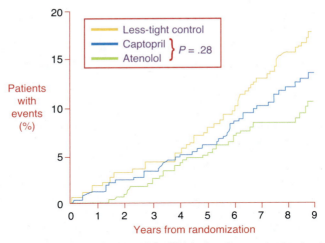

Fig. 3-28 The UKPDS 39. The benefits of β-blocker therapy (reduction in frequency of death related to diabetes) compared with ACE inhibitor-based therapy and "less-tight control of blood pressure" become greater with time (>6 yr follow-up) (From U.K. Prospective Diabetes Study Group. Efficacy of atenolol and captopril in reducing risk of macrovascular and microvascular complications in type-2 diabetes: UKPDS 39. BMJ 1998;317:713–20.)

involving first-line chlorthalidone/second-line atenolol—Table 3-9. In the placebo group, naturally occurring type 2 diabetes at baseline (vs. no diabetes) was associated with a significant 63% excess in cardiovascular mortality over the 14.3-year follow-up.

TABLE 3-9 Drug-induced diabetes, in contrast to spontaneously occurring type 2 diabetes, may not be dangerous to the patient; SHEP study 14-Yr follow-up

Population subset	Effect upon CV mortality (%)
DM2 at baseline in placebo group (vs. no DM2)	+63 (sig)
DM2 at baseline treated with diuretic ± atenolol (vs. placebo)	−31 (sig)
DM2 developing on placebo (vs. no DM2)	+56 (sig)
DM2 developing on diuretic ± atenolol (vs. no DM2)	+4 (NS)

CV, cardiovascular; DM2, type 2 diabetes mellitus; SHEP, Systolic Hypertension in the Elderly Program.

From Kostis JB, Wilson AC, Freudenburger RS, et al, SHEP Collaborative Research Group. Long-term effects of diuretic-based therapy on fatal outcomes in subjects with isolated systolic hypertension with and without diabetes. Am J Cardiol 2005;95:29–35.

Those with naturally occurring diabetes at baseline who were allocated to diuretic±atenolol-based therapy experienced a significant 31% fall in cardiovascular mortality. Naturally occurring type-2 diabetes developing in the placebo group over the whole 14-yr follow-up period was associated with a significant 56% increase in cardiovascular mortality compared with those who did not develop diabetes. In marked contrast, the cardiovascular mortality of diuretic±atenolol-induced type 2 diabetes did not differ from that in those without drug-induced diabetes.

Conclusion: β-blocker/diuretic-induced type 2 diabetes appears not to harm the patient in the long-term compared with naturally occurring type 2 diabetes, which is usually linked to central obesity and an underlying inflammatory process, which does increase cardiovascular mortality. If in doubt, a β-blocker, without ISA or α-blocking activity, which does not induce metabolic changes can be used (e.g., low-dose bisoprolol).

In agreement with these conclusions are results arising from the large ALLHAT study[117] that addressed the issue of diuretic/β-blocker therapy in patients at high risk of developing diabetes (i.e., the metabolic syndrome). The overall trends favoring diuretic-based therapy become even stronger in those with the metabolic syndrome—**Figure 3-29**.

8. Where do angiotensin receptor blockers fit in?

The U.K. NICE committee[13] recommended that in young/middle-aged hypertensive patients ACE inhibitors or ARBs should be preferred first-line choices (not β-blockers). But where is the prospective, randomized, controlled evidence that ARBs will reduce cardiovascular (particularly MI) end-points and death in younger hypertensive patients? Considering that MI is the main cause of death in younger/middle-aged hypertensive patients, being some three times more common than stroke,[41] it is particularly worrying to note that in two meta-analyses,[118] ARBs appear to have no effect upon decreasing the risk of MI (and may even increase the risk!) or cardiovascular points, compared with ACE inhibitors, which do—**Table 3-10**. However, a more recent larger meta-analysis[119] concluded that ARBs did not differ from other therapies (including placebo!) in preventing MI (though all studies were in the elderly, mean age 67 yr).

The effects of ARB in the younger hypertensive patient in whom the risk of MI is high (three times higher than stroke[41]) remain unknown. The high sympathetic nerve activity in younger/

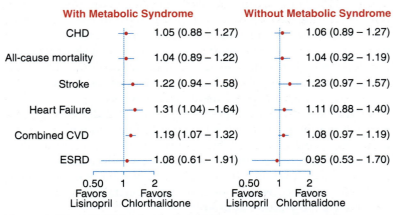

Fig. 3-29 The ALLHAT Study, $N = 33{,}357$. The trends in reducing primary end-points favoring chlorthalidone (second-line β-blocker)–based therapy vs. ACE inhibitor-based therapy in hypertensive patients without the metabolic syndrome become stronger (and sometimes significantly so) in those with the metabolic syndrome. CHD, coronary heart disease; CVD, cardiovascular disease; ESRD, end-stage renal disease. (From Black HR, Davis B, Barzilay J, et al. Metabolic and clinical outcomes in non-diabetic individuals with the metabolic syndrome assigned to chlorthalidone, amlodipine or lisinopril as initial treatment for hypertension. Diabetes Care 2008;31:353–60.)

middle-aged hypertensive patients, with or without the metabolic syndrome or type 2 diabetes, has already been described.[23–26] Unlike ACE inhibitors,[120] ARBs do not reduce sympathetic nerve activity[121] and, indeed, may even increase it in young adults[122,123]—**Figure 3-30** (though, like ACE inhibitors, ARBs can decrease sympathetic nerve activity in cases of renal failure[124]). Such an event, possibly arising from a resetting of the baroreflex due to the marked elevated angiotensin II levels, could well be a reason why ARBs might not reduce (or might even increase) the risk of MI, the main cause of death in younger hypertensive patients.[118]

Thus, a possible conclusion from these data is that antihypertensive agents that further increase already raised sympathetic nerve activity a young/middle-aged diastolic hypertensive patient (i.e., ARB,[122,123] diuretics, and dihydropiridine calcium antagonists[125]) will not reduce the risk of MI, unlike ACE inhibitors and β-blockers that do.

TABLE 3-10 Relative risk of myocardial infarction and cardiovascular death in meta-analyses of angiotensin receptor blockers and angiotensin-converting enzyme inhibitors

	TSUYKI ET AL—ARB (N = 68,711)		STRAUSS & HALL—ARB (N = 55,050)		STRAUSS & HALL—ACE INHIBITORS (N = 150,943)	
	RR (95% CI)	P value	RR (95% CI)	P value	RR (95% CI)	P value
MI	1.03 (0.93–1.113)	.59	1.08 (1.01–1.16)	.03	0.86 (0.82–0.90)	<.0001
CV death	NA	NA	1.01 (0.95–1.07)	.07	0.88 (0.82–0.95)	<.0005

ACE, angniotensin-converting enzyme ARB, angiotensin-receptor blocker; CI, confidence interval; CV, cardiovascular; MI, myocardial infarction; NA, not applicable; RR, relative risk.
From Strauss MH, Hall A. Renin-angiotensin system and cardiovascular risk. Lancet 2007;370:24-5.

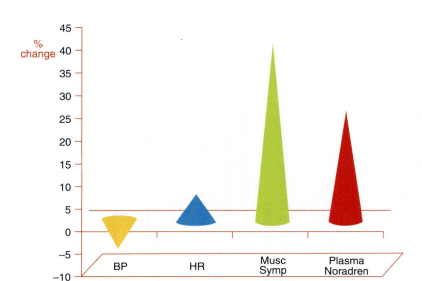

Fig. 3-30 Angiotensin receptor blockers (ARBs) increase sympathetic nerve activity (muscle sympathetic nerve activity and plasma noradrenaline) in young, hypertensive subjects (vs. randomized, cross-over, placebo-controlled, double-blind). BP, blood pressure; HR, heart rate. (From Heusser K, Vithovsky J, Raasch W, et al. Elevation of sympathetic nerve activity by eprosartan in young male subjects. Am J Hypertens 2003;16:658–64.)

9. So how did the U.K. NICE committee get it so wrong?

1. Failure to acknowledge the quite different pathophysiological mechanisms involved in young/middle-aged, probably centrally obese, diastolic hypertensive patients (in whom the high sympathetic drive, heart rate, and cardiac output are ideal for first-line β_1-blockade) and elderly systolic hypertensive patients (in whom first-line β-blockade is inappropriate).
2. Thus, meta-analyses that group together both types of study (young/diastolic and elderly/systolic hypertension) in which β-blockers are given first-line will cloud the issue.
3. Inappropriate attention to (a) surrogate end-points such as blood sugar levels and (b) uncontrolled, observational data regarding drug-induced (combined β-blocker/diuretic) diabetes and cardiovascular events (and cost-effective implications), at the expense of long-term (15-20 yr) prospective, placebo (or surrogate placebo) –controlled studies indicating that drug-induced metabolic changes appear not to be harmful.[44,45,48,126]

4. Ignoring the fact that (a) in the one and only study in which first-line ACE inhibition was compared with first-line β-blockade in younger/middle-aged hypertensive patients (UKPDS 39 study), all the seven primary end-point trends favored the β-blocker, becoming significant after 20 years for all-cause death and (b) ARBs may not prevent MI (main cause of death) in younger middle-aged hypertensive patients.
5. Nonappreciation of the powerful cigarette-smoking interaction that dilutes the significant cardiovascular benefits of first-line nonselective and modestly $β_1$-selective β-blockers in nonsmoking younger/middle-aged diastolic hypertensive patients.

10. Secondary hypertension

A) Renal disease and dialysis patients

Patients with renal failure requiring hemodialysis invariably have hypertension and volume overload. Such patients gain benefit from antihypertensive therapy, with all the main drug classes, including β-blockers, having similar benefit (i.e., an approximate 30% reduction in cardiovascular events[127–129]). This benefit may be due to the fall in BP. However, hemodialysis patients have very high levels of sympathetic nerve activity,[130] as is the case in chronic kidney disease, where it is directly related to cardiovascular mortality,[131] indicating the β-blockade might be highly beneficial in such cases. Particular benefits of β-blockade might be expected in cases of volume overload plus subclinical hypertensive heart failure.[132]

If a β-blocker is used in such cases, choice of an agent that is easily removed by the dialysis process (e.g., atenolol or bisoprolol) would seem sensible.[133]

B) Pheochromocytoma

This has been well reviewed.[134]

A pheochromocytoma is a rare tumor (usually benign) of the chromaffin tissue in the adrenal medulla, and can cause hypertensive crises that may be life-threatening. Noradrenaline is the dominant catecholamine produced, though adrenaline levels are frequently increased.

Giving a nonselective β-blocker such as propranolol alone can induce a marked hypertensive response (SBP > 200 mg Hg) leading to acute pulmonary edema.[135] The hypertensive response is presumably via unbridled α-constriction with high adrenaline levels in the presence of $β_1$- plus $β_2$-blockade. Thus, a nonselective or modestly selective β-blocker should always be given alongside an α-blocker such as phenoxybenzamine. Giving a combined β-/alpha-blocker like labetalol can still be associated with marked hypertensive responses.[136] Probably the best approach is to give a highly $β_1$-selective agent like bisoprolol alongside an α-blocker, where hypertensive interactions with adrenaline do not occur—(see **Figure 3-12**).

C) Hypertension of pregnancy

Hypertension occurs in 5%-10% of pregnancies and can lead to maternal and fetal complications. β-Blockers are generally effective and well tolerated by both mother and fetus[137] as illustrated by the classic randomized, placebo-controlled study of Rubin and coworkers[138] in 120 mothers with late-onset hypertension. BP was well-controlled—**Figure 3-31**—by the β-blocker, which was well-accepted by mother and fetus. Birth weights were the same in both groups, though atenolol was associated with low placental weights. The respiratory distress syndrome occurred significantly less often in the atenolol group. Others[139] have noted low birth weights with all β-blockers, though labetalol may be the exception.[140] In a randomized

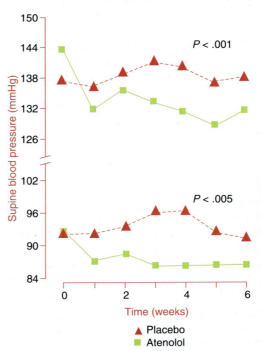

Fig. 3-31 In pregnancy-associated hypertension, atenolol (vs. randomized placebo) effectively controls raised blood pressure. (From Rubin PC, Clark DM, Sumner DJ, et al. Placebo-controlled trial of atenolol in treatment of pregnancy associated hypertension. Lancet 1983;1:431–4.)

comparison between atenolol and methyldopa,[141] the β-blocker was somewhat better at lowering BP, fetal Apgar scores were the same for both drugs, placental weights were lower with atenolol, but fetal hypoglycemia was more common with methyldopa.

The situation is different for hypertension occurring in the first trimester. It is possible, along with diuretics and ACE inhibitors, but unlike calcium antagonists, that β-blockers may be associated with an increase in cardiac malformations[142]

11. Is the choice of β-blocker important in relation to efficacy?

Aspects relating to adverse reactions (including metabolic changes) will be dealt with in the final chapter.

A) Antihypertensive efficacy in young/middle-aged diastolic hypertension

As indicated in the chapter on pharmacology, pure $β_2$-blockade (ICI 118551) induces vasoconstriction and an increase in BP of 7/5 mm Hg (see Pharmacology chapter, ref. 46). Hence, nonselective propranolol is less effective in lowering BP than modestly $β_1$-selective atenolol (see Pharmacology chapter, ref. 47), whereas atenolol, in turn, is less effective than highly $β_1$-selective bisoprolol in controlling 24-hr BP (see Pharmacology chapter, Fig. 1-12[48]). The antihypertensive advantage of bisoprolol over atenolol was particularly noted in smokers[143]—**Figure 3-32a**.

The possession of moderate/high ISA (e.g., pindolol) is associated with good control of daytime BP but little, or no, effect on nocturnal (low sympathetic drive) BP (see Pharmacology chapter, Fig. 1-20[81]).

Thus, the best control of diastolic hypertension in young/middle-aged subjects (which is caused by high sympathetic nerve activity, heart rate, and cardiac output) is via pure $β_1$-blockade.

How does pure $β_1$-blockade (e.g., bisoprolol 5.0 mg) fare against other classes of antihypertensive agents in this younger/middle-aged group? Two classic randomized, cross-over, placebo-controlled studies have answered this question. In a comparison with amlodipine, doxazosin, lisinopril, and bendrofluazide, bisoprolol achieved the lowest mean 24-hr BP and was the most frequent "best" treatment[144]—**Table 3-11, Figure 3-32b**. The second study in 208 middle-aged, hypertensive men comparing 1-month therapy of loasartan, amlodipine, a diuretic, and bisoprolol showed that the

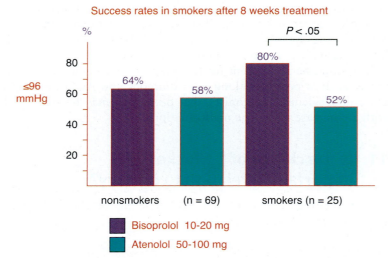

Fig. 3-32a Control of raised blood pressure is better with bisoprolol than with atenolol, particularly in smokers. (From Buhler FR, Berglund G, Anderson OK, et al. Double-blind comparison of the cardioselective beta-blockers bisoprolol and atenolol in hypertension [BIMS]. J Cardiovasc Pharmacol 1986;8:S122–7.)

β-blocker was statistically superior to the other three agents in controlling both systolic and diastolic office BP[145]—**Figure 3-33**—as well as being the best at controlling 24-hr BP during both day and night. These results on BP-control of bisoprolol vs. losartan have been confirmed by others,[146] who also showed that over a 1-year follow-up

TABLE 3-11 β-Blockade (bisoprolol) is superior to other antihypertensive therapies in the younger hypertensive*

Drug	Number of times as "best" treatment	Mean age (yr)	24-hr mean BP (mm Hg)
Amlodipine	5	49	144/95
Doxazosin	4	46	154/102
Lisinopril	10	47	136/89
Bisoprolol	13	43	135/86
Bendrofluazide	2	52	148/99

*24-hr BPs on "best" treatment in younger hypertensives; randomized, double-blind, cross-over design.
BP, blood pressure.
From Deary AJ, Schumann AL, Marfet H, et al. Double-blind, placebo-controlled crossover comparison of five classes of antihypertensive drugs. J Hypertens 2002;20:771–7.

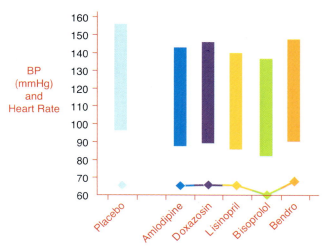

Fig. 3-32b Under randomized, double-blind, cross-over conditions in young/middle-aged (28-55 yr) diastolic hypertensive patients, bisoprolol was the most effective antihypertensive agent compared with the α-blocker doxazosin, the calcium blocker amlodipine, the ACE inhibitor lisinopril, and the diuretic bendrofluazide, dosed for 1 mo each. (From Deary AJ, Schumann AL, Marfet H, et al. Double-blind, placebo-controlled crossover comparison of five classes of antihypertensive drugs. J Hypertens 2002;20:771–7.)

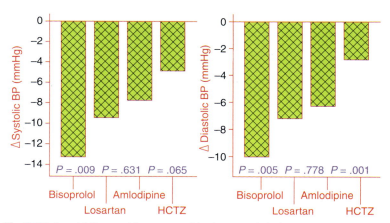

Fig. 3-33 In middle-aged (mean age 50 yr) overweight hypertensive patients, the best control of office blood pressure (BP) and 24-hr ambulatory BP both day and night was with bisoprolol vs. losartan, amlodipine, and a thiazide diuretic (HCTZ). (From Hiltunen TP, Suonsyrja T, Hannila-Handelberg T, et al. Predictors of antihypertensive responses: initial data from a placebo-controlled, randomised, crossover study with four antihypertensive drugs [the GENRES Study]. Am J Hypertens 2007;20:311–8.)

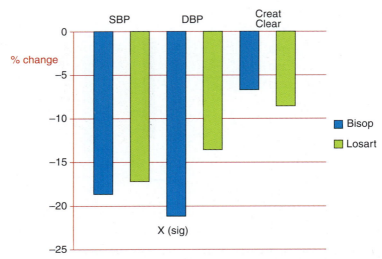

Fig. 3-34 In 72 middle-aged hypertensive patients (mean age 50 yr), bisoprolol is superior to losartan in controlling blood pressure over 1 yr, with no evidence of renoprotection for losartan. Creat Clear, creatine clearance; DBP, diastolic blood pressure; SBP, systolic blood pressure. (From Parrinello G, Paterna S, Torres D, et al. One-year renal and cardiac effects of bisoprolol versus losartan in recently diagnosed hypertensive patients. Clin Drug Invest 2009;29:591–600.)

period, neither agent had significant effects upon creatinine clearance—**Figure 3-34** (i.e., no special "renoprotective" effects of the ARB were apparent). The "renofriendly" property of bisoprolol is likely to be due to the absence of $β_2$-blockade; β-blocker-induced reduction in renal function is predominantly via $β_2$-blockade.[147,148]

B) Effects on central (aortic) hemodynamics in the elderly hypertensive patient

The effects of atenolol upon central hemodynamics have been described earlier in this chapter (i.e., minimal effect upon central SBP and a tendency to increase central PP amplification)—all theoretically bad effects as regards cardiovascular prognosis in the elderly.

β-Blockers with $β_2/β_3$ ISA tend to have more theoretically favorable effects upon central hemodynamics, probably due to vasodilatory actions and lesser falls in heart rate. Celiprolol ($β_2$ ISA) was as effective as enalapril in reducing central pressures.[149] Dilevalol ($β_2$ ISA) was more effective than atenolol in decreasing the augmen-

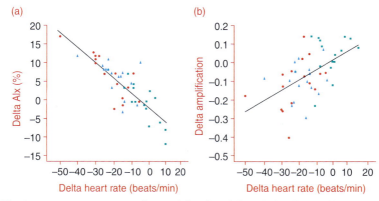

Fig. 3-35 In a comparison of atenolol, nebivolol, and placebo in elderly hypertensive patients, lower heart rates were associated with an increased augmentation index (AIx) and a lower pulse pressure amplification. (From Dhakam Z, Yasmin, McEniery CM, et al. A comparison of atenolol and nebivolol in isolated systolic hypertension. J Hypertens 2008;26:351–6.)

tation index (AIx).[150] Nebivolol (β_2/β_3 ISA), when compared with atenolol, did not increase aortic PP (but did not differ from placebo) but, like atenolol, did increase AIx (vs. placebo) and decrease PP amplification.[150] The change in AIx and PP amplification was related to change in heart rate—**Figure 3-35**.

Whether these effects of β_2/β_3 ISA upon central hemodynamics are clinically relevant are at present unknown. It is possible that the direct effects of β_2/β_3 ISA upon the vulnerable heart (via L-arginine/nitric oxide) may be detrimental.[151]

C) Cigarette smoking interaction

The importance of this interaction cannot be overestimated. As indicated earlier in this chapter, cigarette smoking induces a two-to threefold increase in adrenaline secretion, lasting at least 30 minutes.[46] Because adrenaline is a β_1-, β_2-, and α-receptor stimulant the presence of nonselective (e.g., propranolol) or modestly β_1-selective (e.g., metoprolol and atenolol) will result in unopposed (total or partial) α-constriction, leading to an increase in BP[47] that is marked (30 mm Hg) with nonselective, more modest (9-10 mm Hg) with moderately selective β-blockers, and absent with highly β_1-selective bisoprolol (**see Figure 3-12**). So for a 20/day smoker on a non-, or poorly β_1-, selective β-blocker, the BP will be little different (or maybe considerably higher) from pretreatment levels for most of the day. Hence, the absence of benefit of nonselective and modestly β_1-selective agents in reducing cardiovascular event rate in smokers, whether given first-line in younger/middle-aged hypertensive patients[41-43]—(see **Figures 3-9 and 3-10**)—or second-line in the elderly[66] —(see **Figure 3-22**).

These "out-of-reach" cardiovascular events in smokers receiving nonselective or modestly β_1-selective β-blockers can be brought to "within reach" by the avoidance of β_2-blockade (i.e., lower doses of highly β_1-selective bisoprolol given either first-line to younger/middle-aged hypertensive patients or second-line to a low-dose diuretic in the elderly).

D) Is there a place for β_2-blockade (nonselective agents)?

There is no place for pure β_2-blockade because such a drug (ICI 118,551), owing to vasoconstriction, induces an increase in BP (see Pharmacology chapter). However, hypertension often coexists with other disease entities in which nonselective β-blockers perform better than β_1-selective agents.[152] Such diseases are, for example, migraine, essential tremor, glaucoma, and portal hypertension; under these circumstances, in a nonsmoker, a nonselective β-blocker might be considered in preference to a β_1-selective agent.

SUMMARY AND CONCLUSIONS

1. The role of β-blockers in the treatment of hypertension was thrown into confusion by the 2006 recommendations of the U.K. NICE Committee/British Hypertension Society, namely (a) β-blockers are no longer preferred as routine initial therapy, (b) the combination of β-blocker and diuretic to be discouraged owing to the increased risk of developing diabetes, and (c) in younger patients, first-choice initial therapy should be an ACE inhibitor or ARB.
2. European (ESH)guidelines are much gentler toward β-blockers: (a) all five major classes of antihypertensive agent (including β-blockers) are suitable for first-line therapy, (b) but warn against β-blocker/diuretic combination in patients at high risk of developing type 2 diabetes (i.e., centrally obese or metabolic syndrome), (c) in diabetics, inhibitors of the renin-angiotensin system are favored, and (d) in moderate/severe hypertension, it is permitted to start with fixed low-dose combination products.

3. What are the possible rights and wrongs of the U.K. and European recommendations? Consideration of the pathophysiology of primary hypertension is helpful in understanding the role of β-blockers in the treatment of hypertension.
4. The Framingham Study group and others have linked the development of diastolic hypertension to a younger age, overweight/obesity (particularly central), and a high heart rate and cardiac output. In contrast, isolated systolic hypertension occurs in the elderly and results from aging, poorly compliant arteries.
5. Younger/middle-aged diastolic hypertension, with its link to central obesity, is associated with high sympathetic nerve activity (high noradrenaline production), which is particularly apparent when the metabolic syndrome or type 2 diabetes coexist.
6. The high sympathetic tone is possibly explained by (a) production of adipokinins (e.g., TNF-α and IL-6) by central adipocytes, (b) adipokinins induce an endothelial inflammatory response (linked to high CRP levels), (c) resulting in insulin resistance and high reactive insulin levels, (d) high insulin (and leptin, produced by central adipocytes) levels act centrally, resulting in high sympathetic nerve activity.
7. High noradrenaline activity (chronic $β_1$-stimulation) in younger/middle-aged subjects results in (a) high 24-hr BP, (b) LVH, (c) myocardial necrosis/apoptosis, (d) reduced threshold to ventricular tachycardia/fibrillation (sudden death), (e) increased atheroma formation, (e) stimulation of renal juxtaglomerular apparatus resulting in activation of the renin-angiotensin system, (f) high levels of angiotensin II act centrally resulting in further noradrenaline-release, (g) thus, a vicious circle is set up that, in theory, should be broken by $β_1$-blockade resulting in a reduction in cardiovascular end-points in younger/middle-aged, probably centrally obese, hypertensive patients—what is the evidence for this?
8. There are four key prospective, randomized, controlled, hard-end-points studies in young/middle-aged diastolic hypertensive patients involving nonselective propranolol (MRC) and oxprenolol (IPPPSH), and modestly $β_1$-selective metoprolol (MAPHY) and atenolol (UKPDS 39). The results of the first three (β-blockers vs. placebo or vs. diuretic) can be understood best in the context of the cigarette-smoking/β-blocker interaction.
9. Concentrating on MI (which is the number one cause of death in men), three times more common than stroke in younger hypertensive patients, it is apparent that the 33%-49% reduc-

tion in MI in nonsmokers (70% of total) receiving β-blockers (vs. placebo or diuretic) is negated in smokers (it is the same for stroke with propranolol).

10. The harmful β-blocker/smoking interaction can be explained thus (a) smoking is associated with a threefold increase in adrenaline levels, lasting 30-40 minutes, and (b) adrenaline stimulates $β_1$-, $β_2$-, and α-receptors; thus, in the presence of $β_1$- and $β_2$-blockade, there is unopposed α-constriction resulting in a marked hypertensive response.

11. The nonselective/modestly selective β-blocker/smoking interaction results in an increase of mean BP of about 30 mm Hg for nonselective, 9-10 mm Hg for modestly selective, and zero for highly $β_1$-selective bisoprolol. Thus, the BP levels in a 20/day smoker on non-, or modestly, selective β-blockers, will be at pretreatment, or higher, levels for most of the day.

12. There is a thus a strong case in younger, diastolic hypertensive patients for avoidance of $β_2$-blockade (i.e., choose first-line high $β_1$-selectivity blockers, so that "out-of-reach" cardiovascular events in smokers can be brought to "within-reach"; particularly important in countries with a high smoking-rate such as China).

13. There is only one comparison between first-line ACE inhibitor and β-blocker in younger/middle-aged diastolic hypertensive patients—the UKPDS 39 study comparing atenolol and captopril in obese, type 2 diabetic hypertensive patients.

14. In the UKPDS 38, tight control of BP (either randomized captopril or atenolol) was compared with less-tight (surrogate placebo) control of BP (≤10/5 mm Hg); most of the seven primary end-points were significantly reduced by tight control over a 9- to 10-year period and all seven trends favored the β-blocker over ACE inhibitor treatment; thus, compared with surrogate-placebo, the β-blocker reduced (a) stroke by 50%, (b) peripheral artery disease end-points by 60%, (c) microvascular (eye/kidney) end-points by 45% (no evidence of special ACE inhibitor renoprotection), and (d) heart failure by 65%.

15. After 20 years' follow-up in the UKPDS 38 and 39 study (patients returned to primary care after 10 yr), in those originally allocated to atenolol, there was a significant 23% reduction in all-cause death compared with captopril treatment plus strong trends in reduction of MI and peripheral arterial disease.

16. In the younger/middle-aged diastolic hypertensive patient, reduction in stroke appears related directly to a fall in BP, contrasting with MI, which was reduced only by β-blockade

(vs. diuretic or placebo), in spite of BP control being possibly superior on the diuretic (vs. propranolol). Compared with placebo (Australian study), diuretics reduced stroke by 45% but slightly increased the risk of MI. The case for ARBs has not been made owing to their probable inability to reduce the frequency of MI.

17. In the elderly systolic hypertensive patient, first-line β-blockade (atenolol) has compared poorly vs. comparator agents (diuretic, calcium antagonist, and ARB) in terms of reduced cardiovascular end-points, unless coronary artery disease was also present. Lowering DBP too far in patients with myocardial ischemia can result in an increased risk of MI (J-curve phenomenon).

18. The poor showing of first-line β-blocker (atenolol) in the elderly is undoubtedly due to the modest/absent effect upon central/aortic hemodynamics compared with diuretics, calcium antagonists, and ACE inhibitors. The negative effect of increased magnitude of wave reflection (via absence of vasodilatation) upon augmented SBP and central PP may be responsible, because β-blockers with ISA (e.g., nebivolol, dilevolol, or celiprolol) are less invasive in this respect (the clinical relevance is unknown).

19. In the elderly, β-blockers (atenolol) have been ineffective in reversing LVH, in marked contrast to the younger diastolic hypertensive patient in whom β-blockers are at least as effective as other agents (including ACE inhibitors) in reversing LVH (which arises not only from high BP but also chronic β_1-stimulation from raised noradrenaline levels).

20. β-Blockers given second-line to either diuretics or calcium antagonists have performed well in the elderly of both sex. The low-dose combination of diuretic/β-blocker may even be the desirable combination, in which induced metabolic changes (unlike naturally occurring type 2 diabetes) appear to be clinically unimportant as evidenced in placebo-controlled (or surrogate-placebo) long-term follow-up as long as 15-20 yr (SHEP and UKPDS 38 and 39). If in doubt, a β-blocker that causes no metabolic problem can be used (e.g., by avoidance of β_2-blockade with low-dose bisoprolol). Low-dose fixed combinations may given first-line to those with moderate-severe hypertension (patient compliance improved).

21. The β-blocker/smoking interaction (atenolol) is seen whether the β-blocker is given either first-line or second-line (to diuretic) in the elderly but may be avoided by using high β_1-selectivity.

22. ARBs may be appropriate as first-line agents in the elderly. However, in younger/middle-aged (with high sympathetic nerve

activity), in whom MI is the main cause of death, ARBs may be inappropriate because they appear to increase sympathetic nerve activity and there is doubt as to their ability to reduce the risk of MI (the same situation applies to diuretics and dihydropyridine calcium antagonists, which also increased sympathetic nerve activity).

23. Thus, the NICE committee appear to be wrong in their condemnation of first-line β-blockers in young/middle-aged diastolic hypertensives, particularly when coprescribed with diuretics (metabolic problems), owing to (a) inappropriate meta-analyses including first-line β-blockers in both younger and elderly patients (i.e., ignoring the differing pathophysiologies in the young and elderly hypertensive patient), (b) inappropriate attention to surrogate end-points (e.g., blood sugar, which may be clinically unimportant), (c) nonappreciation of the powerful β-blocker/cigarette smoking interaction in the case of nonselective and modestly $β_1$-selective (e.g., atenolol and metoprolol) agents, and (d) failure to acknowledge the results of UKPDS 39 (the one and only comparison of first-line ACE inhibitor and β-blocker) in which trends in all seven primary end-points favored the β-blocker after 10 years follow-up, becoming significant (23% reduction) after 20 years for all-cause death.

24. In secondary hypertension, β-blockers have a role to play (a) in renal disease and dialysis patients in whom sympathetic nerve activity is very high and β-blockers are as effective as other agents in reducing cardiovascular events; (b) in pheochromocytoma, they are effective when given alongside an α-blocker; (c) in pregnancy hypertension, they are effective and well-tolerated when given in later pregnancy (though placental and fetal weights may be reduced), but in early pregnancy, they may be associated with cardiac abnormalities.

25. β-Blockers are not a homogeneous group of drugs and the choice of β-blocker is all important for optimal efficacy (a) in young/middle-aged diastolic hypertension best control of 24-hr BP is obtained by avoidance of $β_2$-blockade by using low-dose, highly $β_1$-selective bisoprolol that effects pure $β_1$-blockade and is the best way to lower BP not only among β-blockers but also more effective than diuretics, α-blockers, calcium antagonists, ACE inhibitors, and ARBs (no special "renoprotection" noted with ACE inhibitors or ARB), (b) in the elderly, lowering central/aortic augmented SBP and reducing PP is important; agents with $β_2$ or $β_3$ ISA, or α-blockade that cause some vasodilatation and less slowing of the pulse rate may be best in this respect, though

the clinical relevance is unknown and there may be problems with chronic β_3-stimulation on the vulnerable heart, (c) the vitally important cigarette smoking/β-blocker interaction can be avoided by not blocking the β_2-receptor (i.e., high β_1-selectivity with low-dose bisoprolol), thus potentially bringing "out-of-reach" cardiovascular events in smokers to "within reach" of the β-blocker given either as first-line agent in younger diastolic hypertensive patients or as second-line (to diuretic or calcium antagonist) in the older systolic hypertensive patient.

REFERENCES

1. Prichard BNC, Gillam PMS. Use of propranolol in the treatment of hypertension. Br Med J 1964;2:725.
2. Staessen JA, Wang J, Bianchi G, Birkenhager WH. Essential hypertension. Lancet 2003;361:1629–41.
3. MacMahon S, Yan L. Responding to China's hypertensive crisis. Lancet 2009;374:1728–9.
4. Wang TJ, Vasan RS. Epidemiology of uncontrolled hypertension in the United States. Circulation 2005;112:1651–62.
5. Jones DW, Peterson ED. Improving hypertension control rates: technology, people, or systems? JAMA 2008;299:2896–8.
6. Kannel WB, Wolf PA, Verter J, McNamara PM. Framingham study insights on the hazards of elevated blood pressure. JAMA 2008;300:2545–7.
7. Beevers DG. The end of beta-blockers for uncomplicated hypertension? Lancet 2005;366:1510–2.
8. Lindholm LH, Carlberg B, Samuelsson O. Should beta-blockers remain first choice in the treatment of primary hypertension? A meta-analysis. Lancet 2005;366:1545–53.
9. Opie LH. Beta-blockade should not be among several choices for initial therapy of hypertension. J Hypertens 2008;26:161–3.
10. Messerli FH, Bangalore S, Julius S. Should beta-blockers and diuretics remain as first-line therapy for hypertension? Circulation 2008;117:2706–15.
11. Kaplan NM. Beta-blockers in hypertension. Adding insult to injury. J Am Coll Cardiol 2008;52:1490–1.
12. Williams B, Poulter NR, Brown MJ, et al, British Hypertension Society. Guidelines for management of hypertension: report of the fourth working party of the British Hypertension Society, 2004–BHS IV. J Hum Hypertens 2004;18:139–85.
13. NICE Clinical Guidelines 34. Hypertension management of hypertension in primary care. Available at www.nice.org.uk (accessed June 2006)1.
14. Cruickshank JM. New guidelines on hypertension. Lancet 2006;368:641.

15. Cruickshank JM. Are we misunderstanding beta-blockers? Int J Cardiol 2007;120:10–27.
16. 2007 Guidelines for the management of arterial hypertension. The Task Force for the Mmanagement of Arterial Hypertension of the European Society of Hypertension (ESH) and the European Society of Cardiology (ESC). Eur Heart J 2007;28:1462–536.
17. Mancia G, Laurent S, Agabiti-Rosei E, et al. Reappraisal of European guidelines on hypertension management: a European Society of Hypertension Task Force document. J Hypertens 2009;27:2121–58.
18. Franklin SS, Pio JR, Wong ND, et al. Predictors of new-onset diastolic and systolic hypertension. The Framingham Heart Study. Circulation 2005;111:1121–7.
19. Grebla RC, Rodriguez CJ, Borrell LN, Pickering TG. Prevalence and determinants of isolated systolic hypertension among young adults: the 1999–2004 US National Health and Nutrition Examination Survey. J Hypertens 2010;28:15–23.
20. Toprak A, Wang H, Chen W, et al. Relation of childhood risk factors to left ventricular hypertrophy in relatively young adulthood (from the Bogalusa Heart Study). Am J Cardiol 2008;101:1621–5.
21. Rheaume C, Arsenault BJ, Belanger S, et al. Low cardiorespiratory fitness levels and elevated blood pressure. What is the contribution of visceral adiposity? Hypertension 2009;54:91–7.
22. Timpson NJ, Harbord R, Davey-Smith G, et al. Does greater adiposity increase blood pressure and hypertension risk? Hypertension 2009;54:84–90.
23. Drukteinis JS, Roman MJ, Fabsitz RR, et al. Cardiac and systemic haemodynamic characteristics of hypertension and prehypertension in adolescents and young adults. The Strong Heart Study. Circulation 2007;115:221–7.
24. Grassi G, Dell'Oro R, Facchini A, et al. Effect of central and peripheral body fat distribution on sympathetic and baroreflex function in obese hypertensive. J Hypertens 2004;22:2363–9.
25. Huggett RJ, Burns J, Mackintosh AF, Mary DA. Sympathetic neural activation in non-diabetic metabolic syndrome and its further augmentation by hypertension. Hypertension 2004;44:847–52.
26. Huggett RJ, Scott EM, Gilbey SG, et al. Impact of type-2 diabetes mellitus on sympathetic neural mechanisms in hypertension. Circulation 2003;108:3097–4001.
27. Grassi G. Assessment of sympathetic cardiovascular drive in human hypertension. Hypertension 2009;54:690–7.
28. De Simone G, Devereux RB, Daniels SF, et al. Stroke volume and cardiac output in normotensive children and adults. Assessment of relations with body size and impact of obesity. Circulation 1997;95:1837–43.
29. Dunston HP. Obesity and hypertension in Blacks. Cardiovasc Drugs Ther 1990;4:395–402.

30. Zicardi P, Nappo G, Giugliano G, et al. Reduction in inflammatory cytokine concentrations and improvement of endothelial functions in obese women after weight-loss over one year. Circulation 2002;105:804–9.
31. Dandona P, Aljada A, Chaudhuri A, et al. Metabolic syndrome. A comprehensive perspective based on interactions between obesity, diabetes and inflammation. Circulation 2005;111:1448–54.
32. Tack CJ, Smits P, Withelmsen JJ, et al. Effect of insulin on vascular tone and sympathetic nervous system in NIDDM. Diabetes 1996;45: 15–22.
33. Hespel P, Lijnen P, Vanhees L, et al. Beta-adrenoceptors and the regulation of blood pressure and plasma renin during exercise. J Appl Physiol 1986;60:108–13.
34. Marsh AJ, Fontes AF, Killinger S, et al. Cardiovascular responses evoked by leptin acting on neurones in the ventromedial and dorsomedial hypothalamus. Hypertension 2003;42:488–93.
35. Nakamura Y, Ueshema H, Okuda N, et al. Relation of serum leptin to blood pressure of Japanese in Japan and Japanese-Americans in Hawaii. Hypertension 2009;54:1416–22.
36. Henegar JR, Brower GL, Kabour A, Janicki KS. Catecholamine-response to chronic angiotensin II infusion and its role in coronary vascular damage. Am J Physiol 1995;269:H1564–9.
37. Cruickshank JM, Degaute JP, Kuurne T, et al. Reduction of stress/catecholamine-induced cardiac necrosis by beta-1 selective blockade. Lancet 1987;2:585–9.
38. Kramer B, Sautter R, Gulker H, et al. Influence of ISA of beta-blockers on ventricular fibrillation threshold. Circulation 1981;64: A461.
39. Helen P, Lorenzen I, Garbarsch C, Mattiessen ME. Arteriosclerosis in the rabbit aorta induced by noradrenaline. Atherosclerosis 1970;12:125–32.
40. Strand AH, Gudmundsdottir, Os I, et al. Arterial plasma noradrenaline predicts left ventricular hypertrophy independently of blood pressure and body build in men who develop hypertension over 20 years. J Hypertens 2006;24:905–13.
41. Medical Research Council Working Party. MRC trial of treatment of mild hypertension: principal results. Br Med J 1985;291:97–104.
42. IPPPSH Collaborative Group. Cardiovascular risk and risk factors in a randomised trial of treatment-based on the beta-blocker oxprenolol. J Hypertens 1985;3:379–92.
43. Wikstrand J, Warnold T, Tuomilehto J, et al. Metoprolol versus diuretics in hypertension. Morbidity results from MAPHY study. Hypertension 1991;17:579–88.
44. U.K. Prospective Diabetes Study Group. Tight blood pressure control and risk of macrovascular and microvascular complications in type-2 diabetes. UKPDS 38. BMJ 1998;317:703–13.

45. U.K. Prospective Diabetes Study Group. Efficacy of atenolol and captopril in reducing risk of macrovascular and microvascular complications in type-2 diabetes: UKPDS 39. BMJ 1998;317:713–20.
46. Cryer PE, Haymond MW, Satiago JV, Shar SP. Norepinephrine and epinephrine release and adrenergic mediation of smoking-associated hemodynamic and metabolic events. N Engl J Med 1976;295:573–7.
47. Tarnow J, Muller RK. Cardiovascular effects of low-dose epinephrine infusions in relation to the extent of pre-operative beta-blockade. Anaesthesiology 1991;74:1035–43.
48. Holman RR, Paul SK, Bethel MA, et al. Long-term follow-up after tight control of blood pressure in type-2 diabetes. N Engl J Med 2008;359:1565–76.
49. Khan N, McAlister FA. Re-examining the efficacy of beta-blockers for the treatment of hypertension: a meta-analysis. CMAJ 2006;174:1737–42.
50. Wikstrand J. Beta-blockers and cardioprotection—is there any good news from the recent trials? J Clin Pharm Ther 1987;12:347–50.
51. Miall W, Greenberg G (eds). Mild Hypertension: Is There Pressure to Treat? An account of the MRC trial. Cambridge, Cambridge University Press; 1987, pp 101–18.
52. Report by the Management Committee. The Australian Therapeutic Trial in Hypertension. Lancet 1980;1:1261–7.
53. Leren P, Helgeland A. Coronary heart disease and treatment of hypertension. Some Oslo Study data. Am J Med 1986;80(2A):3–6.
54. Blood Pressure Lowering Treatment Trialists Collaboration. Effect of different regimens to lower blood pressure on major cardiovascular events in older and younger adults: meta-analysis of randomised trials. BMJ 2010: doi:10.1136/bmj.39548.738368.BE
55. Law MR, Morris JK, Wald NJ. Use of blood pressure lowering drugs in the prevention of cardiovascular disease: meta-analysis of 147 randomised trials in the context of expectations from prospective epidemiological studies. BMJ 2009;338:1245–53.
56. Kengne A-P, Czernichow S, Huxley R, et al. Blood pressure variables and cardiovascular risk. New findings for ADVANCE. Hypertension 2009;54:399–404.
57. Williams B, Lacy PS, Thom SM, et al. Differential impact of blood-pressure-lowering drugs on central aortic pressure and clinical outcomes: principle results of the CAFE study. Circulation 2006;113:1213–25.
58. Avolio AP, van Bortel LM, Boutouyrie JR, et al. Role of pulse-pressure amplification in arterial hypertension. Experts opinion on review of the data. Hypertension 2009;54:3375–83.
59. Safar ME, Protogarou AD, Blacher J. Statins, central blood pressure, and blood pressure amplification. Circulation 2009;119:9–12.
60. Manisty CH, Zambanini A, Parker KH, et al. Differences in the magnitude of wave reflection account for differential effects of amlodipine- vs atenolol-based regimens pressure (substudy of ASCOT). Hypertension 2009;54:724–30.

61. Cameron JD. Wave intensity and central blood pressure. Hypertension 2009;54:958–9.
62. Robertson JIS. Epidemiology of the renin-angiotensin system in hypertension. In Bulpitt CJ (ed). Epidemiology of Hypertension. Handbook of Hypertension. Amsterdam: Elsevier; 2000, pp 342–89.
63. Feldman RD, Limbird LE, Nadeau J, et al. Alterations in leukocyte beta-receptor affinity with ageing. N Engl J Med 1984;310: 815–9.
64. Buhler FR, Kiowski W. Plasma catecholamines, renin and age and antihypertensive response of men to beta-blockers. In Bevan JA, et al (eds). Vascular Neuroeffector Mechanisms. Proceedings of an International Symposium, Brussels and Wilryk, Belgium, 1978. New York: Raven Press; 1980, 376–83.
65. Coope J, Warrender TS. Randomised trial of treatment of hypertension in primary care (HEP). Br Med J 1986;293:1145–51.
66. Medical Research Council Working Party. MRC trial of treatment of hypertension in older adults: principal results. Br Med J 1992;304: 405–12.
67. Kjeldsen SE, Dahlof B, Devereux RB, et al. Effect of losartan on cardiovascular morbidity and mortality in patients with isolated systolic hypertension and left-ventricular hypertrophy (LIFE). JAMA 2002;288: 1491–8.
68. Dahlof B, Sever P, Poulter N, et al. Prevention of cardiovascular events with an antihypertensive regimen of amlodipine adding perindopril as required versus atenolol adding bendroflumethzide, as required (ASCOT-BPLA); a multicentre randomised controlled trial. Lancet 2005;366:895–906.
69. Fyhrquist F, Dahlorf B, Devereux RB, et al. Pulse-pressure and effects of losartan or atenolol in patients with hypertension and left-ventricular hypertrophy. Hypertension 2005;45:580–5.
70. Pepine CJ, Handberg EM, Cooper-Dehoff RM, et al. A calcium antagonist vs non-calcium antagonist hypertension treatment strategy for patients with coronary artery disease (INVEST). JAMA 2003;290:2805–16.
71. Cruickshank JM, Thorp JM, Zacharias FJ. Benefits and potential harm in lowering high blood pressure. Lancet 1987;1:581–4.
72. Hansson L, Zanchetti A, Carruthers SG, et al, for the HOT Study Group. Effects of intense blood pressure lowering and low-dose aspirin in patients with hypertension: principal results of the Hypertension Optimal Treatment (HOT) randomised trial. Lancet 1998;351:1755–62.
73. Cruickshank JM. The J-curve in hypertension. Curr Cardiol Rep 2003;5:441–52.
74. Morgan T, Lauri J, Bertram D, Anderson A. Effect of different antihypertensive drug classes on central aortic pressure. Am J Hypertens 2004;17:118–23.
75. Mackenzie IS, McEniery CM, Dhakam Z, et al. Comparison of the effects of antihypertensive agents on central blood pressure and arte-

rial stiffness in isolated systolic hypertension. Hypertension 2009;54: 409–13.
76. Williams B, Lacy PS, Thom SM, et al. Differential impact of blood pressure-lowering drugs on central aortic pressure and clinical outcomes (CAFE). Circulation 2006;113:1213–25.
77. Cruickshank JM, Lewis J, Moore V, Dodd C. Reversability of left-ventricular hypertrophy by differing types of antihypertensive therapy. J Hum Hypertens 1992;6:85–90.
78. Fagard RH, Celis H, Thijs L, Wouters S. Regression of left ventricular mass by antihypertensive treatment. A meta-analysis of randomised comparative studies. Hypertension 2009;54:1084–91.
79. Sugishita Y, Aida K, Ohtsukas, Yamaguchi I. Ventricular wall stress revisited. A keystone of cardiology. Jpn Heart J 1994;35:517–87.
80. Burns J, Sivananthan MV, Ball SG, et al. Relationship between central sympathetic drive and MRI imagery determined left-ventricular mass in essential hypertension. Circulation 2007;115:1999–2005.
81. Agabiti-Rosei E, Marcia G, O'Rourke MF, et al. Central blood pressure measurements and antihypertensive therapy. A consensus document. Hypertension 2007;50:154–60.
82. Schulman SP, Weiss JL, Becker LC, et al. The effects of antihypertensive therapy on left-ventricular mass in elderly patients. N Engl J Med 1990;322:1350–6.
83. Buus NH, Bottcher M, Jørgensen CG, et al. Myocardial perfusion during long-term ACE-inhibition or beta-blockade in patients with essential hypertension. Hypertension 2004;44:1350–6.
84. Schneider MP, Klingbeil AV, Delles C, et al. Effects of irbesartan versus atenolol on left-ventricular mass and voltage. Hypertension 2004;44:61–6.
85. Devereux RB, Dahlof B, Gerdts E, et al. Regression of hypertensive left-ventricular hypertrophy by losartan compared to atenolol (LIFE Study). Circulation 2004;110:146–62.
86. Cruickshank JM, Higgins TJ, Pennart K, et al. The efficacy and tolerability of antihypertensive treatment based on atenolol in the prevention of stroke and the regression of LVH. J Hum Hypertens 1987;1:87–93.
87. Fogari R, Zoppi A, Poletti L, et al. Chronic beta-1 blockade and control of left-ventricular hypertrophy in hypertension. Int J Clin Pharmacol Ther Toxicol 1987;25:334–41.
88. Otterstadt JE, Froeland G, Soeyland AK, et al. Changes in left-ventricular dimensions and systolic function in 100 mildly hypertensive men during one year's treatment with atenolol vs hydrochlorthiazide and amiloride. J Intern Med 1992;231:493–501.
89. Rosatti F, Lunardi M, Mangrella M, et al. Effect of atenolol and ramipril on regression of left-ventricular hypertrophy. Adv Ther 1995;12:147–55.
90. Franz IW, Behr V, Ketelhut R, Tonnesmann V. Decreasing the antihypertensive dosage during long-term treatment and complete regression of LVH. Dtsch Med Wochenschr 1996;121:472–7.

91. de Teresa E, Gonzalez M, Camacho-Vasquez C, Tabuenca MJ. Effects of bisoprolol on LVH in hypertension. Cardiovasc Drugs Ther 1994;8:837–43.
92. Matuszewska G, Marek B, Kajdanuik D, et al. The importance of bisoprolol in prevention of LVH in patients with long-term L-thyroxin suppressive therapy. Endokrynol Pol 2007;58:384–96.
93. Goss P, Routaut R, Herreo G, Dallocchio M. Beta-blockers vs ACE-inhibition in hypertension: effects on left-ventricular hypertrophy. J Cardiovasc Pharmacol 1990;16:S 145–50.
94. Motz W, Vogt M, Scheler S, et al. Improvement of coronary reserve following regression of hypertrophy resulting from blood pressure lowering with a beta-blocker. Dtsch Med Wochen 1993;118:535–40.
95. Gottdiener JS, Reda DJ, Massie BM, et al. Effect of single-drug therapy on reduction of left-ventricular mass in mild to moderate hypertension. Circulation 1997;95:2007–14.
96. Reims HM, Oparil S, Kjeldsen SE, et al. Losartan benefits over atenolol in non-smoking hypertensive patients with left-ventricular hypertrophy (LIFE study). Blood Press 2004;13:376–84.
97. Fu Q, Zhang R, Witkowski S, et al. Persistent sympathetic activation during chronic antihypertensive therapy: a potential mechanism for long-term morbidity? Hypertension 2005;45:513–21.
98. Meredith PA, Elliot HL. Dichydropridine calcium channel blockers; basic pharmacological similarities but fundamental therapeutic differences. J Hypertens 2004;22:1641–8.
99. SHEP Cooperative Research Group. Prevention of stroke by antihypertensive drug treatment in older persons with isolated systolic hypertension. JAMA 1991;265:3255–64.
100. The ALLHAT Officers and Coordinators for the ALLHAT Collaborative Research Group. Major outcomes in high-risk hypertensive patients randomised to ACE-inhibitor or calcium channel blocker vs diuretic. JAMA 2002;288:2981–97.
101. Boger-Megiddo I, Heckbert SR, Weiss NS, et al. Myocardial infarction and stroke associated with diuretic-based two drug antihypertensive regimens: population based case-control study. BMJ 2010;340:303.
102. Schlienger RG, Kraenzlin ME, Meier CR. Use of beta-blockers and risk of fractures. JAMA 2004;292:1326–32.
103. Brown MJ, Palmer CR, Castaigne A et al. Morbidity and mortality in patients randomised to double-blind treatment with a long-acting calcium channel blocker or diuretic in the International Nifedepine GITS study. Intervention as a Goal in Hypertension Treatment (INSIGHT). Lancet 2000;356:366–72.
104. Turnbull F, Woodward M, Neal B, et al. Do men and women respond differently to blood pressure lowering treatment? Eur Heart J 2008;29:2669–80.
105. Gupta K, Arshad S, Poulter NR. Compliance, safety and effectiveness of fixed-dose combinations of antihypertensive agents. A meta-analysis. Hypertension 2010;55:399–407.

106. Frishman WH, Burris JF, Mroczek WJ, et al. First-line therapy option with low-dose bisoprolol fumarate and low dose hydrochlorothiazide with stage I and stage II systemic hypertension. J Clin Pharmacol 1995;35:182–8.
107. Neutel JM, Rolf CN, Valentine SN, et al. Low dose combination therapy at first-line treatment of mild to moderate hypertension the efficacy and safety of bisoprolol/6.25 mg HCTH versus amlodipine, enalapril and placebo. Cardiovasc Rev Rep 1996;17:33–45.
108. Papademetriou V, Neutel J, Naravan P, et al. Comparison of bisoprolol and low-dose hydrochlorothiazide with losartan alone and in combination with hydrchlorothiazide, in the treatment of hypertension: a double-blind randomised, placebo controlled trial. Cardiovasc Rev Rep 1998;19:1-8.
109. Lewin AJ, Lueg MC, Targum S, et al. A clinical trial evaluating the 24 hour effects of bisoprolol 5/hydrochlorothiazide 6.25 mg combination in patients with mild to moderate hypertension. Clin Cardiol 1993;16:732–6.
110. Cruickshank JM, Prichard BNC (eds). Beta-Blockers in Clinical Practice. 2nd ed. Edinburgh: Churchill Livingstone; 1994, pp 87–258.
111. Dominguez LJ, Barbagello M, Jacober SJ, et al. Bisoprolol and captopril effects on insulin receptor tyrosine kinase activity in essential hypertension. Am J Hypertens 1997;10:1349–55.
112. Fogari R, Zoppi A. The clinical benefits of beta-1 selectivity. Rev Contemp Pharmacother 1997;8:45–54.
113. Seguchi H, Nekamura H, Aosaki N, et al. Effects of carvediolol on serum lipids in hypertensive and normotensive subjects. Eur J Clin Pharmacol 1990;38 (suppl 2):S139–42.
114. Ehmer B, van der Does R, Rudorf J. Influence of carvedilol on blood glucose and glycohaemoglobin A-1 in non-insulin-dependent diabetes. Drugs 1988;36 (suppl 6):136–40.
115. Poirer L, Cleroux J, Nadeau A, Lacourcier Y. Effects of nebivolol and atenolol on insulin sensitivity and haemodynamics in hypertensive patients. J Hypertens 2001;19:1429–35.
116. Cushiman WC. Systolic hypertension in the elderly. Safe treatment with low-dose thiazide diuretics. Postgrad Med 1993;94: 143–8.
117. Black HR, Davis B, Barzilay J, et al. Metabolic and clinical outcomes in non-diabetic individuals with the metabolic syndrome assigned to chlorthalidone, amlodipine or lisinopril as initial treatment for hypertension. Diabetes Care 2008;31:353–60.
118. Strauss MH, Hall A. Renin-angiotensin system and cardiovascular risk. Lancet 2007;370:24-5.
119. Volpe M, Tocci G, Sciarretta S, et al. Angiotensin ll receptor blockers and myocardial infarction: an updated analysis of randomised clinical trials. J Hypertens 2009;27:941–6.
120. Cerasola G, Cottone S, D'Ignoto G, et al. Effects of enalapril maleate on blood pressure renin-angiotensin-aldosterone system, and

peripheral sympathetic activity in essential hypertension. Clin Ther 1987;9:390–9.
121. Krum H, Lambert E, Windebank E, et al. Effect of angiotensin II receptor blockade on autonomic nervous system function in patients with essential hypertension. Am J Physiol Heart Circ Physiol 2006;290: H1706–12.
122. Heusser K, Vithovsky J, Raasch W, et al. Elevation of sympathetic nerve activity by eprosartan in young male subjects. Am J Hypertens 2003;16:658–64.
123. Moltzer E, Raso FU, Karamermer Y, et al. Comparison of candesartan versus metoprolol for treatment of systemic hypertension after repaired aortic coarctation. Am J Cardiol 2010;105:217–22.
124. Klein IH, Ligtenbergh G, Oey PL, et al. Enalapril and losartan reduce sympathetic hyperactivity in patients with chronic renal failure. Am Soc Nephrol 2003;14:425–30.
125. Giles TD, Sander GE, Roffidal LC, et al. Comparison of nitrendipine and hydrochlorthiazide for systemic hypertension. Am J Cardiol 1987;60:103–6.
126. Kostis JB, Wilson AC, Freudenburger RS, et al, SHEP Collaborative Research Group. Long-term effects of diuretic-based therapy on fatal outcomes in subjects with isolated systolic hypertension with and without diabetes. Am J Cardiol 2005;95:29–35.
127. Agarwal R, Sinha AD. Cardiovascular protection with antihypertensive drugs in dialysis patients. Hypertension 2009;53:860–6.
128. Heerspink HJ, Ninomiya T, Zoungas S, et al. Effect of lowering blood pressure on cardiovascular events and mortality in patients on dialysis; a systematic review and meta-analysis of randomised, controlled trials. Lancet 2009;373:1009–15.
129. Norris K, Bourgoigne J, Gassman J, et al. Cardiovascular outcomes in the African American Study of Kidney Diseases and Hypertension (AASK) Trial. Am J Kidney Dis 2006;48:739–51.
130. Horl MP, Tepel M. Drug therapy for hypertension in haemodialysis patients. Minerva Med 2005;96:277–85.
131. Penne EL, Neumann J, Kleen IH, et al. Sympathetic hyperactivity and clinical outcome in chronic kidney disease patients during standard treatment. J Nephrol 2009;22:208–15.
132. Tomson CR. Blood pressure and outcome in patients on dialysis. Lancet 2009;373:981–2.
133. Cruickshank JM, Prichard BNC (eds). Beta-Blockers in Clinical Practice. 2nd ed. Edinburgh: Churchill Livingstone; 1994, pp 287–9.
134. Cruickshank JM, Prichard BNC (eds). Beta-Blockers in Clinical Practice. 2nd ed. Edinburgh: Churchill Livingstone; 1994, pp 765–9.
135. Sloand EM, Thompson BT. Propranolol-induced pulmonary oedema and shock in a patient with phaeochromachtoma. Arch Intern Med 1908;144:173–4.
136. Briggs RS, Birtwell AJ, Pohl JE. Hypertensive response to labetalol in phaemchromocytoma. Lancet 1978;1:1045–6.

137. Podymow T, August P. Update on the use of anti-hypertensive drugs in pregnancy. Hypertension 2008;51:960–9.
138. Rubin PC, Clark DM, Sumner DJ, et al. Placebo-controlled trial of atenolol in treatment of pregnancy associated hypertension. Lancet 1983;1:431–4.
139. Dubois D, Petitcolas J, Temperville B, et al. Beta-blocker therapy in 125 cases of hypertension during pregnancy. Clin Exp Hypertens Hypertens Pregnancy 1983;B2:41–59.
140. Lardoux H, Gerard H, Blazquez G, et al. Hypertension in pregnancy: evaluation of two beta-blockers atenolol and labetalol. Eur Heart J 1983;4 (suppl G):35–40.
141. Thorley KJ. Randomised trial of atenolol and methyldopa in pregnancy related hypertension (abstract). Clin Exp Hypertens 1984;B3.
142. Caton AR, Bell EM, Druschel CM, et al. Anti-hypertensive medication use during pregnancy and the risk of cardiovascular malformations. Hypertension 2009;54:63–70.
143. Buhler FR, Berglund G, Anderson OK, et al. Double-blind comparison of the cardioselective beta-blockers bisoprolol and atenolol in hypertension (BIMS). J Cardiovasc Pharmacol 1986;8:S122–7.
144. Deary AJ, Schumann AL, Marfet H, et al. Double-blind, placebo-controlled crossover comparison of five classes of antihypertensive drugs. J Hypertens 2002;20:771–7.
145. Hiltunen TP, Suonsyrja T, Hannila-Handelberg T, et al. Predictors of antihypertensive responses: initial data from a placebo-controlled, randomised, crossover study with four antihypertensive drugs (the GENRES Study). Am J Hypertens 2007;20:311–8.
146. Parrinello G, Paterna S, Torres D, et al. One-year renal and cardiac effects of bisoprolol versus losartan in recently diagnosed hypertensive patients. Clin Drug Invest 2009;29:591–600.
147. Wilkinson R. Beta-blockers and renal function. Drugs 1982;23:195–206.
148. Nakamura A, Imaizumi A, Yangawa Y, et al. Beta-2 adrenoceptor activation attenuates endotoxin-induced acute renal failure. J Am Soc Nephrol 2004;15:316–25.
149. Boutouyrie P, Bussy C, Hayoz D, et al. Local pulse-pressure and regression of arterial wall hypertrophy. Circulation 2000;101:2601–6.
150. Dhakam Z, Yasmin, McEniery CM, et al. A comparison of atenolol and nebivolol in isolated systolic hypertension. J Hypertens 2008;26:351–6.
151. Schulman SP, Becker LC, Kass DA, et al. L-Arginine therapy in acute myocardial infarction. JAMA 2006;295:58–64.
152. Cruickshank JM, Prichard BNC (eds). Beta-Blockers in Clinical Practice. 2nd ed. Edinburgh: Churchill Livingstone; 1994, pp 765–905.

β-Blockers and Cardiac Arrhythmias

CHAPTER 4

INTRODUCTION

This topic has been well reviewed.[1] Antiarrhythmic drugs have been classified by Vaughan Williams[2] into classes I (A-C), II, III, and IV—**Table 4-1**. Antiarrhythmic drugs may also be classified according to their site of action[3]—**Table 4-2**.

Class I drugs have local anesthetic properties and the depolarization of the cardiac cell membrane is depressed by restricting entry of the fast sodium current, thus reducing the rise of phase O of the action potential and depresses the rate of phase 4 diastolic depolarization, so reducing automaticity. Class A agents lengthen the duration of the action potential, class B shorten it, and class C have no effect.

Class II drugs (β-blockers) antagonize catecholamine actions upon the conduction system—that is, in the intact heart sympathetic stimulation leads to (i) an increase in pacemaker activity at all levels, (ii) atrioventricular (AV) conduction is increased and the refractory period of the AV node is shortened, (iii) the rate of diastolic depolarization of automatic cells is increased, thus increasing pacemaker activity, and (iv) there is nonuniformity of the recovery of the refractory period, thus lowering the threshold for ventricular fibrillation.

All β-blockers occupy and antagonize the $β_1$-receptor, and the electrophysiological effects arising from this are demonstrated by the highly $β_1$-selective β-blocker bisoprolol—that is, prolonged sinoatrial (SA) and AV nodal conduction and refractory periods; R-R and PR intervals increased; QTc intervals shortened and QT and T-wave dispersion decreased (see later).

Some β-blockers have additional antiarrhythmic properties. Sotalol has an additional class III action (see later), and propranolol has membrane stabilizing activity (class I antiarrhythmic, "quinidine-like"), but this property is expressed only at exceedingly high dosage.[4]

Class III drugs prolong the duration of the action potential with resulting prolongation of the effective refractory period; they also depress phase 4 depolarization.

Class IV agents inhibit the slow inward calcium-mediated current and accelerate phases 2 and 3 of the action potential. These drugs influence the AV node and may have value in blocking one limb (or both) of a reentry circuit.

1. Clinical management of arrhythmias with β-blockers

β-Blockers can be effective in the treatment and prevention of both supraventricular and ventricular arrhythmias, particularly if the arrhythmia is linked to increased sympathetic nerve activity (i.e., exercise, stress, emotion) or myocardial ischemia.

TABLE 4-1 Classification (Vaughan Williams) of antiarrhythmic drugs

	Class I	Class II	Class III	Class IV
A	Quinidine	β-adrenoceptor blocking agents	Amiodarone	Verapamil
	Procainamide		Disopyramide	
	Disopyramide		Bretylium	
	Ajmaline		Sotalol	
B	Lignocaine			
	Mexiletine			
	Aprindine			
	Phenytoin			
	Tocainide			
	Ethmozin			
C	Encainide			
	Lorcainide			
	Flecainide			

TABLE 4-2 Site of action of antiarrhythmic compounds

Sinus node, atrium	Atrioventricular node	Anomalous pathways	Ventricle
β-blockers	Digoxin	Disopyramide	Lignocaine
Digoxin	Verapamil	Amiodarone	Disopyramide
Verapamil	β-blockers	Procainamide	Tocainide
Procainamide		Quinidine	Mexiletine
Disopyramide			Phenytoin
Amiodarone			Procainamide
Quinidine			Quinidine
			Amiodarone

From Hillis WS, Whiting B. Antiarrhythmic drugs. Br Med J 1983;286:13332–6.

A) Supraventricular arrhythmias

Such arrhythmias are invariably not life-threatening but can markedly affect the quality of life; thus, they frequently need active treatment. The expected response of supraventricular arrhythmias to treatment with β-blockers is shown in **Table 4-3**.[5]

i) Ectopic supraventricular tachycardia

Ectopic supraventricular tachycardia (SVT) is often associated with high sympathetic nerve activity and is thus suited to β-blockade.[6] Children with this condition respond well to sotalol.[7]

TABLE 4-3 Expected response of supraventricular cardiac arrhythmias to treatment with β-blockers

Supraventricular arrhythmia	Response to β-blockers
Sinus tachycardia	Excellent
Paroxysmal supraventricular tachycardia (including WPW syndrome)	Good—both elective and prophylactic
Chronic ectopic supraventricular tachycardia	Good—sinus rhythm sometimes restored
Atrial fibrillation	Ventricular rate reduced—sinus rhythm rarely restored
Atrial flutter	Ventricular rate reduced—sinus rhythm sometimes restored

WPW, Wolff-Parkinson-White.
From Singh BN, Jewitt DE. Beta-blockers in cardiac arrhythmias. Cardiovasc Drugs 1977;2:119–59.

Digoxin toxicity also causes ectopic SVT and can respond well to propranolol.[8,9] However, AV block can be exacerbated by β-blockade, so phenytoin is thus preferred by many physicians.

ii) Reentrant, paroxysmal, arrhythmias involving the atrioventricular node

a) Paroxysmal supraventricular tachycardia —excluding WPW syndrome

In modern times, catheter ablation, a safe/high-success rate technique, is an alternative to preventive pharmacotherapy.[10]

Intravenous β-blocker therapy can be highly successful,[11] well illustrated by a study involving metoprolol[12]—**Table 4-4**.

Similar benefits have been observed with intravenous bisoprolol (5 mg) in terms of arrhythmia termination and prevention of induced arrhythmia.[13]

Prophylactic oral β-blocker therapy can be extremely effective, particularly when the arrhythmia is emotion-/exercise-provoked.[8] Several β-blockers without intrinsic sympathetomimetic activity (ISA; propranolol, atenolol, nadolol) have proved effective,[1] even in children[14]—**Table 4-5**. In resistant cases, sotalol (containing class III action, as well as β-blockade) can be effective, but because it prolongs the QT interval, ventricular irritability and torsades de points (ventricular tachycardia [VT]) can be precipitated.[15]

b) Paroxysmal supraventricular tachycardia — arising from preexcitation syndromes, including the WPW syndrome

The so-called preexcitation syndromes have been well reviewed.[16] Accessory tracts bypass the normal pathways linking the atria and the ventricles—**Figure 4-1**. The classic bypass tract was called the "bundle of Kent." These events are reflected in the electrocardiogram (ECG) by a short PR interval and a preexcitation, or delta, wave—(see **Figure 4-1**.)

To abort the acute arrhythmia, first-line therapy is usually intravenous adenosine,[17] because β-blockers are not always effective.[18] However, intravenous propranolol can be highly effective[19]—**Figure 4-2**—with IV sotalol suitable for resistant cases.[20]

Oral β-blockade is a first-line choice for prophylactic therapy,[18] particularly in children— (see **Table 4-5**). A good long-term response can be predicted by the effects of oral sotalol upon programmed stimulation.[21] However, chronic use of oral sotalol, though highly

TABLE 4-4 Effect of intravenous metoprolol in patients with supraventricular tachyarrhythmias

Type of SVT	Total number of patients	Number of patients converted to sinus rhythm	HR reduced > 25% and/or to < 100 beats/min	HR reduced > 10% and to < 150 beats/min but not > 25% or to < 100 beats/min	Number of nonresponders
Paroxysmal atrial tachycardia	28	16 (57%)	18 (64%)	3 (11%)	7 (25%)
Atrial flutter	35	8 (23%)	22 (63%)	3 (9%)	10 (28%)
Atrial fibrillation	79	10 (13%)	56 (71%)	19 (24%)	4 (5%)

HR, heart rate; SVT, supraventricular tachyarrhythmia.
From Rehnqvist N. Clinical experience with intravenous metoprolol in supraventricular tachyarrhythmias. Ann Clin Res 1981;13(suppl 30):68–72.

TABLE 4-5 Antiarrhythmic effects of oral propranolol in arrhythmias in childhood

Type of arrhythmia	Response rate
Sinus tachycardia (hyperthyroidism)	2/2
SVT with:	
WPW	6/8
Concealed anomalous pathway	7/9
Automatic ectopic focus	6/8
Undetermined mechanism	3/5
Atrial flutter	1/3
Atrial fibrillation	1/1
Ventricular premature beats	1/3
Ventricular tachycardia (prolonged QT interval)	1/1
Tachycardia/brachycardia syndrome	0/1
WPW	28/41

WPW, Wolff-Parkinson-White.
From Gillette PC, Garson A, Enterovic E, et al. Oral propranolol treatment in infants and children. J Pediatr 1978;92:141–4.

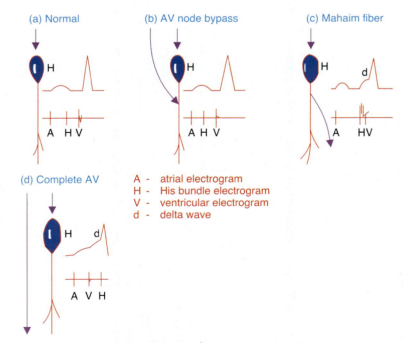

Fig. 4-1 Paroxysmal supraventricular tachycardia. Types of accessory pathway in preexcitation syndromes. (From Gallagher JJ, Pritchett EL, Sealey WC, et al. The pre-excitation syndromes. Progr Cardiovasc Dis 1978;20:285–327.)

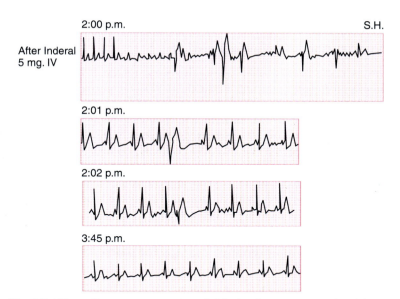

Fig. 4-2 Effect of intravenous propranolol (Inderal) on paroxysmal atrial tachycardia in a patient with Wolff-Parkinson-White syndrome. (From Cruickshank JM, Prichard BNC. Beta-Blockers in Clinical practice. 2nd ed. Edinburgh: Churchill Livingstone; 1994, p 720.)

effective, is in 2%-4% of cases associated with VT/fibrillation (torsades de pointes), even in children.[22] Thus, in children, classic β-blockade is appropriate,[23] keeping sotalol for resistant cases.[24]

iii) Atrial fibrillation

Atrial fibrillation (AF) is the most frequently occurring sustained cardiac arrhythmia, and its prevalence doubles with each decade of age after 50 years, approaching 10% in those over 80 years[25]. Hypertension is the most common risk factor for AF, with a relative risk (RR) of 1.4 to 2.1.[25] However, with the less commonly occurring heart failure situation, the RR for AF is much greater at 6.1 to 17.5.[26]

a) Young patients

Lone AF occurs in those younger than 60 years with no cardiovascular disease and has an excellent prognosis. Wolff-Parkinson-White (WPW) syndrome needs to be ruled out as a cause of the AF because β-blockade can precipitate ventricular fibrillation in such cases.[27]

b) Older patients

Hypertension and prevention of AF

This is not a well-studied area. However, in the LIFE (Losartan Intervention for Endpoint Reduction) study comparing first-line atenolol and losartan, the appearance of AF was reduced by 33% in those allocated to the losartan group.[28] In a nested case-control study of 4661 treated hypertensive patients with AF compared with 18,642 hypertensive (no AF) controls, compared with long-term calcium blocker therapy, there was a significant reduction in the frequency of AF of 25% with angiotensin-converting enzyme (ACE) inhibitors, 29% with angiotensin receptor blockers (ARBs), and 21% with β-blockers[29]—Table 4-6a.

Treatment and maintenance therapy for paroxysmal or sustained AF

Paroxysmal AF often has a diurnal distribution, with daytime episodes being linked to increased sympathetic nerve activity. Such patients respond particularly well to β_1-blockade—81% of patients (elderly, often with hypertension) on bisoprolol had improved quality of life with no longer ECG evidence of AF over a 2-year follow-up period.[30] In such patients, either rate control or rhythm-control results in a similar prognosis in terms of all-cause death and cardiovascular morbidity.[31]

TABLE 4-6A Risk of developing atrial fibrillation in hypertensive patients treated with angiotensin-converting enzyme inhibitors, angiotensin receptor blockers, or β-blockers, compared with treatment with calcium blockers

	ACE inhibitor (OR)	ARB (OR)	BB (OR)
Incidence of AF vs. calcium blockers	0.75 (0.65-0.87)	0.71 (0.57-0.89)	0.79 (0.67-0.92)
Statistically significant	Yes	Yes	Yes

ACE, angiotensin-converting enzyme; AF, atrial fibrillation; ARB, angiotensin receptor blocker; BB, β-blocker; OR, odds ratio.
From Schaer BA, Schneider C, Jick SS, et al. Risk for incidental atrial fibrillation in patients who receive antihypertensive drugs: a nested control study. Ann Intern Med 2010;152:78–84.

TABLE 4-6B Effects of randomized bisoprolol and sotalol on the reappearance of atrial fibrillation post-cardioversion

	QT duration (ms)	AF at 1 Yr (%)	Torsade de pointes (VT) (n)
Bisoprolol 5 mg (n = 64)	Pre = 370 1 mo = 381	42	0
Sotalol 80 mg (n = 64)	Pre = 375 1 mo = 407	41	2

AF, atrial fibrillation; VT, ventricular tachycardia.
From Plewan A, Lehman G, Ndrepepa J, et al. Maintenance of sinus rhythm after electrical cardioversion of persistent AF: sotalol vs bisoprolol. Eur Heart J 2001;22:1504–10.

For sustained AF, electocardioversion may be deemed necessary. In a large study (N = 665), patients with AF were randomized to placebo, amiodarone, and sotalol; both the β-blocker and the amiodarone facilitated the conversion to sinus rhythm compared with placebo.[32] The presumption that sotalol is superior to other β-blockers in AF has been seriously questioned. In a study of 128 cases of AF who came to cardioversion,[33] patients were randomized to either bisoprolol 5 mg or sotalol 80 mg bid, and at 1 year, about 40% of patients had returned to AF in both drug groups—**Table 4-6b**—but 2 patients had experienced torsades de pointes on sotalol. Thus, the need for sotalol in such cases has been questioned.[34] Bisoprolol and carvedilol were similar in maintaining sinus rhythm post-AF cardioversion, though the trend favored carvedilol.[35]

For those who remain in AF, or are unsuited to electoconversion, rate control is important, and this is best achieved with a combination of digoxin with either a β-blocker or a rate-limiting calcium antagonist.[36]

The elderly are often unsuited to electoconversion, particularly when the bradytachycardia syndrome is present. In such cases, a permanent pacemaker is necessary[37] accompanied by appropriate drug therapy; both sotalol and classic β-blockers are equivalent in decreasing hospitalization and the need for atrial cardioversion shocks.[38]

c) Postoperative (coronary artery bypass graft) AF

AF is a frequent complication post-coronary artery bypass graft (CABG).[39] It occurs in about 20%-50% of cases, mostly on the second or third postoperative day and results in an increase in adverse events and hospital stay.

TABLE 4-6C Effect of bisoprolol plus magnesium vs. control on post-coronary artery bypass graft atrial fibrillation

	Postop AF (%) - all	Postop AF—Elderly (>65 Yr) (%)	Days in Hospital
Bisoprolol + Mg	20	17	7
Control	42	65	9
P value	.03	.001	.02

AF, atrial fibrillation; MG, magnesium.
From Behmanesh S, Tossios P, Homedan H, et al. Effect of prophylactic bisoprolol plus magnesium on the incidence of AF after CABG: results of randomised controlled trial. Curr Med Res Open 2006;22:1443–50.

Compared with control, postoperative carvedilol reduced the risk of post-CABG AF by over 50%[40] and appears to be superior to metoprolol in this respect.[41-43] Metoprolol has also proved inferior to β_1-selective betaxolol given post-CABG.[44] Bisoprolol (plus magnesium), like carvediolol, has also reduced the rate of post-CABG AF by about 50%,[45] being particularly beneficial in the elderly and reducing the time spent in hospital—**Table 4-6c**. Sotalol, with additional class III antiarrhythmic action, has been reported to be superior to classic β-blockers in preventing post-CABG AF.[46] However, in a large, randomized trial comparing post-CABG oral amiodarone (like sotalol also with class III action) versus oral bisoprolol, the highly β_1-selective β-blocker was at least as effective as amiodarone in suppressing AF and superior in reducing the heart rate of AF[47]—**Table 4-7**.

TABLE 4-7 In 200 post-coronary artery bypass graft cases, randomized oral bisoprolol (2.5 mg) was at least as effective as oral amiodarone in reducing the risk of atrial fibrillation and superior in controlling the heart rate in atrial fibrillation

	Risk of post-CABG AF (%)	Heart rate of post-CABG AF (beats/min)
Bisoprolol	12.7	125
Amiodarone	15.3	144

AF, atrial fibrillation; CABG, coronary artery bypass graft.
From Sleilaty G, Madi-Jebara S, Yazigi A, et al. Post-operative oral amiodarone versus oral bisoprolol as prophylaxis against AF after CABG: a prospective, randomised trial. Int J Cardiol 2009;137:116–22.

d) Heart failure and AF

AF is common in systolic heart failure, occurring in 5% of mild cases, 10%-26% in moderate cases, and up to 50% of severe cases[48]. The early appearance of AF augers badly for prognosis[48].

A meta-analysis has shown that β-blockers decrease the risk of AF in heart failure by 27%:[49] this trend was similar in all trials except SENIORS (see β-Blockers and Heart Failure chapter), which involved nebivolol (with $β_3$ ISA).

How best to treat patients with heart failure plus AF? Certainly in patients with an implantable cardioverter defibrillator (ICD), the fewest shocks occurred in those on amiodarone compared with sotalol, which in turn was associated with fewer shocks than traditional β-blockers.[50] However, the important question is how traditional β-blockers affect mortality in patients with heart failure and AF. A large study of such patients ($N = 1269$) compared the effects of digoxin, β-blocker, β-blocker plus digoxin versus a control group.[51] The β-blocker alone or combined with digoxin was associated with a 40% reduction in mortality compared with no effect with digoxin versus control, and the benefit was observed in both ischemic and

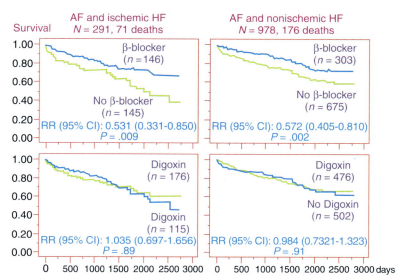

Fig. 4-3 Patients with atrial fibrillation (AF) in ischemic and nonischemic heart failure (HF). β-Blockade significantly reduces death rate in both types of HF, in contrast to digoxin, which does not. CI, confidence interval; RR, relative risk. (From Fauchier L, Grimard C, Pierre B, et al. Comparison of beta-blocker and digoxin alone and in combination for management of patients with AF and heart failure. Am J Cardiol 2009;103:248-54.)

nonischemic patients—**Figure 4-3**. This result is important in the context of the question "Which is the important factor in heart failure plus AF, rhythm or rate control?" Three large randomized, prospective trials[48] concluded that the same mortality results occurred with rhythm and rate control approaches. Thus, the unpleasant adverse reactions of some antiarrhythmic drugs (e.g., amiodarone) can be avoided. However, in an important minority of patients, particularly younger and physically active people and those who have symptoms while in rapid, irregular AF, the rhythm control method may be preferred—now attainable by radiofrequency ablation techniques in selected cases.[52]

iv) Post-myocardial infarction supraventricular arrhythmias

Elective management can be successful as evidenced by intravenous practolol[53]—**Table 4-8**. Prophylactic management can also

TABLE 4-8 Effects of intravenous practolol on cardiac arrhythmias due to acute myocardial infarction in 75 patients

		RESPONSE WITHIN 15 MIN		
Arrhythmia	Number of patients	Return to SR	Ventricular rate ↓ < 100 beats/min with or without SR	No response
Atrial fibrillation	18	5	14	4
Atrial flutter or tachycardia	13	8	12	1
Nodal tachycardia	4	2	2	2
Ventricular fibrillation	5	3*	0	2
Ventricular tachycardia	16	7	7	9
Ventricular extrasystoles	24	13†	0	9

*Plus DC shock, ineffective before practolol.
†In a further two patients, the frequency of extrasystoles was reduced to 25% of control value.
DC, direct current; SR, sinus rhythm.
From Jewitt D, Croxon R. Practolol in the management of cardiac dysrhythmias following myocardial infarction and cardiac surgery. Postgrad Med J 1971; 47(suppl):25–9.

be effective. A randomized study involving intravenous followed by oral atenolol showed a significant reduction in the frequency of AF and SVT.[54]

v) Others

a) Hypertrophic obstructive cardiomyopathy

SVTs respond well to either β-blockade or verapamil.[55]

b) Pacemaker-induced

Such SVTs respond well to β-blockade.[56]

c) Stroke or head injury

Poststroke arrhythmias respond well to intravenous followed by oral propranolol.[57]

In a double-blind, randomized, placebo-controlled study of 114 cases of acute head injury, intravenous followed by oral atenolol significantly reduced the risk of SVT[58]—Figure 4-4.

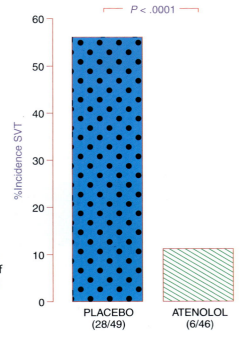

Fig. 4-4 In a placebo-controlled study of patients with acute head injury, intravenous followed by oral atenolol significantly reduced the occurrence of supraventricular tachycardia (SVT) during Holter monitoring. (Cruickshank JM, Degaute JP, Kuurne T, et al. Reduction of stress/catecholamine-induced cardiac necrosis by beta-1 selective blockade. Lancet 1987;2:585–9.)

d) Postural tachycardia syndrome

Postural tachycardia syndrome (POTS) is a disorder of chronic orthostatic (standing) intolerance, occurring mainly in women of child-bearing age. Symptoms that occur on standing are palpitations, light-headedness, chest discomfort, shortness of breath, blurred vision, and mental clouding and are relieved by sitting or lying down. Standing is associated with heart rate increases of about 30 beats/min, but no fall in blood pressure, and elevated plasma noradrenaline.

A randomized, placebo-controlled, cross-over study with propranolol 20 mg and 80 mg[59] showed clearly that propranolol 20 mg significantly reduced symptoms, with no benefit in increasing the dose—**Figure 4-5**.

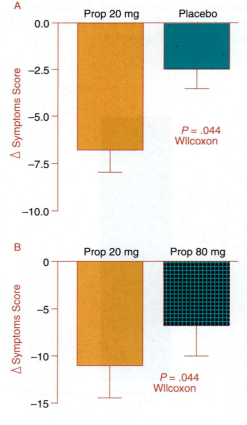

Fig. 4-5 In a placebo-controlled study of patients with postural tachycardia syndrome, low-dose propranolol significantly attenuated the tachycardia and improved symptoms (blurring of vision, palpitations, shortness of breath, and lightheadedness). (From Raj SR, Black BK, Biaggioni I, et al. Propranolol decreases tachycardia and improves symptoms in the postural tachycardia syndrome. Circulation 2009;120: 725–34.)

B) Ventricular arrhythmias

The presence of ventricular arrhythmias has a more sinister implication than SVTs. Even the presence of simple ventricular premature beats (VPBs) in the post-myocardial infarction (MI) period was associated with a doubling of mortality.[60] Patients who experienced death during Holter monitoring did so usually with ventricular fibrillation (VF), with the terminal episode invariably preceded by complex VPBs.[61]

The expected response to ventricular arrhythmias to treatment with β-blockers is shown in **Table 4-9**.

i) Idiopathic ventricular arrhythmias and β-blockers

a) Ventricular tachycardia

This topic has been reviewed.[1] Sustained VT requires cardioversion. Inducible VT can be prevented by low-dose propranolol in about 25% of cases, with no added action of high doses.[62] Even better results have been reported with sotalol.[63]

Exercise-induced paroxysmal VT responds very well to propranolol,[8,11] and even when not precipitated by exercise, good results can occur from both oral propranolol[8] and atenolol.[64] Children with normal hearts, who have exercise-induced VT, respond well to atenolol.[65]

TABLE 4-9 Expected response of ventricular arrhythmias to treatment with β-blockers

Ventricular arrhythmia	Response
Ventricular premature beats	Poor, unless related to digitalis toxicity, exercise or stress, ischemic heart disease, mitral valve prolapse, or the long QT syndrome
Ventricular tachycardia (sustained)	Fair, but good when due to digitalis toxicity, exercise or stress, or the long QT syndrome
Paroxysmal ventricular tachycardia	Good, particularly in cases unresponsive to other antiarrhythmic therapy
Ventricular fibrillation	Good if: 1. Due to digitalis toxicity or sympathomimetic amines, or 2. Refractory to initial defibrillation

Modified from Singh BN, Jewitt DE. Beta-blockers in cardiac arrhythmias. Cardiovasc Drugs 1977;2:119–59.

b) Ventricular fibrillation

Stress or exercise-induced VF has been well described, particularly in children, and responds well to propranolol.[11,66] Such patients, of course, require implantation of an automatic defibrillator, and of 10 such cases on nadolol versus 10 on no β-blocker, only 4 required shocks in the nadolol group compared with all 10 on no β-blocker.[67]

ii) Post-myocardial infarction ventricular arrhythmias

High catecholamine levels and tachycardia after acute MI predispose to ventricular arrhythmias,[11] and the number of arrhythmias markedly increases in the absence of β-blockade.[68]

a) Acute myocardial infarction

Elective intravenous (uncontrolled) practolol can be effective in terminating ventricular arrhythmias[53]—(see **Table 4-8**)—as can propranolol.[8]

Prophylactic β-blockade can be effective, particularly in threatened infarction[69]—**Figure 4-6**, in which intravenous followed by oral atenolol was effective in suppressing ventricular arrhythmias compared with control. Propranolol vs. placebo was shown to prevent VF.[70] Surprisingly, in the large, early intervention studies with atenolol (ISIS-1 [First International Study of Infarct Survival])[71] and metoprolol (MIAMI [Metoprolol in Acute Myocardial Infarction]),[72] there was no reduction in VF. However, in the vast COMMIT (Clopidogrel and Metoprolol in Myocardial Infarction Trial),[73] intravenous followed by oral metoprolol effected a significant 17% reduction in VF (though there was no significant reduction in death rate and a 30% increase in carcinogenic shock).

In patients with acute MI who underwent percutaneous coronary intervention (PCI) of the affected artery, pre-/postprocedure oral metoprolol or carvedilol were similar in their preventive actions regarding ventricular arrhythmias as assessed by Holter monitoring.[74]

b) Late-intervention—prophylactic

β-Blockers do reduce the risk of sudden death as shown in the two large late-intervention studies involving propranolol (BHAT [β-blocker Heart Attack Trial])[75] and timolol.[76] Though it is not possible to ascribe all this benefit to arrhythmia prevention, propranolol was shown to reduce ventricular arrhythmias compared

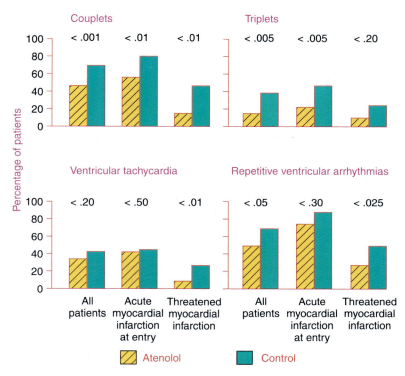

Fig. 4-6 Effect of intravenous, followed by oral, atenolol on ventricular arrhythmias following acute or threatened myocardial infarction. There was a significant reduction of extrasystoles in all patients and ventricular tachycardia/repetitive ventricular arrhythmias in those with threatened infarction. (From Rossi PR, Yusuf S, Ramsdale D, et al. Reduction of ventricular arrhythmias by early I.V. atenolol in suspected acute myocardial infarction. Br Med J 1983;286:506–10.)

with placebo[77]—**Figure 4-7**. It has been suggested that postinfarct ventricular arrhythmias are more likely in the presence of hypokalemia, and thus, nonselective β-blockers may be more effective than $β_1$-selective β-blockers in arrhythmia suppression. However, nonselective sotalol, which did increase serum potassium levels, was no different from atenolol in suppressing postinfarct ventricular arrhythmias.[78]

Some post-MI patients experience an "electrical storm" associated with multiple VF episodes; such patients respond well to β-blockade and survival is improved compared with those who receive class I antiarrhythmic agents.[79]

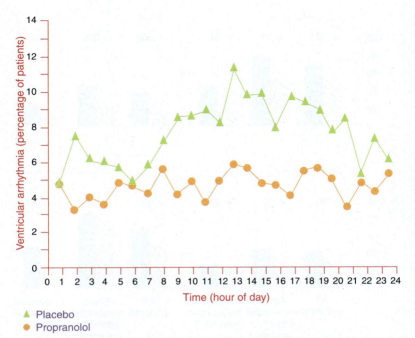

▲ Placebo
● Propranolol

Fig. 4-7 β-blocker Heart Attack Trial (BHAT) late intervention post-myocardial infarction. Oral propranolol (vs. placebo) significantly reduced the frequency of ventricular arrhythmias (extrasystoles and ventricular tachycardia) over 24 hr after 6 wk therapy. (From Lichstein E, Morganroth J, Harrist R, Hubble E. Effect of propranolol and ventricular arrhythmias. The BHAT experience. Circulation 1983;67[suppl I]:I5–10.)

iii) Others

a) Digitalis toxicity

Digitalis has a low therapeutic index and induced ventricular arrhythmias are not uncommon, necessitating drug withdrawal and/or giving potassium.

β-Blockers can be highly effective in such cases with good results arising from intravenous followed by low-dose oral propranolol,[8] though severe bradycardia, or even asystole, can occur.[11]

b) Mitral valve prolapse

Mitral Valve Prolapse (MVP) is not uncommon, occurring mainly in young women. The Framingham survey indicated that 17% of women in their 20s had MVP,[80] with symptoms such as chest discomfort, palpitations, light-headedness, or syncope. VPBs were noted in 45% and VT in 6%, and sudden death (VF) can occur.[81]

Such cases often respond well to β-blockade,[82] particularly in the presence of an implanted pacemaker.[83]

c) Long QT syndrome

This syndrome comprises a long QT interval in the ECG and is associated with syncopal attacks, or sudden death, associated with ventricular arrhythmias.[84] It is thought to be due to a neural input imbalance between the right and the left cardiac sympathetic nerves,[84] leading to a geographical heterogeneity in the rate of ventricular repolarization. Syncopal attacks tend to be triggered by stress, emotion, fright, or exercise.

β-Blockers, such as propranolol, shorten the QTc and are the drugs of choice in the treatment of this syndrome.[85] Sometimes, heart block complicates the picture[86]—**Figure 4-8**—necessitating both demand pacing plus β-blocker. Though controlled studies are absent, it has

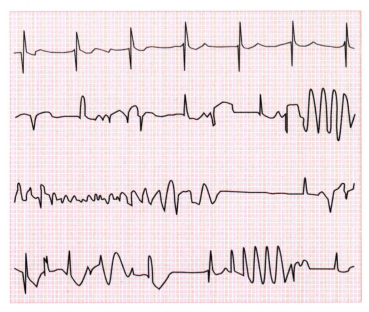

Fig. 4-8 This 13-year-old patient with the long QT interval syndrome, showing runs of ventricular tachycardia/fibrillation on electrocardiogram, responded well to propranolol plus demand right ventricular pacing. (From Crawford MH, Karliner JS, O'Rourke RA, Friedman WF. Prolonged Q-T interval syndrome. Chest 1975;68:369–71.)

been estimated that β-blockers markedly reduce the mortality rate.[84] However, it is now recognized that there are different phenotypic expressions of the long QT syndrome and not all respond that well to β-blockade.[87] Those that remain symptomatic in spite of β-blocker therapy would now also receive an implantable cardiovertor-defibrillator or left cervicothoracic sympathetic denervation.[88]

d) Hypertrophic obstructive cardiomyopathy

Patients with HOCM are prone to ventricular arrhythmias and sudden death.[89] Such ventricular arrhythmias, though often stress/poststress-induced,[90] appear to respond poorly to β-blockade (propranolol)[91] unless combined with other antiarrhythmic agents.[92]

There are no randomized, controlled, prospective studies to scientifically assess the role of β-blockade, though the strong impression is that β-blockade improves both symptoms and prognosis.[93] Management has evolved over the years;[94] medical therapy should be tried first, comprising high dosage of β-blockade, verapamil, and/or disopyramide; only when this approach fails should invasive procedures involving dual chamber pacing, septal ablation, or surgery be considered.

e) Pacemakers and arrhythmias

Pacemaker-induced ventricular arrhythmias may be effectively suppressed by β-blockade.[8] In modern times, patients at high risk of life-threatening ventricular arrhythmias could well have an ICD inserted.[94] When such patients experience an ICD shock, it is often unpleasant and quality of life is impaired. Such patients experience fewer shocks when on β-blockers.[94] Not only is quality of life improved by β-blockade in such patients, but prognosis (nonrandomized data) also appears best in those receiving β-blockers.[95]

f) Anesthesia, surgery, and arrhythmias

The role of sympathetic stimulation in the occurrence of sudden death during/post surgery is well known.[1] Halothane sensitizes the myocardium to catecholamimines and, alongside adrenaline, can precipitate VT, as can cyclopropane. The situation is exacerbated if there has been recent β-blocker withdrawal, possibly resulting in VF,[96] which is responsive to propranolol administration—**Table 4-10**. The sensible approach, particularly in cardiac surgery, is not to discontinue β-blocker therapy preoperation[97]—**Table 4-11**. Such an approach would make postoperative VF, responsive to β-blockade,[98] less likely, thus improving prognosis.[99]

TABLE 4-10 Intraoperative life-threatening arrhythmias in 239 cardiac surgical patients: response to propranolol 0.4-1.0 mg intravenously

Arrhythmia	Number of patients	Success rate (%)
Sinus, atrial or tachycardia	46	100
Ventricular tachycardia	12	100
Multifocal VPBs	2	100
Atrial premature beats	4	100
VPBs (simple)	29	68
Acute atrial fibrillation	10	100
Chronic atrial fibrillation	58	72
Ventricular fibrillation	78	100

VPBs, ventricular premature beats.
From Romagnoli A, Sabawala PB. Effect of Propranolol Withdrawal on Subsequent Anaesthesia and Surgery. 4th Asian and Australian Congress on Anaesthesia Singapore 1974, pp 150–1.

TABLE 4-11 Effects of preoperative propranolol continuance or discontinuance upon intraoperative (coronary bypass) complications (between induction of anesthesia and institution of cardiopulmonary bypass)

Complication	Control (%) ($n = 41$)	Group B: Propranolol therapy discontinued (%) ($n = 40$)	Group A: Propranolol therapy continued (%) ($n = 38$)
Bradycardia (<50 beats/min)	5	8	0
Hypotension (<80% control systolic)	20	20	18
Atrial arrhythmias	5	3	0
Ventricular arrhythmias	7	20*	3
ST changes (>2 mV)	24	43†	13
Patients with one or more complication	51*	70†	26

*Significantly higher than group A ($P < .05$).
†Significantly higher than group A ($P < .01$).
From Slogoff S, Keats AS, Ott E. Pre-operative propranolol therapy and aortocoronary bypass operation. JAMA 1978;240:1487–90.

g) Catecholaminergic mono-/polymorphic ventricular tachycardia

This condition has no underlying morphological abnormality of the heart, may be familial, and is linked to VT/VF and sudden death, often precipitated by exercise. It can affect children and young adults[100,101] or older subjects[102–104] and responds well to β-blockade[100–103] ±verapamil[104] and to automatic ICD.

An allied condition, arrhythmogenic right ventricular cardiomyopathy, also responds well to an ICD and β-blockade plus/minus amiodarone.[105]

2. Is the choice of β-blocker important?

A) $β_1$-blockade

The antiarrhythmic activity of β-blockers resides mainly in their $β_1$-blocking property.[1] Certainly, polymorphic varieties of the $β_1$-receptor, compared with the $β_2$-receptor, are associated with a 10-fold increase in life-threatening ventricular arrhythmias.[106] The highly $β_1$-selective agent bisoprolol was successful, compared to ACE inhibition, in preventing sudden death in heart failure.[107] Bisoprolol is also highly effective in SVT[13] and AF[30] prevention, being as effective as sotalol[33] and amiodarone[47] in this latter respect. Atenolol, though only moderately $β_1$-selective, is highly effective in preventing postinfarction ventricular arrhythmias.[69]

Thus, $β_1$-blockade has powerful anti-supraventricular and -ventricular arrhythmic properties and should be the first β-blocking choice, avoiding the problems of $β_2$-blockade (e.g., bronchospasm), ISA (lack of efficacy), class III (sotalol can induce torsades de pointes), and α-blockade (postural hypotension and sexual dysfunction).

B) $β_2$-blockade

$β_2$-Stimulation can prolong the QT interval and trigger ventricular arrhythmias,[108] particularly in the presence of hypokalemia.[109] However, the clinical relevance of these observations in support of $β_2$-blockade is not strong.[110]

C) Intrinsic sympathomimetic activity

In the postinfarction period, β-blockers with ISA are less effective than those without ISA (see Chapter 2). Certainly, a high degree of ISA, as with pindolol, can lower the threshold to VF.[111] In heart failure, nebivolol, with β_3 ISA, was the only β-blocker not to reduce the risk of AF.[49] Thus, ISA is not a desirable feature for arrhythmia prevention.

D) Additional class III activity—sotalol

Though sotalol can be highly effective in the treatment of supraventricular[7] and ventricular[63] arrhythmias, it usually offers no advantages over β_1-blockade.[33] However, unlike ordinary β-blockers, it can, in 2%-4% of cases, induce torsades de pointes (VT/VF),[22] see example[112]—**Figure 4-9**—even at low dose.[113] Thus, some would not recommend using sotalol[34] or would keep it only for resistant cases.[20,24]

E) α-Blockade (in addition to β-blockade)

Both α_1- and α_2-blockade can reduce atrial arrhythmias by about 30%[114] and may have contributed to the superiority of carvedilol over metoprolol in preventing post-CABG AF.[41-43] However, α_2-blockade appears to increase the risk of VT linked to ischemia,[115] though doxazosin does reduce the risk of VF in heart failure.[113]

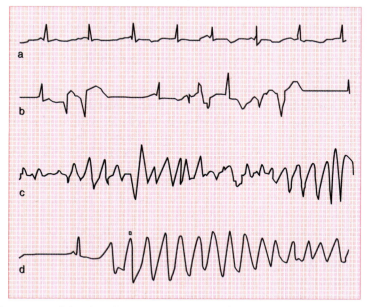

Fig. 4-9 Sotalol-induced ventricular tachycardia (torsades de pointes) in a patient with the long QT syndrome. Arrhythmia occurred after the second tablet of sotalol 160 mg. (see mark on trace d) (From McGibbon JK, Pocock WA, Barlow JB, et al. Sotalol, hypokalaemia, syncope and torsades de pointes. Br Heart J 1984;51:157–62.)

Carvedilol, like other β-blockers, is effective in reducing the risk of postinfarction atrial and ventricular arrhythmias.[116]

F) Additional class I activity

Propranolol is known to possess membrane stabilizing activity, or "quinidine-like" properties. Such properties come under the heading of class IA antiarrhythmic action—(see **Table 4-2**). However, this acute antiarrhythmic action comes into play only at blood levels of propranolol many times greater than occur with normal propranolol dosage.[4]

SUMMARY AND CONCLUSIONS

1. β-Blockers belong to class II antiarrhythmic agents and antagonize the effects of increased sympathetic nerve activity that (a) increase pacemaker activity, (b) increase AV conduction and shorten the refractory period of the AV node, (c) increase the rate of diastolic depolarization of automatic cells, thus increasing pacemaker activity, (d) provide nonuniformity of recovery of the refractory period, thus lowering the threshold of VF.
2. SVTs often respond well to β-blockers. This includes ectopic SVTs and reentrant, paroxysmal SVTs, including WPW syndrome, in which prevention is especially good if the SVT is provoked by exercise, emotion, or stress.
3. The most commonly experienced supraventricular arrhythmia is AF, particularly in the elderly. (a) Paroxysmal AF, particularly if stress-induced, responds well to $β_1$-blockade, with most patients remaining in sinus rhythm (SR). (b) β-Blockers facilitate conversion to SR via electrocardioversion and control heart rate in those who remain in AF. (c) In AF requiring a pacemaker, fewer shocks are needed in the presence of a β-blocker. (d) Postoperative (particularly CABG) AF is markedly reduced by β-blockers. (e) In heart failure, β-blockers (no ISA) are effective in reducing the risk of AF, and in those with AF, mortality is significantly reduced (rate control is as effective as conversion to SR). (f) β-Blockers also reduce the risk of AF in both postinfarction patients and hypertensive patients (significantly more so than calcium blockers).
4. Other conditions susceptible to SVT/AF that benefit from β-blockers are (a) HOCM, (b) pacemaker-induced, (c) stroke/head injury, and (d) postural tachycardia syndrome.
5. Idiopathic VT and VF, particularly if exercise-/stress-induced, can be prevented by β-blockers. Those requiring ICDs experience fewer unpleasant shocks.

6. Postinfarction ventricular arrhythmias can be both terminated and prevented by β_1-blockade.
7. Other conditions linked to VT/VF: (a) digitalis toxicity-induced ventricular arrhythmias can respond well to β-blockers; (b) MVP, common in young women, is linked to VT and sudden death, which can be prevented by β-blockers, with or without pacemaker; (c) long QT syndrome is linked to ventricular arrhythmias and sudden death, which appear to respond to β-blockers with a shortened QT interval and fewer deaths (though some phenotypes do not); (d) HOCM cases are prone to sudden death and appear to benefit from β-blockers, with or without pacemaker; (e) pacemaker-induced ventricular arrhythmias often respond well to β-blockers; (f) anesthesia-/surgery-induced ventricular arrhythmias often respond well to β-blockers; do not stop β-blockers presurgery; (g) catecholaminergic mono-/polymorphic VT and arrhythmogenic right ventricular cardiomyopathy respond well to β-blocker±pacemaker.
8. Choice of β-blocker is important: (a) β_1-blockade (e.g., bisoprolol) is the main component of the β-blocker antiarrhythmic property and should be the first choice; (b) ISA (e.g., pindolol [β_1 and β_2] and nebivolol [β_3]) may diminish efficacy; (c) β_2-blockade (e.g., propranolol) may be useful if hypokalemia is a factor, but the clinical relevance is still undecided and metabolic disturbance and bronchospasm may be problematic; (d) α_1-blockade (e.g., carvedilol) may have additional benefits in preventing AF, but some patients (particularly the elderly) may experience postural hypotension; (e) class III antiarrhythmic activity (e.g., sotalol) can produce additional efficacy, but induced torsades de pointes (VT/VF) is a problem; thus, sotalol should be kept "in reserve."

REFERENCES

1. Cruickshank JM, Prichard BNC. Beta-Blockers in Clinical Practice. 2nd ed. Edinburgh: Churchill Livingstone; 1994, pp 705–63.
2. Vaughan Williams EM. Classification of arrhythmia drugs. In Sandoe E, Flensted-Jensen E, Olsen K (eds). Symposium on Cardiac Arrhythmias, Elsinore, Denmark, April 23-25, 1970. Sodertalje, Sweden: AB Astra.
3. Hillis WS, Whiting B. Antiarrhythmic drugs. Br Med J 1983;286: 13332–6.
4. Duff HJ, Mitchell LB, Wyse G. Antiarrhythmic efficacy of propranolol: comparison of low and high serum concentrations. J Am Coll Cardiol 1986;8:969–75.

5. Verrier RL. Mechanisms of behaviourally induced arrhythmias. Circulation 1987;76:I 48–56.
6. Singh BN. Clinical aspects of antiarrhythmic actions of beta-blockers: part 1. Pattern of response of common arrhythmias. N Z Med J 1973; 78:482–6.
7. Colloridi V, Perri C, Ventriglia F, Critelli G. Oral sotalol in paediatric atrial ectopic tachycardia. Am Heart J 1992;123:254–6.
8. Gibson DG, Sowton E. The use of beta-blockrs in dysrhythmias. Prog Cardiovasc Dis 1969;12:16–39.
9. Theilen EO, Wilson WR. Beta-blockers in the treatment of cardiac arrhythmias. Med Clin North Am 1968;52:1017–29.
10. Medi C, Kalman JM, Freedman SB. Supraventricular tachycardia. Med J Aust 2009;190:255–60.
11. Singh BN, Jewitt DE. Beta-blockers in cardiac arrhythmias. Cardiovasc Drugs 1977;2:119–59.
12. Rehnqvist N. Clinical experience with intravenous metoprolol in supraventricular tachyarrhythmias. Ann Clin Res 1981;13(suppl 30): 68–72.
13. Van den Ven LL, Crijns HJ, de Muinck ED, et al. Electophysiological and antiarrhythmic effects of I.V. bisoprolol in atrioventricular nodal re-entry tachycardia. Curr Ther Res 1996;57:950–7.
14. Gillette PC, Garson A, Enterovic E, et al. Oral propranolol treatment in infants and children. J Pediatr 1978;92:141–4.
15. Millar RN. Efficacy of sotalol in controlling re-entrant supraventricular tachycardias. Cardiovasc Drugs Ther 1990;4 (suppl 3):625–9.
16. Gallagher JJ, Pritchett EL, Sealey WC, et al. The pre-excitation syndromes. Progr Cardiovasc Dis 1978;20:285–327.
17. Langan MN. The acute treatment of supraventricular tachycardia. Mt Sinai J Med 1997;64:142–5.
18. Prystowsky EN, Greer S, Packer DL, et al. Beta-blocker therapy for the Wolff-Parkinson-White syndrome. Am J Cardiol 1987;60:46D–50D.
19. Cruickshank JM, Prichard BNC. Beta-Blockers in Clinical Practice. 2nd ed. Edinburgh: Churchill Livingstone; 1994, p 720.
20. Nathan AW, Hellestrand KJ, Bexton RS, et al. Electrophysiological effects of sotalol—just another beta-blocker? Br Heart J 1982;47: 515–20.
21. Kunz K-P, Schluter M, Kuck K-H. Sotalol in patients with Wolff-Parkinson-White syndrome. Circulation 1987;75:1050–7.
22. Sasse M, Paul T, Bergmann P, Kallfeiz HC. Sotalol-associated torsades de pointes tachycardia in a 15 month-old child. Pacing Clin Electrophysicol 1999;21:143.
23. Luedtke SA, Kuhn RJ, McCaffrey FM. Pharmacological management of supraventricular tachycardias in children. Part 1: WPW and atrioventricular node re-entry. Ann Pharmacother 1997;31:1227–43.
24. Ratnasamy C, Rossique-Gonzalez M, Young ML. Pharmacological therapy in children with atrioventricular re-entry: which drug? Curr Pharm Des 2008;14:753–61.

25. Kannel WB, Wolf RA, Benjamin EJ, Levy D. Prevalence, incidence, prognosis and predisposing conditions for atrial fibrillation. Am J Cardiol 1998;82:2N–9N.
26. Healy JS, Conolly SJ. Atrial fibrillation: hypertension as a causative agent, risk factor for complications and potential therapeutic target. Am J Cardiol 2003;91:9G–14G.
27. Kim RJ, Gerling BR, Kouo AT, Greenberg ML. Precipitation of ventricular fibrillation by intravenous diltiazem and metoprolol in a young patient with occult WPW syndrome. Pacing Clin Electophys 2008;31: 776–9.
28. Watchtell K, Lehto M, Gerdts E, et al. Angiotensin II receptor blockade reduces new-onset atrial fibrillation and subsequent stroke compared to atenolol (LIFE). J Am Coll Cardiol 2005;45:712–9.
29. Schaer BA, Schneider C, Jick SS, et al. Risk for incidental atrial fibrillation in patients who receive antihypertensive drugs: a nested control study. Ann Intern Med 2010;152:78–84.
30. Ishiguro H, Ikeda T, Abe A, et al. Antiarrhythmic effect of bisoprolol, a highly selective beta-1 blocker, in patients with paroxysmal atrial fibrillation. Int Heart J 2008;49:281–93.
31. Ogawa S, Yamashita T, Yamazaki T, et al. Optimal treatment strategy for patients with paroxysmal–atrial fibrillation: J-RHYTHM Study. Circ J 2009;73:242–8.
32. Singh SN, Tang XC, Deda D, Singh BN. Systematic electrocardioversion for atrial fibrillation and role of antiarrhythmic drugs (SAFE-T trial). Heart Rhythm 2009;6:152–5.
33. Plewan A, Lehman G, Ndrepepa J, et al. Maintenance of sinus rhythm after electrical cardioversion of persistent AF: sotalol vs bisoprolol. Eur Heart J 2001;22:1504–10.
34. Coumel P. Sotalol: a fool's deal? Eur Heart J 2001;22:1370–3.
35. Katritisis DG, Panagiotakos DB, Karvouni E, et al. Comparison of effectiveness of carvedilol versus bisoprolol for maintenance of sinus rhythm after cardioversion of persistent AF. Am J Cardiol 2003;92:1116–9.
36. Nikolaudon T, Channer KS. Chronic atrial fibrillation: a systematic review of medical heart rate control management. Postgrad Med J 2009;85:303–12.
37. Aronow WS. Management of atrial fibrillation in the elderly. Minerva Med 2009;100:3–24.
38. Capucci A, Botto G, Molon G, et al. The DAPHNE study: a randomised trial comparing sotalol versus beta-blockers to treat symptomatic AF in patients with the bradytachycardia syndrome implanted with anti-tachycardia pacemaker. Am Heart J 2008;156:373.e1–8.
39. Rostagno C. Recent developments in pharmacologic prophylaxix of AF in patients undergoing surgical revascularization. Cardiovasc Haemat Agents Med Chem 2009;7:137–46.
40. Tsuboi J, Kawazoe K, Izumoto H, Okabayashi H. Postoperative treatment with carvedilol prevents paroxysmal AF after CABG. Circulation 2008;72:588–91.

41. Haghjoo M, Saravi M, Hashemi MJ, et al. Optimal beta-blocker for prevention of AF after a-pump CABG; carvedolol versus metoprolol. Heart Rhythm 2007;4:1170–4.
42. Acikel S, Bozlas H, Guitekin B, et al. Comparison of the efficacy of metoprolol and carvedilol for preventing AF after CABG. Int J Cardiol 2008;126:108–13.
43. Celik T, Iyisoy A, Jata B, et al. Beta-blockers for the prevention of AF after CABG: carvedilol versus metoprolol. Int J Cardiol 2009;135:393–6.
44. Iluita L, Christodorescu R, Filpescu D, et al. Prevention of postoperative AF with beta-blocker in CABG: betaxilol versus metoprolol. Interact Cardiovasc Thorac Surg 2009;9:89–93.
45. Behmanesh S, Tossios P, Homedan H, et al. Effect of prophylactic bisoprolol plus magnesium on the incidence of AF after CABG: results of randomised controlled trial. Curr Med Res Open 2006;22: 1443–50.
46. Patel A, Dunning J. Is sotalol more effective than standard beta-blockers for the prophylaxis of AF during cardiac surgery? Interact Cardiovasc Thorac Surg 2005;4:147–50.
47. Sleilaty G, Madi-Jebara S, Yazigi A, et al. Post-operative oral amiodarone versus oral bisoprolol as prophylaxis against AF after CABG: a prospective, randomised trial. Int J Cardiol 2009;137:116–22.
48. Anter E, Jessup M, Callans AJ. Atrial fibrillation and heart failure. Treatment considerations for a dual epidemic. Circulation 2009;119: 2516–25.
49. Nsr IA, Bouzamondo A, Hulot JS, et al. Prevention of atrial fibrillation onset by beta-blocker treatment in heart failure: a meta-analysis. Eur Heart J 2007;28:457–62.
50. Lee CH, Nam GB, Park HG, et al. Effect of antiarrhythmic drugs on inappropriate shocks in patients with implantable cardioverter defibrillators. Circ J 2008;72:102–5.
51. Fauchier L, Grimard C, Pierre B, et al. Comparison of beta-blocker and digoxin alone and in combination for management of patients with AF and heart failure. Am J Cardiol 2009;103:248–54.
52. Betts T, Mitchell A. Is rate more important than rhythm in treating atrial fibrillation? BMJ 2009;339:664–5.
53. Jewitt D, Croxon R. Practolol in the management of cardiac dysrhythmias following myocardial infarction and cardiac surgery. Postgrad Med J 1971;47(suppl):25–9.
54. Yusuf S, Sleight P, Rossi P, et al. Reduction in infarct size, arrhythmias and chest pain by early intravenous beta-blockade in suspected acute myocardial infarction. Circulation 1983;67(suppl 1):I32–41.
55. Milazzotto F, Ceci V, Remei E, et al. Treatment of HOCM: comparison between verapamil and pindolol (abstract). VIII Europ Congr Cardiol, Paris, 1980, 0350.
56. Jachuck SJ. Implanted-pacemaker-induced dysrhythmia and its management. Postgrad Med J 1973;49:14–17.

57. Mizroch S, Harter L, Fields D. Stroke, tachyarrythmias and propranolol. JAMA 1978;239:1394–5.
58. Cruickshank JM, Degaute JP, Kuurne T, et al. Reduction of stress/catecholamine-induced cardiac necrosis by beta-1 selective blockade. Lancet 1987;2:585–9.
59. Raj SR, Black BK, Biaggioni I, et al. Propranolol decreases tachycardia and improves symptoms in the postural tachycardia syndrome. Circulation 2009;120:725–34.
60. Coronary Drug Project. Prognostic importance of premature beats following myocardial infarction. JAMA 1973;223:116–24.
61. Nikolic G, Bishop RC, Singh JB. Sudden death recorded during Holter monitoring. Circulation 1982;66:218–25.
62. Duff HJ, Roden DM, Brorson L, et al. Electrophysiological actions of high plasma concentrations of propranolol in human subjects. J Am Coll Cardiol 1983;2:1134–40.
63. Senges J, Lengfelder W, Jauernig R, et al. Elecctrophysiological testing in assessment of therapy with sotalol for sustained VT. Circulation 1984;69:577–84.
64. Heng MK, Zimmer I. Reduction of ventricular arrhythmias by atenolol. Am Heart J 1985;109:1273–80.
65. Trippel DL, Gillette PC. Atenolol in children with ventricular arrhythmias. Am Heart J 1990;119:1312–6.
66. Wennevold A, Sandoe E. Paroxysmal VF in children. Acta Med Scand 1977;202:425–7.
67. Leclercq JF, Leenhardt A, Coumel P, Slama R. Efficacy of beta-blocking agents in reducing the number of shocks in patients with implanted with first-generation automatic defibrillators. Eur Heart J 1992;13:1180–4.
68. Piccini JP, Hranitzky PM, Kilaru R, et al. Relation of mortality to failure to prescribe beta-blockers in patients with sustained ventricular tachycardia and fibrillations following acute myocardial infarction (VALIANT). Am J Cardiol 2008;102:1427–32.
69. Rossi PR, Yusuf S, Ramsdale D, et al. Reduction of ventricular arrhythmias by early I.V. atenolol in suspected acute myocardial infarction. Br Med J 1983;286:506–10.
70. Norris RM, Brown MA, Clark ED, et al. Prevention of ventricular fibrillation during acute myocardial infarction by I.V. propranolol. Lancet 1984;2:883–6.
71. ISIS-1 Collaborative Group. Randomised trial of I.V. atenolol among 16,027 cases of suspected myocardial infarction. Lancet 1986;2:57–66.
72. MIAMI Trial Research Group. Metoprolol in acute myocardial infarction. A randomised, placebo-controlled international trial. Eur Heart J 1985;6:199–226.
73. COMMIT. Early intravenous and oral metoprolol in 45,852 patients with acute MI: randomised, controlled trial. Lancet 2005;366:1622–32.

74. Toly R, Witt M, Schwarz B, et al. Comparison of carvedilol and metoprolol in patients with acute myocardial infarction undergoing primary coronary intervention—the PASSAT Study. Clin Res Cardiol 2006;95:31–41.
75. Beta-blocker Heart Attack Research Group. A randomised trial of propranolol in patients with acute myocardial infarction. JAMA 1982;247:1707–14.
76. Norwegian Multicentre Study Group. Timolol-induced reduction in mortality and re-infarction in patients surviving acute myocardial infarction. N Engl J Med 1981;304:801–7.
77. Lichstein E, Morganroth J, Harrist R, Hubble E. Effect of propranolol and ventricular arrhythmias. The BHAT experience. Circulation 1983; 67(suppl I):I5–10.
78. Cobb LA, Werner JA. Editorial: Antiarrhythmic therapy, ventricular premature depolarisation and sudden death: the tip of the ice-berg. Circulation 1969;59:864–5.
79. Nademanee K, Taylor R, Bailey WE. Treating electrical storm: sympathetic versus advanced cardiac life-support-guided therapy. Circulation 2000;102:742–7.
80. Savage DD, Garrison RJ, Devereux RB, et al. Mitral valve prolapsed in the general population. The Framingham Study. Am Heart J 1983;106:571–6.
81. Pocock WA, Bosaman CK, Chester E, et al. Sudden death in primary valve prolapse. Am Heart J 1984;107:378–82.
82. Winkle RA, Lopez MG, Goodman DJ, et al. Propranolol for patients with mitral valve prolapse. Am Heart J 1977;93:422–7.
83. Richie JL, Hammermeister KE, Kennedy JW. Refractory VT and VF in a patient with mitral valve prolapse: successful control with overdrive. Am J Cardiol 1976;37:314–6.
84. Schwartz PJ, Periti M, Malliani A. The long Q-T syndrome. Am Heart J 1975;89:378–90.
85. Milne JR, Ward DE, Spurrell RA, Camm AJ. The long Q-T syndrome: effect of drugs and left stellate ganglion block. Am Heart J 1982;104:194–8.
86. Crawford MH, Karliner JS, O' Rourke RA, Friedman WF. Prolonged Q-T interval syndrome. Chest 1975;68:369–71.
87. Priori SG, Napolitano C, Schwartz PJ, et al. Association of long Q-T syndrome loci and cardiac events among patients treated with beta-blockers. JAMA 2004;292:1341–4.
88. Goldenberg I, Moss AJ. Long Q-T syndrome. J Am Coll Cardiol 2008;51:2291–300.
89. McKenna WJ, England D, Doi YL, et al. Arrhythmia in hypertrophic cardiomyopathy. I. Influence on prognosis. Br Med J 1981;46:168–72.
90. Losse B, Christoph I, Borggrefe M, Koniger HH. Risk of stress-induced ventricular arrhythmias in HOCM. Z Kardiol 1984;73:304–12.

91. McKenna WJ, Chetty S, Oakley CM, Goodwin JF. Arrhythmia in HOCM: exercise and 48-hour ambulatory ECG assessment with and without beta-blockers. Am J Cardiol 1980;45:1–5.
92. Canedo MI, Frank MI, Abdulla AM. Management of potentially life-threatening arrhythmias in HOCM. Clin Res 1979;27:768.
93. Frank MJ, Abdulla AM, Canedo MI, Saylors RE. Long-term medical management of HOCM. Am J Cardiol 1978;42:993–1001.
94. Page WC. Antiarrhythmic drugs for all patients with an ICD? JAMA 2006;295:211–3.
95. Lai HM, Aronow WS, Kruger A, et al. Effect of beta-blockers, ACE inhibitors, ARB and satins on mortality of patients with ICDs. Am J Cardiol 2008;102:77–8.
96. Romagnoli A, Sabawala PB. Effect of Propranolol Withdrawal on Subsequent Anaesthesia and Surgery. 4th Asian and Australian Congress on Anaesthesia Singapore 1974, pp 150–1.
97. Slogoff S, Keats AS, Ott E. Pre-operative propranolol therapy and aortocoronary bypass operation. JAMA 1978;240:1487–90.
98. Romagnoli A, Sabawala PB. Propranolol in recurrent ventricular fibrillation (abstract). Clin Pharmacol Ther 1974;15:217.
99. Mehta RH, Starr AZ, Lopes RD, et al (APEX AMI Investigators). Incidence of and outcomes associated with VT and VF in patients undergoing primary PTCI. JAMA 2009;301:1779–89.
100. Fazio G, Novo G, Sutera L, et al. Sympathetic tone and ventricular tachycardia. J Cardiovasc Med 2008;9:963–6.
101. Tan JH, Scheinman MM. Exercise-induced polymorphic ventricular tachycardia in adults without structural disease. Am J Cardiol 2008;101:1142–6.
102. Aronow WS. A focus on when and when not to use antiarrhythmic drugs in treating ventricular arrhythmias and indications for the use of automatic implantable cardioverter defibrillators. Geriatrics 2008;63:20–8.
103. Hayashi M, Denjoy K, Extramiana F, et al. Influence and risk-factors of arrhythmic events in catecholaminergic polymorphic ventricular tachycardia. Circulation 2009;119:2426–34.
104. Rosso R, Kalman JM, Rogowski O, et al. Calcium channel blockers and beta-blockers versus beta-blockers alone for preventing exercise-induced arrhythmias in catecholaminergic polymorphic ventricular tachycardia. Heart Rhythm 2007;4:1149–54.
105. Boldt LH, Haverkamp W. Arrhythmic right ventricular cardiomyopathy: diagnosis and risk stratification. Herz 2009;34:290–7.
106. Ulucan C, Cetintas V, Tetik A, et al. Beta-1 and beta-2 receptor polymorphisms and idiopathic ventricular arrhythmias. Cardiovasc Electrophysiol 2008;19:1053–8.
107. Willenheimer R. The current role of beta-blockers in chronic heart failure: with special emphasis on the CIBIS III trial. Eur Heart J 2009;11(suppl A):A15–20.

108. Lowe MD., Rowland E, Brown MJ, Grace AA. Beta-2 adrenergic receptors mediate important electrophysiological effects in the human ventricular myocardium. Heart 2001;86:45–51.
109. Struthers AD, Reid JC, Whitesmith R, Roger JC. The effect of cardioselective and non-selective beta-blockers on the hypokalaemic and cardiovascular responses to adrenomedullary hormones in man. Clin Sci 1983;65:143–7.
110. Editorial. Adrenaline and potassium: everything in flux. Lancet 1983;2:1401–3.
111. Raeder EA, Verrier RL, Lown B. Intrinsic sympathomimetic activity and the effects of beta-blockers on vulnerability to ventricular fibrillation. J Am Coll Cardiol 1983;1:1442–6.
112. McKebbin JK, Pocock WA, Barlow JB, et al. Sotalol, hypokalaemia, syncope and torsades de pointes. Br Heart J 1984;51:157–62.
113. Di Bianco R, Parker JO, Chakko S, et al. Doxazosin for the treatment of chronic congestive heart failure. Am Heart J 1991;121:372–80.
114. Richer LP, Vinet A, Kus T, et al. Alpha adrenoceptors blockade modifies naturally induced atrial arrhythmias. Am J Physiol Regul Intrgr Comp Physiol 2008;295:R1175–80.
115. Amar DO, Xing D, Martins JB. Alpha-2 adrenergic antagonism enhances risk of VT during ischaemia. Scand Cardiovasc J 2007;41:378–85.
116. McMurray J, Kober L, Robertson M, et al. Antiarryththmic effects of carvedilol after acute myocardial infarction (CAPRICORN). J Am Coll Cardiol 2005;45:525–30.

β-Blockers and Heart Failure

CHAPTER 5

INTRODUCTION

In developed countries, about 2% of the adult population have heart failure (HF), though this frequency increases to 6%-10% over the age of 65 years.[1] Men are more vulnerable than women[2]—**Figure 5-1**. The lifetime risk of developing HF is about 20% for both men and women, increasing to 40% in the presence of hypertension.[3] Though the incidence of HF has declined somewhat in the last 50 years or so (particularly in women),[4] probably due to the increased prescribing of angiotensin-converting inhibitors (ACE) inhibitors and β-blockers, the burden (hospital admissions) is predicted to increase between the years 2010 and 2030, especially in the elderly.[5]

1. Two main types of HF pathophysiology

A) Systolic HF with reduced ejection fraction

Pathophysiological mechanisms underlying heart failure with reduced ejection fraction (HFREF) have changed over the years. In developed countries, coronary artery disease (CAD) is responsible for about 65% of HFREF.[6] However, in the elderly, 75% have a past history of hypertension.[7] Obesity is now a recognized risk factor, doubling the risk of developing HFREF.[8] The postmyocardial remodeling process that can lead to HFREF is shown in **Figure 5-2**.[7]

In idiopathic dilated cardiomyopathy (DCM) stimulating autoantibodies to the $β_1$-receptor are detected in about one third of cases and are associated with a threefold increase in mortality.[9]

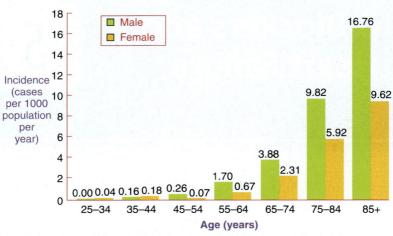

Fig. 5-1 Incidence of heart failure in the United Kingdom, by sex and age group. N = 220. (From Wood DA. Preventing clinical heart failure: the rationale and scientific evidence. Heart 2002;88:15–22.)

Such stimulating autoantibodies induce cardiomyocyte apoptosis[10] and can be antagonized by β_1-blockade (bisoprolol).[11]

The prognosis for HFREF patients newly admitted to the hospital is poor, with a 1-year survival of only 57%, falling to 27% after 5 years.[12] The worst prognosis occurs in patients who are old, with low systolic blood pressure, high respiratory rate, and poor renal function.[13] Southern Asians are more likely than whites to be admit-

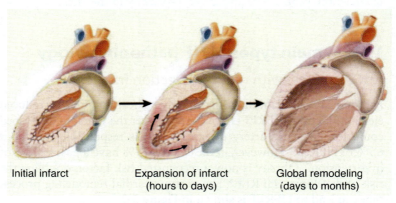

Fig. 5-2 Left ventricular remodeling following a myocardial infarction (sometimes leading on to systolic heart failure (heart failure with reduced ejection fraction [HFREF]). (From Jessup M, Brozena S. Heart failure. N Engl J Med 2003;348:2007–18.)

ted to the hospital with HFREF but have a similar prognosis.[14] Even asymptomatic patients with HFREF have a poor prognosis.[15]

B) Diastolic HF with normal ejection fraction

About 50% of HF cases have so-called diastolic HF.[10] Because diastolic HF is usually associated with some degree of regional systolic dysfunction, it is now termed "heart failure with normal ejection fraction (HFNEF)." Typical characteristics of patients with HFNEF and HFREF are shown in **Table 5-1**.[7]

It is thus apparent that HFNEF and HFREF are quite different medical conditions,[16] particularly in their response to β-blockers.[17] The morphological[7]—**Figure 5-2** and **5-3**—and microscopic changes

TABLE 5-1 Characteristics of patients with diastolic and systolic heart failure

Characteristic	Diastolic heart failure	Systolic heart failure
Age	Frequently elderly	All ages, typically 50-70 yr
Sex	Frequently female	More often male
Left ventricular ejection fraction	Preserved or normal, approximately ≥ 40%	Depressed, approximately ≤ 40%
Left ventricular cavity size	Usually normal, often with concentric left ventricular hypertrophy	Usually dilated
Left/ventricular hypertrophy on electrocardiography	Usually present	Sometimes present
Chest radiography	With or without cardiomegaly	Congestion and cardiomegaly
Gallop rhythm present	Fourth heart sound	Third heart sound
Coexisting conditions		
Hypertension	+++	++
Diabetes	+++	++
Previous myocardial infarction	+	+++
Obesity	+++	+
Chronic lung disease	++	0
Sleep apnea	++	++
Long-term dialysis	++	0
Atrial fibrillation	+ (usually paroxysmal)	+ (usually persistent)

From Jessup M, Brozena S. Heart failure. N Engl J Med 2003;348:2007–18.

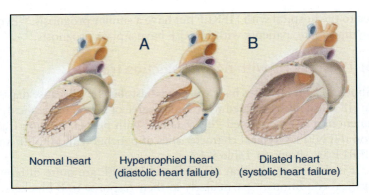

Fig. 5-3 Left ventricular remodeling. A, Typically elderly, isolated systolic hypertension (wide pulse pressure). B, Typically middle-aged, overweight/obese, diastolic ± systolic hypertension (normal pulse pressure) (From Jessup M, Brozena S. Heart failure. N Engl J Med 2003;348:2007–18.)

in the two conditions[17] are shown in **Table 5-2**. The prognosis of HFNEF is either similar to[18] or better than[19] HFREF.

Thus, a typical case of HFNEF would be an elderly female with a history of systolic hypertension, concentric left ventricular hypertrophy (LVH) (as opposed to eccentric LVH in HFREF), with a small left ventricular cavity.[20] Such patients have a stiff left ventricle with increased end-diastolic and pulmonary artery pressure during exercise,[21] resulting in effort intolerance, increase sympathetic nerve activity, and raised brain naturetic peptide.[22]

2. β-Blockers and mortality in HFREF (systolic HF)

A) History

It is counterintuitive that β-blockers should be beneficial to patients with HFREF. β-Blockers possess negative inotropic properties, and the acute effect in patients with HFREF is to apparently worsen the hemodynamic situation by causing a fall in left ventricular contractility and cardiac output.[23] Indeed, even very low doses of propranolol were known sometimes to precipitate severe low-output heart failure in frail, elderly patients with ischemia.[24]

However, chronic dosing of β-blockers to patients with HFREF results in beneficial hemodynamic changes producing increases in effort tolerance and ejection fraction and a small increase in blood pressure.[25] Thus, $β_1$-blockade (bisoprolol) results in a 45% increase

TABLE 5-2 Morphological, microscopic, resting and dynamic functional changes in heart failure with normal ejection fraction and heart failure with reduced ejection fraction

Parameters	HFNEF	HFREF
Microscopic and Neuroendocrine Features		
Cardiac cell hypertrophy	Increased	Minimal
Resting tension of cardiomyocytes	Increased	Decreased
Myofilament density	Preserved	Decreased
Titin N2B/N2BA ratio	Increased	Decreased
Interstitial collagen	Increased	Decreased
MMP-1/TIMP-1 ratio	Little changed	Decreased
Patterns of peptide growth factor induction	Different	Different
β-Receptor down-regulation and/or myocardial β-adrenergic receptor desensitization (postsynaptic)	Present	Present
Norepinephrine	Increased	Increased
B-type natriuretic peptide	Increased	More increased
Resting Echocardiographic Parameters		
LV cavity size	Normal or decreased	Increased
LV shape and geometry	Little changed	Spherical
LV mass index	Increased	Increased
LV mass to cavity ratio	Increased	Normal or decreased
Relative wall thickness	Increased	Normal
End-diastolic volume/wall stress	Normal or decreased	Increased
End-systolic volume/wall stress	Normal	Increased
LV ejection fraction	Normal	Decreased
Longitudinal velocity/strain	Decreased	More decreased
Radial strain	Decreased	More decreased
LV twist (torsion)	Normal or decreased	Decreased
LV twisting rate	Normal or decreased	Decreased
LV untwisting rate	Normal or decreased with/without delayed onset	Decreased

HFNEF, heart failure with normal ejection fraction; HF, heart failure with reduced ejection fraction; LV, left ventricular; MMP-1, matrix metalloproteinase-1; TIMP-1, tissue inhibitor of metalloproteinases-1.

From Yip GW-K, Frenneaux M, Sanderson JE. Heart failure with a normal ejection fraction: new developments. Heart 2009;95:1549–52.

TABLE 5-3 Bisoprolol improves effort tolerance over 1 year in moderate CCF

Parameter	BISOPROLOL		PLACEBO	
	Baseline (%)	1 Year	Baseline (%)	1 Year
EF (%)	25.0	36.2*	27.0	26.2
Exercise time (min)	9.1	11.4	9.2	9.9
Watts	117.9	146.1*	116.2	127.0

*$P < .05$.
CCF, congestive cardiac failure; EF, ejection fraction.
From Dubach P, Myers J, Bonetti P, et al. Effects of bisoprolol fumarate on left-ventricular size, function and exercise capacity in patients with heart failure. Am Heart J 2002;143:676–83.

in ejection fraction and 24% increase in effort tolerance (watts) vs. placebo, after 1 year's therapy[26]—**Table 5-3**.

The first indication that β-blockers might be beneficial in terms of morbidity/mortality, came from two postinfarction studies[27,28] showing that patients with a history of HF did better than those without HF on propranolol or timolol than on placebo in terms of fewer cardiovascular events—**Figure 5-4**. Exciting results were also forthcoming from a placebo-controlled study on nonischemic patients with idiopathic DCM[29] in which only 2 patients on metoprolol deteriorated to the extent of requiring a cardiac transplant compared with 19 receiving placebo.

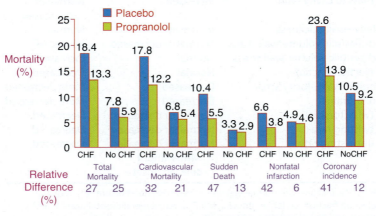

Fig. 5-4 β-blocker Heart Attack Trial (BHAT). Effect of propranolol in postinfarction cases upon morbidity and mortality in relation to the presence or absence of congestive heart failure (CHF). (From Chadda K, Goldstein S, Byington R, Curb JD. Effect of propranolol after acute myocardial infarction in patients with congestive heart failure. Circulation 1986;73:503–10.)

The scene was thus set for large, randomized, placebo-controlled studies to assess the usefulness of β-blockers in patients with HFREF.

B) Large randomized placebo-controlled studies involving β-blockers in systolic HF (HFREF), with a predefined end-point of all-cause death; all patients on background of ACE inhibitor therapy

Results are shown in **Table 5-4**[30] and **Figure 5-5**.[30] Positive results were observed only with β-blockers without intrinsic sympathomimetic activity (ISA)—that is, bisoprolol, carvedilol, and metoprolol,[31–33] in which the reduction in all-cause death was a significant 34%-35%. Particularly notable was a 42% reduction in sudden death with bisoprolol in the CIBIS (Cardiac Insufficiency

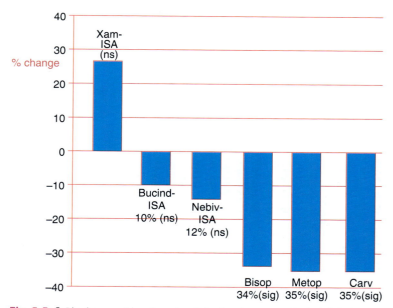

Fig. 5-5 β-Blockers and hard-end-point, placebo-controlled trials in heart failure. Intrinsic sympathomimetic activity (ISA) reduces efficacy (all-cause death). Bisop (bisoprolol), Metop (metoprolol), and Carv (carvedilol) reduced all-cause death by a significant 34%-35%. In contrast, β-blockers with ISA—i.e., Xam (xamoterol), Bucind (bucindolol), and Nebiv (nebivolol)—had insignificant effects on reducing all-cause death. ns, not significant; sig, significant. (From Cruickshank JM. Are we misunderstanding beta-blockers? Int J Cardiol 2007;120:10–27.)

TABLE 5-4 Placebo-controlled heart failure trials involving β-blockers—effects on all-cause death

	Study	BB	ISA	HF severity	Number of patients	All-cause mortality (%)	Statistical significance
Positive Trials	CIBIS II[31]	Bisoprolol (highly β_1-selective)	No	Moderate/severe	2649	↓34	Yes
	MERIT[32]	Metoprolol succinate (moderately β_1-selective)	No	Mild/moderate	3991	↓34	Yes
	COPERNICUS[33]	Carvedilol (non-selective + α-blocker)	No	Severe	2289	↓35	Yes
Negative Trials	Xamoterol[34]	Xamoterol (β_1-selective)	43% β_1 ISA	Moderate/severe	516	↑249	(Yes)
	BEST[35]	Bucindolol (weak α-blocker + nonselective)	25% ISA	Moderate/severe	2708	↓10	No
	SENIORS[36]	Nebivolol (β_1-selective)	Both β_2 and β_3 ISA	Moderate/severe	2128	↓12	No

BB, β-blocker; BEST, Beta-blocker Evaluation of Survival Trial; CIBIS II, Cardiac Insufficiency Bisoprolol Study; CAPERNICUS, Carvedilol Prospective Randomised Cumulative Survival Study; HF, heart failure; ISA, intrinsic sympathomimetic activity; MERIT, Metoprolol Rendomised Intervention Trial; SENIORS, Study of Effects of Nebivolol Intervention on Outcomes and Rehospitilisation in Seniors with Heart Failure.
From Cruickshank JM. Are we misunderstanding beta-blockers? Int J Cardiol 2007;120:10–27.

Bisoprolol Study) II.[31] The common property of the three effective β-blockers was $β_1$-blockade, indicating that $β_1$-blockade is the active ingredient responsible for reducing all-cause death.

In contrast, the negative, or nonsignificant, results in reducing all-cause death[34–36] were associated with β-blockers that contained ISA, involving the $β_1$- (xamoterol[34]), $β_1$- and $β_2$- (bucindolol[35]), and $β_2$- and $β_3$- (nebivolol[36]) receptors.

C) Do all patients with HFREF benefit from $β_1$-blockade?

In CIBIS II[31] with bisoprolol, patients whose HF was due to ischemia gained particular benefit. In MERIT–HF (Metroprolol Randomised Intervention Trial), involving metoprolol succinate, elderly (>65 yr) patients obtained at least the same benefit as younger patients in terms of lives saved and hospitalization avoided.[37] Indeed, for all three major positive studies involving carvedilol, metoprolol, and bisoprolol, there was no significant difference in the relative risk reduction in mortality between elderly and nonelderly HF patients.[38] In MERIT-HR, black patients benefited to the same extent as white patients.[39] Patients with atrial fibrillation benefit from β-blockade, with or without digoxin, to the tune of a 42% reduction in mortality.[40]

There has been a good deal of debate regarding women with HF and their response to therapy. A large overview regarding ACE inhibitors suggested that women with systolic HF gained little benefit.[41] It is different for β-blockers, in which a pooling of data from MERIT-HF (metoprolol), CIBIS II (bisoprolol), and CAPERNICUS (Carvedilol Prospective Randomised Cumulative Survival Study) (carvedilol) indicated comparable survival benefit for both sexes.[41] However, it should be borne in mind that the good results with β-blockers were with a selected group of women with systolic HF (HFREF). Older women, usually with hypertension, are prone to concentric LVH and diastolic HF (HFNEF), for which, at present, there is no known treatment (including β-blockers) (see later).

D) Why does ISA markedly diminish the efficacy of β-blockers in the treatment of systolic HF?

Importantly, the fall in heart rate is less with β-blockers with ISA (thus the work of the heart is reduced less). Xamoterol, which increased mortality vs. placebo by 249%, actually increases resting heart rate for about two thirds of the 24-hour period[42]—**Figure 5-6**. The fall in heart rate with bucindolol (nonsignificant 10% fall

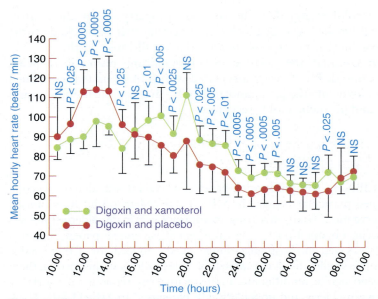

Fig. 5-6 Effect of chronic oral xamoterol (high ISA) upon 24-hour heart rate in patients with moderate heart failure plus atrial fibrillation. For much of the 24 hours, xamoterol increased heart rate. NS, not significant. (From Molajo AO, Coupe MO, Bennett DH. Effect of Corwin (ICI 118,587) on resting and exercise heart rate and exercise tolerance in digitalised patients with chronic atrial fibrillation. Br Med J 1984;52:392–5.)

in all-cause mortality) and nebivolol (nonsignificant 12% fall in all-cause mortality) was only 8-9 beats/min[35,36] compared with the 13-14 beats/min with the non-ISA β-blockers bisoprolol, metoprolol, and carvedilol.[31-33]

Bucindolol, which reduced all-cause death by a nonsignificant 10%, displays about 25% ISA,[43] acting mainly through the $β_1$-receptor.[44] But this β-blocker also appears to cause a marked sympatholytic action,[45] suggestive of $α_2$-stimulation of presynaptic receptors, which appears to be potentially harmful in severe systolic HF (HFREF). In the BEST (Beta-blocker Evaluation of Survival Trial),[35] high baseline noradrenaline levels in the placebo group were associated with increased mortality; by contrast, bucindolol-induced falls in noradrenaline levels were also associated with an increased mortality (probably by removing the sustaining noradrenaline support in severe HF, as occurs with the $α_1$-/$α_2$-agonist clonidine.[46]

Nebivolol, which reduced all-cause mortality by a nonsignificant 12%, possesses ISA, which acts via the $β_3$-receptors in the vascular

TABLE 5-5 Acute post-myocardial infarction patients, randomized to placebo vs. L-arginine; trial stopped due to excess deaths in L-arginine group

	Placebo (%)	L-Arginine (%)	P value
Mortality	0.0	8.6	.01

From Schulman SP, Becker LC, Kass DA. L-Arginine therapy in acute myocardial infarction. JAMA 2006;295:58–64.

endothelium[47] and the heart,[48] resulting in nitric oxide (NO) release. NO causes potentially advantageous vasodilatation and vascular protection, but its direct effects upon the heart are more problematical. In the normal heart, β_3-stimulation is potentially beneficial in contrast to the failing heart, in which it is possibly harmful.[49] In the severely failing heart, there is β_3-receptor up-regulation,[49] and β_3-stimulation has a negative inotropic effect leading to myocardial dysfunction.[49,50] Indeed, in the postinfarction period, L-arginine (substrate for NO synthase) significantly increased mortality vs. placebo[51]—Table 5-5.

E) Other placebo-controlled HF studies involving β-blockers

The U.S. Carvedilol Trial Program[52] involved 1094 HF cases, but mortality was not a prespecified primary end-point; there was a significant 65% reduction in mortality with carvedilol vs. placebo.

The CAPRICORN (Carvedilol Post-Infarction Survival Control in left ventricular dysfunction) study[53] involved postinfarct patients with impaired left ventricular function; there was a significant 23% reduction in all-cause death with carvedilol vs. placebo.

A study in children/adolescents with HF[54] showed that carvedilol did not differ from placebo, though all trends, including all-cause mortality, favored the β-blocker.

F) Comparative (nonplacebo) studies involving β-blocker

i) COMET study—carvedilol vs. metoprolol tartrate

COMET (Carvedilol Or Metoprolol European Trial),[55] a double-blind, randomized study comparing metoprolol tartrate and carvedilol in 3029 moderate/severe HF cases, showed that over a 6-year follow-up period, all-cause mortality was significantly lower (17%) on carvedilol.

This result stimulated severe criticism,[56,57] the nub of which related to dose and plasma half-lives. In the original MERIT-HF study,[32] metoprolol succinate was given as a controlled-release/extended-release formula (metoprolol CR/XL), which was dosed up to 200 mg daily, lowering heart rate by 14 beats/min and reducing all-cause mortality by 34% vs. placebo (the same as the 34%-35% reduction with bisoprolol[31] and carvedilol[33]). By contrast, in the COMET study,[55] short-acting metoprolol tartrate was used, dosed up to 100 mg daily and lowering heart rate by only 11 beats/min. Thus, the poor result for short-acting metoprolol tartrate in the COMET study could be readily explained by too-low a dose rendering inadequate β-blockade over 24 hours.

ii) CIBIS III study—first-line bisoprolol vs. first-line enalapril

The CIBIS III study[58] addressed the issue of whether a β-blocker given first-line would be "not inferior" to first-line ACE inhibition in patients with mild/moderate HF; the two drugs were combined after 6 months. First-line bisoprolol proved "not inferior" to first-line enalapril in reducing the primary end-point of all-cause mortality or hospitalization and was at least as well tolerated as enalapril. In a prespecified subgroup analysis, patients with a very low ejection fraction (<28%) fared significantly better on bisoprolol than on enalapril. Sudden death was a significant 46% less common after 1 year in the first-line β-blocker group[59]—**Figure 5-7**.

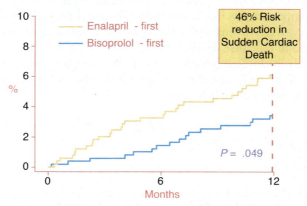

Fig. 5-7 Cardiac Insufficiency Bisoprolol Study (CIBIS) III. In heart failure patients, first-line bisoprolol therapy significantly reduced the frequency of sudden death by 46% vs. first-line enalapril therapy. (From Willenheimer R. The current role of beta-blockers in chronic heart failure: with special emphasis on the CIBIS III trial. Eur Heart J 2009;11(suppl A):A15–20.)

3. Mechanism of action of β-blockers in moderate/severe systolic HF (HFREF)

This topic has already been discussed,[30] and possible mechanisms involve

1. Slowing of heart rate leading to (a) reduction in cardiac work and oxygen requirement and (b) prolonged diastolic coronary filling time.
2. Antiventricular arrhythmic activity.
3. Up-regulation of cardiac $β_1$-receptors.
4. Inhibition of the renin-angiotensin system.
5. Increase in brain natriuretic factor (BNP).
6. Beneficial effects on left ventricular remodeling,[60] resulting in improved left ventricular volumes and ejection fraction.
7. Antagonism of stimulatory $β_1$-receptor autoantibodies.
8. Restoration of calcium release channel/cardiac ryanodin receptor (Ry R2) function,[61] probably linked to a reduction in the risk of sudden cardiac death.[62]
9. Inhibition of catecholamine-induced necrosis/apoptosis/inflammation.

The last two mechanisms (8 and 9), involving the ryanodine receptor and catecholamine-induced cardiac damage, are arguably the most important and involve both the β1- and the $β_2$-cardiac receptors. Chronic stimulation of the $β_1$-receptor induces myocardial myocyte apoptosis/necrosis via a cyclic adenosine monophosphate (c-AMP)-dependent process, whereas chronic stimulation of the $β_2$-receptor inhibits myocardial apoptosis/necrosis via a Gi-coupled pathway.[63] The implication is that $β_2$-blockade would be potentially harmful—**Figure 5-8**.

Certainly, $β_1$-blockade in humans has been shown to prevent cardiac necrosis (assessed postmortem) under randomized, placebo-controlled conditions.[64] In an acute head injury study, high plasma noradrenaline levels related to cardiac damage as assessed by CK-MB (MB isoenzyme of creatine kinase) enzymes blood levels and atenolol reduced CK-MB enzyme blood levels over 1 week by about 80%—**Figure 5-9**. In that study, postmortem hearts of $β_1$-blocked patients were free of cardiac necrotic lesions in contrast to non-β-blocked hearts, which displayed many necrotic lesions in the subendocardial region. Such $β_1$-stimulatory myotoxic effects can also be prevented by highly $β_1$-selective bisoprolol.[65] $β_1$-Blockade may be acting by stabilizing the ryanodine receptor on the cardiac sarcoplasmic reticulum, thus preventing excessive calcium release and

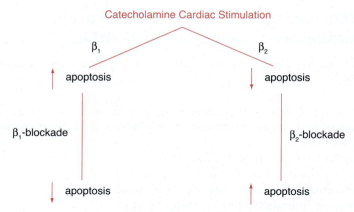

Fig. 5-8 Effect of chronic β_1- and β_2-stimulation upon cardiac muscle apoptosis/necrosis and the action of β_1- and β_2-blockade. (From Communal C, Singh K, Sawyer DB, Colucci WS. Opposing effects of beta-1 and beta-2 adrenergic receptors on cardiac myocyte apoptosis. Circulation 1999;100:2210–2.)

related poor myocardial function and increased risk of ventricular fibrillation.[66] Specific β_2-blockade (ICI 118, 551) has been shown to induce a marked negative inotropic effect upon isolated myocytes

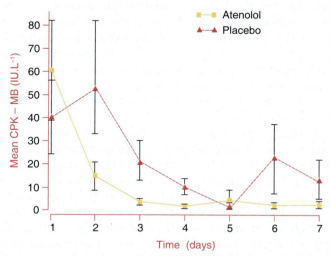

Fig. 5-9 In patients with acute head injury, intravenous followed by oral atenolol significantly reduced cardiac damage (plasma MB isoenzyme of creatinine phosphokinase [CPK-MB] levels) vs. placebo, over 1 week. (From Cruickshank JM, Degaute JP, Kuurne T, et al. Reduction in stress-/catecholamine-induced cardiac necrosis by beta-1 selective blockade. Lancet 1987;ii:585–9.)

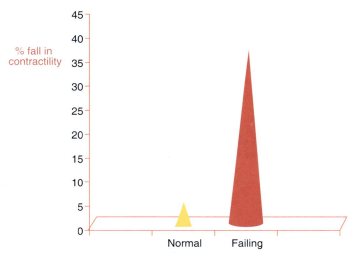

Fig. 5-10 Effect of pure β_2-blockade (ICI 118,551) on the contractility of isolated cardiac myocytes from normal and failing human hearts. (From Gong H, Hong S, Koch WJ, et al. Specific beta-2 blocker ICI 118,551 actively decreases contraction through a Gi-coupled form of the beta-2 AR in myocytes from failing human heart. Circulation 2002;105:2497–503.)

from failing human hearts[67]—**Figure 5-10**; this action is direct and quite independent of inhibiting external β_2-stimulation.

The clinical implications of the preceding are illustrated in the following section.

4. End-stage systolic HF and the salutary effect of specific β_2-stimulation plus specific β_1-blockade

End-stage HF, in spite of optimal medical therapy, requires urgent cardiac transplantation. However, transplantation has a 10%-20% 1-year mortality with only 15% survival after 20 years[68] In addition, the quality of survival is markedly impaired owing to the problems associated with immunosuppression.

There is now a potential alternative to cardiac transplantation.[69] Fifteen patients with end-stage HF (nonischemic cardiomyopathy), aged 15-56 years and a mean ejection fraction of only 12%, were surviving only with the aid of an implanted left ventricular assist device, inotropic drugs, ACE and angiotensin receptor blocker (ARB) inhibitors, spironolactone, and carvedilol. In order to test

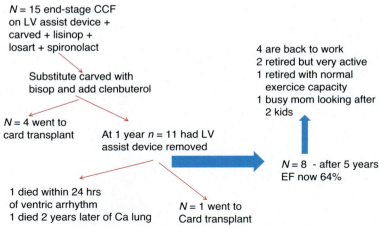

Fig. 5-11 End-stage heart failure in 15 congestive cardiac failure (CCF) patients (mean ejection fraction [EF] 12%) on left ventricular (LV) assist device. Dramatic benefit resulted from combination of β_1-blockade (bisoprolol [bisop]) and β_2-stimulation (clenbuterol). Ca, cancer; card, cardiac; carved, carvedilol; lisinop, linisopril; losart, losartan; spironolact, spironolactone; ventric arrhythm, ventricular arrhythmia. (From Birks EJ, Tansley PD, Hardy J, et al. Left ventricular assist device and drug therapy for the reversal of heart failure. N Engl J Med 2006;355:1873–84.)

the β_1-blockade plus β_2-stimulant idea for reducing cardiac apoptosis/necrosis,[63] carvedilol was exchanged for highly β_1-selective bisoprolol, followed by the addition of the β_2-stimulant clembuterol (nonselective carvedilol would have inhibited its action on the β_2-receptors). **Figure 5-11** illustrates subsequent events. Four of the 15 gained no benefit from the new therapy and underwent cardiac transplantation (1 died). After 1 year, the remaining 11 had the implanted left ventricular assist device removed; 1 died within 24 hours (arrhythmia), one died 2 years later of lung cancer, and 1 received a cardiac transplant 33 months later. The remaining 8 (53% of the original number) were followed-up for 4 years and all had a normal effort tolerance and were leading normal lives with an ejection fraction of 64%.

These remarkable results require confirmation in further studies.

5. Diastolic HF (HFNEF)

Such a heart is illustrated in (see **Figure 5-3**) and its characteristics, compared with systolic HF, are listed in (see **Tables 5-1 and 5-2**).

TABLE 5-6 Hazard ratios (95% confidence interval) for 1-year outcomes in elderly patients with heart failure, β-blocker vs. no β-blocker therapy, by left ventricular functional status

End-point	LV systolic dysfunction, $N = 3001$	Preserved LV systolic function, $N = 4153$
Mortality	0.77 (0.68-0.87)	0.94 (0.84-1.07)
Readmission	0.89 (0.80-0.99)	0.98 (0.90-1.06)
Mortality or readmission	0.87 (0.79-0.96)	0.98 (0.91-1.06)

*Adjusted for baseline age, sex race, HF etiology, LVEF, systolic blood pressure, smoking, signs of congestion, laboratory values, discharge medications, in-hospital invasive procedures, and history of diabetes and cardiovascular, neurological, pulmonary, and renal diseases.
LV, left ventricular; LVEF, left ventricular ejection fraction.
From Jondeau G, Neuder Y, Eicher J-C, et al. B-CONVINCED: Beta-blocker CONtinuation Vs Interruption in patients with Congestive heart failure hospitilisED for decompensation. Eur Heart J 2009;30:2186–92.

As already mentioned,[18] about 50% of all HF comprises diastolic failure (HFNEF), with a similar[18] or better[19] prognosis to that of systolic HF.

How best to treat HFNEF remains, at present, a mystery owing to an absence of randomized, controlled trials.[16]

However, a clue to the possible role (or nonrole) of β-blockers was given in a recent large prospective observational study.[70] Elderly patients with systolic HF discharged on β-blockers showed a significant 23% reduction in 1-year mortality compared with no benefit in diastolic HF patients on β-blockers—**Table 5-6**. Another observational study has indicated that β-blockers seem to increase the risk of hospitalization in women with HFNEF.[71]

The experience with ACE inhibitors is also not promising.[72] Certainly, ARB inhibitors appear not to be useful. In a study of 4128 HFNEF cases (CHARM [Candesartan in Heart Failure—Failure Assessment of Reduction in Mortality and Morbidity program] [73]), candasartan did not differ from placebo in reducing morbidity and mortality from cardiovascular disease.

6. Contraindications to β-blockers in congestive cardiac failure

There are absolute and relative contraindications.[74]

A) Absolute contraindications

1. Advanced heart block, unless a permanent pacemaker is present.
2. Sinus bradycardia of less than 50 beats/min, unless a pacemaker is present.
3. Systolic blood pressure of less than 85 mm Hg. However, it cannot be stated too forcibly that in patients with worsening HF, which could involve a systolic blood pressure less than 85 mm Hg, β-blockers should not be stopped, thus avoiding excess mortality at a later date.[75,76]
4. Asthma or labile reversible airways disease (though use of a highly $β_1$-selective agent, at low dose, like bisoprolol may be tried [in a hospital environment])—see section on Adverse Reactions.

B) Relative contraindications

1. Chronic obstructive pulmonary disease (COPD) is usually not a problem even for nonselective β-blockers.[77]
2. Peripheral vascular disease is usually quoted as a relative contraindication—almost certainly wrongly (see Chapter 2 on Ischemia).

7. HF—prevention

Because coronary heart disease/myocardial infarction (see Fig. 5-2) and hypertension are the two main contributors to the appearance of HF, is there any evidence to suggest that the administration of β-blockers in these two conditions results in a reduction in the frequency of HF?

A) Myocardial infarction

i) Early intervention (intravenous followed by oral)

In the large COMMIT (Clopidogrel and Metoprolol in Myocardiat Infarction Trial)[78] involving 45,852 cases of acute infarction, there was a 30% excess of cardiogenic shock, mainly on days 0-1, in those randomized to metoprolol vs. placebo. Thus, β-blockade should be administered only to those who are hemodynamically stable.

ii) Late intervention (oral β-blocker started a few days postevent and continued for several years)

A meta-analysis[79] showed a small, significant excess (5.9% vs. 5.4%) of HF in those randomized to the β-blocker. There is thus no evidence from randomized studies that β-blockers prevent HF

TABLE 5-7 Admission for heart failure in relation to β-blocker dose in 8232 elderly post-myocardial infarction patients with no history of heart failure

β-Blocker dose	Total (8232)	Heart failure (%)	Adjusted risk ratio	Statistical significance
No β-blocker	3551	9.2%	1.0	—
Low dose	1635	3.9%	0.48	Yes
Medium dose	2443	4.4%	0.58	Yes
High dose	603	6.0%	0.78	No

From Rochon PA, Tu JV, Anderson GM, et al. Rate of heart failure and 1-year survival for older people receiving low-dose beta-blocker therapy after myocardial infarction. Lancet 2000;356:639–44.

after late intervention postmyocardial infarction. However, a large, albeit observational, survey of older (men aged 75 yr) postinfarct cases discharged from the hospital showed that the dose of β-blocker is important in terms of readmission to the hospital for HF.[80] In 8232 postinfarct patients with no history of HF, dispensing of a β-blocker was associated with a significant 43% reduction in subsequent admission for HF. However, the β-blocker dose was important because admission rate was a significant 53% higher on the high-dose vs. low-dose group—**Table 5-7**. These data require confirmation under prospective, randomized conditions.

B) Hypertension

i) First-line β-blockade in younger/middle-aged diastolic hypertensive patients

HF was not usually a prespecified primary or secondary end-point, except in the UKPDS (U.K. Prospective Diabetes Study)[81,82] involving overweight/obese hypertensive patients with type 2 diabetes. In UKPDS 38,[81] tight control of blood pressure (first-line atenolol or captopril) was compared with less-tight control; the difference was 10.5 mm Hg. **Table 5-8** shows the effect of tight-control (overall), tight-control with atenolol and captopril individually vs. less-tight-control. It is apparent that the prime contribution to the 56% reduction in HF was the β-blocker.[82]

ii) Second-line β-blocker (first-line diuretic) in elderly systolic hypertensive patients

In the SHEP (Systolic Hypertension in the Elderly Program) placebo-controlled study[83] in 4736 elderly patients with isolated systolic

TABLE 5-8 Effect of tight control vs. less-tight control of blood pressure (difference 10/5 mm Hg) in young/middle-aged, obese hypertensive patients with type 2 diabetes, and the contribution of atenolol and captopril, in reducing the frequency of heart failure

Treatment (vs. less-tight control of BP)	% Reduction in heart failure (vs. less-tight control)	Statistical significance
Tight control (either atenolol or captoptil)	56	$P < .01$
Atenolol-based	60	—
Captopril-based	50	—

BP, blood pressure.
From U.K. Prospective Diabetes Study Group. Efficacy of atenolol and captopril in reducing risk of macrovascular and microvascular complications in type 2 diabetes: UKPDS 39. BMJ 1998;317:713–20.

hypertension, first-line diuretic/second-line atenolol was associated with a significant 49% reduction in the frequency of HF vs. placebo. In patients with a previous myocardial infarction, the reduction was 80%.

In the large ALLHAT (Antihypertensive and Lipid-Lowering Treatment to Prevent Heart Attack Trial) study involving 33,357 elderly hypertensive patients,[84] diuretic-based (β-blocker second-line) therapy was significantly superior to both calcium antagonist- (amlodipine) and ACE inhibitor- (lisinopril) based therapy in preventing HF. A follow-up analysis of that study[85] showed that the diuretic-/β-blocker-based therapy was significantly superior to ACE inhibitor-, calcium antagonist-, and alpha-blocker-based therapy in reducing the frequency of diastolic HF (HFNEF) and significantly superior to calcium antagonist- and α-blocker-based therapy in reducing the frequency of systolic HF (HFREF)—**Table 5-9** and **Figure 5-12.**

iii) LVH, the remodeling process and HF: implications for role of β-blockers

LVH is a powerful predictor of HF[86]—**Table 5-10**. However, not all forms of LVH are dangerous. Appropriate LVH, with normal wall stress, is typically associated with athletes and is compatible with a normal life span.[87] Inadequate LVH has a high wall stress that is linked to high blood pressure and has a poor prognosis in terms of cardiovascular events.[88] Inappropriate LVH has a low wall stress and is not associated with high blood pressure but is closely linked to neurohumoral activation[87] and has a poor prognosis, particularly regarding HF. Thus, inappropriate LVH is associated

TABLE 5-9 Diuretic/β-blocker combination best for heart failure prevention; hazard ratios (95% confidence interval) for new heart failure in elderly systolic hypertensive patients after initial therapy with chlorthalidone (second-line β-blocker), by type of heart failure and comparator drug—ALLHAT

Comparator drug	Heart failure with preserved ejection fraction (95% CI)	Systolic HF with low ejection fraction (95% CI)
Lisinopril	0.74 (0.56-97)	1.07 (0.82-1.40)
Amlodipine	0.69 (0.53-0.91)	0.74 (0.59-0.94)
Doxazosin	0.53 (0.38-0.73)	0.61 (0.47-0.79)

ALLHAT, Antihypertensive and Lipid-Lowering Treatment to Prevent Heart Attack Trial; CI, confidence interval; HF, heart failure.
From Davis BR, Kostis JM, Simpson LM, et al, ALLHAT Collaborative Research Group. Heart failure with preserved and reduced left-ventricular ejection fraction in the Antihypertensive and Lipid-Lowering Treatment to Prevent Heart Attack Trial. Circulation 2008;118:2259–67.

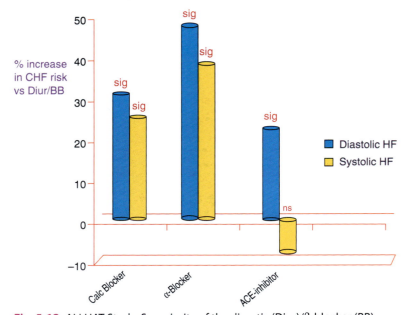

Fig. 5-12 ALLHAT Study. Superiority of the diuretic (Diur)/β-blocker (BB) combination (vs. calcium [Calc] blocker, angiotensin-converting enzyme [ACE] inhibitor and α-blocker-based therapy) in preventing heart failure (HF) in elderly hypertension. CHF, congestive heart failure; sig, significant. (From Davis BR, Kostis JM, Simpson LM, et al, ALLHAT Collaborative Research Group. Heart failure with preserved and reduced left-ventricular ejection fraction in the antihypertensive and lipid-lowering treatment to prevent heart attack trial. Circulation 2008;118:2259–67.)

TABLE 5-10 Framingham—hypertension and congestive cardiac failure

1	Lifetime risk of CCF	= 20%
2	Lifetime risk of CCF in hypertensive patients	40% men; 60% women
3	RR of CCF with LVH (ECG)	RR = 15.0 (~4 for CHD; ~6 for stroke)

CCF, congestive cardiac failure; ECG, electrocardiogram; LVH, left ventricular hypertrophy; RR, risk ratio.
From Anderson K, Wilson PW, Odell PM, Kannel WB. An updated coronary risk profile—a statement for health professions. Circulation 1991;83:356–62.

with very high levels of sympathetic nerve activity,[89] particularly in the heart.[90,91] The high sympathetic activity levels are particularly associated with increased left ventricular wall thickening[90]—**Figure 5-13**. Such hearts, under the influence of chronic β_1-stimulation, go on to develop apoptosis, necrosis, inflammation, fibrosis, and myofibrillar linkage breakdown, resulting in a remodeled left ventricle with dilated systolic HF.[92] This harmful process can be prevented by β_1-blockade.[93] Interestingly, angiotensin II-induced cardiac fibrosis acts via noradrenaline release and can be modified by β_1-blockade as well as ACE inhibition.[94]

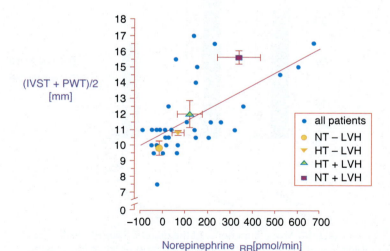

Fig. 5-13 Relationship between cardiac release of noradrenaline and left ventricular mass. HT, hypertensive; IVST, inter ventricular septal thickness; LVH, left ventricular hypertrophy; NT, normotensive; PWT, posterior wall thickness; RR, relative risk. (From Kelm M, Schafer S, Mingers S, et al. Left-ventricular mass is linked to cardiac noradrenaline in normotensive and hypertensive patients. J Hypertens 1996;14:1365–7.)

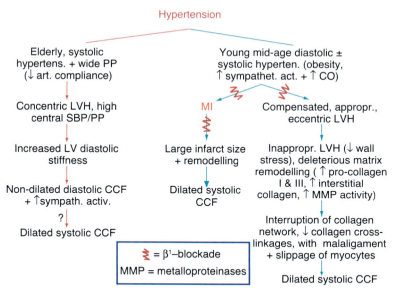

Fig. 5-14 Model for the development of heart failure (both systolic/HFREF [SBP] and diastolic/HFNEF [heart failure with normal ejection fraction; DBP]) in hypertensive patients. CCF, congestive cardiac failure; CO, cardiac output; LV, left ventricular; LVH, left ventricular hypertrophy; PP, pulse pressure. (From Cruickshank JM. Are we misunderstanding beta-blockers? Int J Cardiol 2007;120:10–27.)

LVH in elderly isolated systolic hypertension, resulting from poor vascular compliance,[95] is associated with a high central augmented systolic pressure.[96] Such LVH is usually concentric and leads on to a stiff, inelastic left ventricle, shortness of breath, and diastolic HF (HFNEF).

A model for the development of HF resulting from diastolic hypertension in young/middle-aged and systolic hypertension in the elderly is shown in **Figure 5-14**. Also shown are possible ways that β_1-blockade may intervene in the remodeling process and the prevention of HF.

β-Blockers have had a poor image as agents to reverse LVH. An overview has indicated that β-blockers reverse LVH only modestly compared with ACE inhibitors.[97] However, such analyses took no account of age. For example, atenolol has a total absence of efficacy in reversing LVH (probably concentric) in elderly patients with isolated systolic hypertension[98] (but does when given second-line to a diuretic as in the SHEP study[99]). In stark contrast, atenolol is highly effective in reversing LVH (probably eccentric) in younger/middle-aged hypertensive patients, whether assessed by electrocardiogram

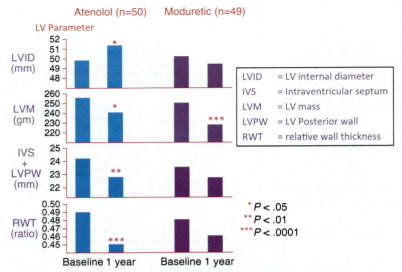

Fig. 5-15 Comparison of atenolol and diuretic in reversal of left ventricular hypertrophy (LVH) in younger diastolic hypertensive patients over 1 year. Atenolol is superior in regressing posterior wall and septal thickness. (From Otterstad JE, Froeland G, Soeyland AK, et al. Changes in left-ventricular dimensions and systolic function in 100 mildly hypertensive men during one year's treatment with atenolol vs hydrochlorthiazide and amiloride. J Intern Med 1992;231:493–501.)

(ECG)[100] or echocardiography,[101] as is metoprolol.[102] Compared with a diuretic, atenolol was particularly effective in reducing posterior wall and septal thickness[101]—**Figure 5-15**. Bisoprolol is also highly effective in reducing LVH in younger/middle-aged hypertensive patients,[103,104] with improvement of diastolic function and coronary flow reserve[105]—**Figure 5-16**. Importantly, bisoprolol is at least as effective as the ACE inhibitor enalapril in reversing echocardiographic LVH[106]—**Figure 5-17**.

8. Choice of β-blocker for the treatment of systolic HF (HFREF)

Clearly, β-blockers containing ISA (i.e., xamoterol, bucindolol, nebivolol) would be inappropriate because they have failed to significantly reduce all-cause mortality in HF patients—(see **Table 5-4**).

The three β-blockers without ISA that have achieved a significant 34%-35% decrease in all-cause mortality are bisoprolol,[31]

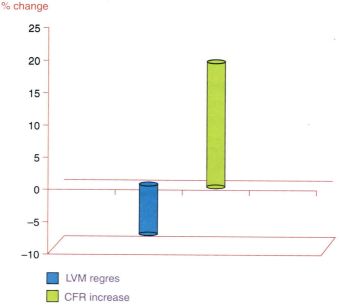

Fig. 5-16 Bisoprolol effective in regressing left ventricular mass (LVM) and increasing coronary flow reserve (CFR) in 10 hypertensive patients with coronary artery disease. (From Motz W, Vogt M, Scheler S, et al. Improvement in coronary reserve following regression of hypertrophy resulting from blood pressure lowering with a beta-blocker. Dtsch Med Wochenschr 1993;118:535–40.)

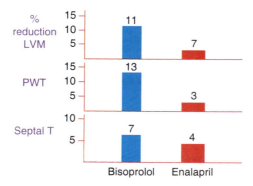

Fig. 5-17 Bisoprolol at least as effective as enalapril in reversing left ventricular hypertrophy (LVH) in 56 middle-aged hypertensive patients (mean age 50 yr), over 6 months. LVM, left ventricular mass; PWT, posterior wall thickness; Septal T, septal thickness. (Goss P, Routaut R, Herreo G, Dallochio M. Beta-blockers vs ACE-inhibition: effects on left-ventricular hypertrophy. J Cardiovasc Pharmacol 1990;16:S145–50.)

metoprolol,[32] and carvedilol[33]—(see **Table 5-4**). First-line bisoprolol has also proved to be at least as good as the first-line ACE inhibitor enalapril in reducing all-cause death and superior in reducing sudden death[59]—(see **Figure 5-7**.)

There is thus now a genuine choice of first-line agent, ACE inhibitor or β-blocker, for the treatment of systolic HF (HFREF). Clearly $β_1$-blockade, the common, shared property of bisoprolol, metoprolol, and carvedilol, is the active ingredient as regards β-blocker efficacy in HFREF.[107]

The additional property shared by metoprolol and carvedilol, $β_2$-blockade, has not been shown to be of benefit in the treatment of HF. Indeed, $β_2$-blockade can induce bronchospasm (see next chapter) and inhibits the cardiac apoptosis/necrosis benefit of $β_2$-stimulation in end-stage HF.[63]

α-Blockade (prazosin) has shown no survival benefit in patients with HF (HFREF).[108] Indeed, when given to HF patients with prostatic hypertrophy, $α_1$-blockers increased hospital admissions for worsening HF.[109] Of relevance may be the ability of $α_1$-blockade (doxazasin) to induce cardiac apoptotic changes.[110] Thus, the presence of $β_1$-blockade may be necessary to prevent this potential harmful effect of $α_1$-blockade.[109]

Certainly, the additional property of class III antiarrhythmic effect (i.e., sotalol) is not helpful. Indeed, the reverse is the case as shown in the SWORD Study (Survival With Oral D-Sotalol).[111] The SWORD study was a randomized, placebo-controlled study involving D-sotalol (unlike L-sotalol, it has no β-blocking activity, only class III antiarrhythmic action) in 3121 patients with ischemic heart failure; the study was stopped prematurely owing to a significant excess of deaths in the D-sotalol group.

As pointed out in a recent heart failure review,[112] the potential harmful effects of ISA, $β_2$-blockade, class III antiarrhythmic activity, and $α_1$-blockade (including postural hypotension—see next chapter) can be avoided by the choice of pure $β_1$-blockade (i.e., low-dose bisoprolol).

SUMMARY AND CONCLUSIONS

1. The lifetime risk of developing HF is about 20% (40% if hypertension is present). With increasing longevity in the developed world, the burden of HF (hospitalization) is set to increase from the years 2010 to 2030.
2. Coronary heart disease and hypertension are the two main causes of HF in the developed world: coronary heart disease

(and obesity) in the case of systolic HF (HFREF) and systolic hypertension in the case of diastolic HF (HFNEF), which occurs mainly in the elderly.
3. β-Blockers have become the cornerstone (alongside ACE inhibitors) in the treatment of systolic HF (HFREF). Bisoprolol, metoprolol, and carvedilol (all on an ACE inhibitor background) have reduced all-cause death by 34%-35%. The presence of ISA (xamoterol, bucindolol, and nebivolol) markedly diminishes efficacy (reduction in all-cause death) in the treatment of systolic HF.
4. First-line bisoprolol has proved "noninferior" to first-line enalapril in reducing all-cause death and superior in reducing the risk of sudden death.
5. The main mode of action of β-blockers in treating systolic HF is inhibition of chronic $β_1$-stimulation–induced myocardial apoptosis/necrosis/inflammation. The combination of pure $β_1$-blockade (low-dose bisoprolol) and pure $β_2$-stimulation (clenbuterol, which also suppresses apoptosis) may prove invaluable in the treatment of end-stage systolic HF, rendering cardiac transplantation unnecessary.
6. The appropriate treatment of diastolic HF (HFNEF) has yet to be determined.
7. β-Blockade is effective in the prevention of HF linked to previous hypertension. As first-line therapy in the treatment of diastolic hypertension in young/middle-aged subjects, the risk of HF is reduced by about 60% (UKPDS 39). When given as second-line therapy (to first-line diuretics) in the elderly systolic hypertensive patient, the risk of HF is reduced by about 50% (SHEP), being superior to α-blocker-, ACE inhibitor-, and calcium blocker-based therapies (ALLHAT).
8. β-Blockers are highly effective in reversing LVH—a precursor of HF—in young/middle-aged diastolic hypertensive patients, being superior to diuretics and at least as good as ACE inhibitors (bisoprolol). LVH in the elderly systolic hypertensive patient is not reversed by β-blockade, unless given as second-line to first-line diuretic therapy.
9. In the treatment of systolic HF (HFREF) choice of β-blocker is important. ISA markedly diminishes efficacy (xamoterol, bucindolol, nebivolol). β-Blockers without ISA—bisoprolol, metoprolol, and carvedilol—all reduce all-cause death by 34%-35%, the active ingredient being $β_1$-blockade ($β_2$-blockade, class III antiarrhythmic activity, and α-blockade do not contribute to activity).

REFERENCES

1. McMurray JJ, Pfeffer MA. Heart failure. Lancet 2005;365:1877–89.
2. Wood DA. Preventing clinical heart failure: the rationale and scientific evidence. Heart 2002;88:15–22.
3. Lloyd-Jones DM, Larson MG, Leep EP, et al. Lifetime risk of developing congestive heart failure. The Framingham Heart Study. Circulation 2002;106:3068–72.
4. Levy D, Kenchaiah S, Larson MG, et al. Long-term trends in the incidence of and survival with heart failure. N Engl J Med 2002;347:1397–402.
5. Stewart S, MacIntyre K, Capewell S, Mc Murray JJ. Heart failure and the aging population an increasing burden in the 21st century? Heart 2003;89:49–53.
6. Gheorghiade M, Sopko G, De Luca L, et al. Navigating the crossroads of coronary artery disease and heart failure. Circulation 2006;114:1202–13.
7. Jessup M, Brozena S. Heart failure. N Engl J Med 2003;348:2007–18.
8. Kenchaiah S, Evans JC, Levy D, et al. Obesity and the risk of heart failure. N Engl J Med 2002;347:305–13.
9. Stork S, Boivin V, Horf R, et al. Stimulating autoantibodies directed against the cardiac beta-1 adrenergic receptor predict increased mortality in idiopathic cardiomyopathy. Am Heart J 2006;152:697–704.
10. Jane-wit D, Altuntas CZ, Johson JM, et al. Beta-1 adrenergic receptor autoantibodies mediate dilated cardiomyopathy by agonistically inducing cardiomyocyte apoptosis. Circulation 2007;116:399–410.
11. Jahns R, Boivin V, Siegmund C, et al. Autoantibodies activating human beta-1 adrenergic receptors are associated with reduced cardial function in chronic heart failure. Circulation 1999;99:649–54.
12. Blackledge HM, Tomlinson J, Squire IB. Prognosis for patients newly admitted to hospital with heart failure: survival trends in 12,220 index admissions in Leicestershire 1993–2001. Heart 2003;89:615–20.
13. Lee DS, Austin PC, Rouleau JL, et al. Predicting mortality among patients hospitalized for heart failure. JAMA 2003;290:2581–7.
14. Blackledge HM, Newton J, Squire IB. Prognosis for South Asian and white patients newly admitted to hospital with heart failure in the United Kingdom historical cohort study. BMJ 2003;327:526–30.
15. Wong TJ, Evans JC, Benjamin EJ, et al. Natural history of asymptomatic left ventricular systolic dysfunction in the community. Circulation 2003;108:977–82.
16. Yip GW-K, Frenneaux M, Sanderson JE. Heart failure with a normal ejection fraction: new developments. Heart 2009;95:1549–52.
17. Hamdani N, Paulus WJ, van Heerebeek L, et al. Distinct myocardial effects of beta-blocker therapy in heart failure with normal and reduced ejection fraction. Eur Heart J 2009;30:1863–72.
18. Tribouilloy C, Rusinaru D, Mahjoub H, et al. Prognosis of heart failure with preserved ejection fraction: a 5 year prospective population-based study. Eur Heart J 2008;29:339–47.

19. Vasan RS. Diastolic heart failure. BMJ 2003;327:1181–2.
20. Aurigemma GP, Gaasch WH. Diastolic heart failure. N Engl J Med 2004;351:1097–105.
21. Westermann D, Kasner M, Steendijk P, et al. Role of left ventricular stiffness in heart failure with normal ejection fraction. Circulation 2008;117:2051–60.
22. Kitzman DW, Little WC, Brubaker PH. Pathophysiological characterization of isolated diastolic heart failure in comparison to systolic heart failure. JAMA 2002;288:2144–50.
23. Haber HL, Simek CL, Gimple LW. Why do patients with congestive heart failure tolerate the initiation of beta-blocker therapy? Circulation 1993;88:1610–9.
24. Greenblatt DJ, Koch-Weser J. Adverse reactions of propranolol in hospitalised medical patients: a report from the Boston Collaborative Drug Surveillance Program. Am Heart J 1973;86:478–84.
25. Ertl G, Neubauer S, Gaudron P, et al. Beta-blockers in cardiac failure. Eur Heart J 1994;15(suppl c):16–24.
26. Dubach P, Myers J, Bonetti P, et al. Effects of bisoprolol fumarate on left-ventricular size, function and exercise capacity in patients with heart failure. Am Heart J 2002;143:676–83.
27. Chadda K, Goldstein S, Byington R, Curb JD. Effect of propranolol after acute myocardial infarction in patients with congestive heart failure. Circulation 1986;73:503–10.
28. Norweigian Multicentre Study Group. Timolol-induced reduction in mortality and reinfarction in patients surviving acute myocardial infarction. N Engl J Med 1081;304:801–7.
29. Waagstein F, Bristow MR, Swedberg K, et al. Beneficial effects of metoprolol in idiopathic dilated cardiomyopathy. Metolpolol in Dilated Cardiomyopathy (MDC) Trial Study Group. Lancet 1993;342:1441–6.
30. Cruickshank JM. Are we misunderstanding beta-blockers? Int J Cardiol 2007;120:10–27.
31. CIBIS-II investigators and committee. The Cardiac Insufficiency Bisoprolol Study II (CIBIS-II): a randomised trial. Lancet 1999;353:9–13.
32. The MERIT-HR Investigators. Effect of metoprolol CR/XL in chronic heart failure. Metoprolol CR/XL Randomised Intervention Trial in Congestive Heart Failure (MERIT-HR). Lancet 1999;35:2001–7.
33. Packer M, Coats AJ, Fowler MB, et al. Effect of carvedilol on survival in severe chronic heart failure. N Engl J Med 2001;344:1651–8.
34. Xamoterol in Severe Heart Failure Study Group. Xamoterol in severe heart failure. Lancet 1990;336:1–6.
35. The Beta-blocker Evaluation of Survival Trial Investigators. A trial of the beta-blocker bucindolol in patients with advanced chronic heart failure. N Engl J Med 2001;344:1659–67.
36. Flather MD, Shibata MC, Coats AJ, et al. Randomised trial to determine the effect of nebivolol on mortality and cardiovascular hospital admissions in elderly patients with heart failure (SENIORS). Eur Heart J 2005;26:215–25.

37. Deedwania PC, Gottlieb S, Ghali JK, et al, for the MERIT-HF Study Group. Efficacy, safety and tolerability of beta-adrenergic blockade with metoptolol CR/XL in elderly patients with heart failure. Eur Heart J 2004;25:1300–9.
38. Dulin BR, Haas SJ, Abraham WT, Krum H. Do elderly systolic heart failure patients benefit from beta-blockers to the same extent as the non-elderly? Meta-analysis of > 12,000 patients in large-scale clinical trials. Am J Cardiol 2005;95:896–8.
39. Goldstien S, Dedwania P, Gottlieb S, Wikstrand J, for the MERIT-HF Study Group. Metoprolol CR/XL in black patients with heart failure (from the Metoprolol CR/XL Randomised Intervention Trial in Chronic Heart Failure). Am J Cardiol 2003;92:478–80.
40. Fauchier L, Grimard C, Pierre B, et al. Comparison of beta-blocker and digoxin alone and in combination for management of patients with atrial fibrillation and heart failure. Am J Cardiol 2009;103:248–54.
41. Wenger NK. Women, heart failure and heart failure therapies. Circulation 2002;105:1526–8.
42. Molajo AO, Coupe MO, Bennett DH. Effect of Corwin (ICI 118,587) on resting and exercise heart rate and exercise tolerance in digitalised patients with chronic atrial fibrillation. Br Med J 1984;52:392–5.
43. Andreka P, Aiyar N, Olson LC, et al. Bucindolol displays intrinsic sympathomimetic in congestive heart failure (MERIT-HF). Lancet 1999;353:2001–7.
44. Maack C, Bohm M, Vlaskin L, et al. Partial agonist activity of bucindolol is dependent on the activation state of the human beta-1 adrenergic receptor. Circulation 2003;108:348–53.
45. Brostow MR, Krause-Steinrauf H, Nuzzo R, et al. Effect of baseline or changes in adrenergic activity on clinical outcomes on the Beta-blocker Evaluation of Survival Trial. Circulation 2004;110:1437–42.
46. Floras JS. The "unsympathetic" nervous system of heart failure. Circulation 2002;105:1753–5.
47. Dessy C, Moniotte S, Ghisdal P, et al. Endothelial beta-3 adrenoceptors mediate vaso-relaxation of human coronary microarteries through nitric oxide and endothelium-dependent hyperpolarisation. Circulation 2004;110:948–54.
48. Maffei A, Di Pardo A, Carangi R, et al. Nebivolol induces nitric oxide release in the heart through inducible nitric oxide synthase activation. Hypertension 2007;50:652–6.
49. Moniotte S, Kobzik L, Feron O, et al. Upregulation of beta-3 adrenoceptors and altered contractile response to inotropic amines in human failing myocardium. Circulation 2001;103:1649–55.
50. Gauthier C, Leblais V, Kobzik L, et al. The negative inotropic effect of beta-3 adrenoceptor stimulation is mediated by activation of a nitric oxide synthase pathway in human ventricle. J Clin Invest 1998;102:1377–84.
51. Schulman SP, Becker LC, Kass DA. L-Arginine therapy in acute myocardial infarction. JAMA 2006;295:58–64.

52. Packer M, Bristow MR, Cohn JM, et al. The effect of carvedilol on morbidity and mortality in patients with chronic heart failure. N Engl J Med 1996;334:1349–55.
53. The CAPRICORN Investigators. Effect of carvedilol on outcome after myocardial infarction in patients with left-ventricular dysfunction: the CAPRICORN randomised trial. Lancet 2001;357:1385–90.
54. Shaddy RE, Boucek MM, Hsu DT, et al. Carvedilol for children and adolescents with heart failure. JAMA 2007;298:1171–9.
55. Poole-Wilson PA, Swedberg K, Cleland JG, et al. Comparison of carvedilol and metoprolol on clinical outcomes in patients with chronic heart failure in the Carvedilol Or Metoprolol European Trial (COMET): randomised controlled trial. Lancet 2003;362:7–13.
56. Dargie HJ. Beta-blockers in heart failure. Lancet 2003;362:2–3.
57. Correspondence. COMET: a proposed mechanism of action to explain the results and concerns about dose. Lancet 2003;362:1076–8.
58. Willenheimer R, van Velduisen JJ, Silke B, et al. Effect on survival and hospitalisation of initiating treatment of chronic heart failure with bisoprolol followed by enalapril, as compared with the opposite sequence. Results of the Randomised Cardiac Insufficiency Study (CIBIS III). Circulation 2005;112:2426–35.
59. Willenheimer R. The current role of beta-blockers in chronic heart failure: with special emphasis on the CIBIS III trial. Eur Heart J 2009;11(suppl A):A15–20.
60. Bellenger NG, Rajappan K, Rahman SL, et al. Effect of carvedilol on left-ventricular remodelling in chronic stable heart failure: a cardiovascular magnetic resonance study. Heart 2004;90:760–4.
61. Reicken S, Wehrens HT, Vest JA, et al. Beta-blockers restore calcium-release channel function and improve cardiac muscle performance in human heart-failure. Circulation 2003;107:2459–66.
62. Brown DA, Cascio WE. "Leaky" ryanodine receptors and sudden cardiac death. Cardiovasc Res 2009;84:343–4.
63. Communal C, Singh K, Sawyer DB, Colucci WS. Opposing effects of beta-1 and beta-2 adrenergic receptors on cardiac myocyte apoptosis. Circulation 1999;100:2210–2.
64. Cruickshank JM, Degaute JP, Kuurne T, et al. Reduction in stress-/catecholamine-induced cardiac necrosis by beta-1 selective blockade. Lancet 1987;ii:585–9.
65. Tan LB, Burniston, Clark WA, et al. Characterisation of adrenoceptor involvement in skeletal and cardiac myotoxicity induced by sympathomimetic agents. J Cardiovasc Pharmacol 2003;41:518–25.
66. Reiken S, Gabujakova M, Gaburjakova J, et al. Beta-adrenergic receptor blockers restore cardiac calcium release channel (ryanodine receptor) structure and function in heart failure. Circulation 2001;104:2843–8.
67. Gong H, Hong S, Koch WJ, et al. Specific beta-2 blocker ICI 118,551 actively decreases contraction through a Gi-coupled form of the beta-2 AR in myocytes from failing human heart. Circulation 2002;105:2497–503.

68. Anyanwu A, Treasure T. Prognosis after heart transplantation. Transplants alone cannot be the solution for end stage heart failure. BMJ 2003;326:509–10.
69. Birks EJ, Tansley PD, Hardy J, et al. Left ventricular assist device and drug therapy for the reversal of heart failure. N Engl J Med 2006;355: 1873–84.
70. Henandez AF, Hammill BG, O'Connor CM, et al. Clinical effectiveness of beta-blockers in heart failure: findings from the OPTIMIZE-HF Registry. J Am Coll Cardiol 2009;53:184–92.
71. Farasat SM, Bolger DT, Shetty V, et al. Effect of beta-blocker therapy on rehospitalization-rates in women versus men with heart failure and preserved ejection fraction. Am J Cardiol 2010;105:229–34.
72. Voors AA, de Jong M. Treating diastolic heart failure. Heart 2008;94: 971–2.
73. Yusuf S, Pfeffer MA, Swedberg K, et al. Effect of candesartan in patients with chronic heart failure and preserved left-ventricular ejection fraction: the CHARM-Preserved Trial. Lancet 2003;363:777–81.
74. Gheorghiade M, Colucci WS, Swedberg K. Beta-blockers in chronic heart failure. Circulation 2003;107:1570–5.
75. Jondeau G, Neuder Y, Eicher J-C, et al. B-CONVINCED: Beta-blocker CONtinuation Vs Interruption in patients with Congestive heart failure hospitilisED for decompensation. Eur Heart J 2009;30:2186–92.
76. Swedberg K. Beta-blockers in worsening heart failure: good or bad? Eur Heart J 2009;30:77–9.
77. Shelton RJ, Rigby AS, Cleland JG, Clark AL. Effect of a community heart failure clinic on uptake of beta-blockers by patients with obstructive airways disease and heart failure. Heart 2006;92:331–6.
78. COMMIT (Clopidogrel and Metoprolol in Myocardial Infarction Trial). Early intravenous and oral metoprolol in 45,852 patients with acute myocardial infarction; randomised placebo-controlled trial. Lancet 2005;366:1622–32.
79. Yusuf S, Peto R, Lewis J, et al. Beta-blockade during and after myocardial infarction: an overview of the randomised trials. Progr Cardiovasc Dis 1985;27:335–71.
80. Rochon PA, Tu JV, Anderson GM, et al. Rate of heart failure and 1-year survival for older people receiving low-dose beta-blocker therapy after myocardial infarction. Lancet 2000;356:639–44.
81. U.K. Prospective Diabet4s Study Group. Tight blood pressure control and risk of macrovascular and microvascular complications in type 2 diabetes: UKPDS 38. BMJ 1998;317:703–13.
82. U.K. Prospective Diabetes Study Group. Efficacy of atenolol and captopril in reducing risk of macrovascular and microvascular complications in type 2 diabetes: UKPDS 39. BMJ 1998;317:713–20.
83. Kostis JB, Davis BR, Cutler J, et al. Prevention of heart failure by antihypertensive drug treatment in older persons with isolated systolic hypertension. SHEP Cooperative Research Group. JAMA 1997;278: 212–6.

84. The ALLHAT Officers and coordinators for the ALLHAT Collaborative Research Group. Major outcomes in high-risk hypertensive patients randomised to angiotensin–converting enzyme inhibitor or calcium channel blocker vs diuretic. JAMA 2002;288:2981–97.
85. Davis BR, Kostis JM, Simpson LM, et al, ALLHAT Collaborative Research Group. Heart failure with preserved and reduced left-ventricular ejection fraction in the antihypertensive and lipid-lowering treatment to prevent heart attack trial. Circulation 2008;118:2259–67.
86. Anderson K, Wilson PW, Odell PM, Kannel WB. An updated coronary risk profile—a statement for health professions. Circulation 1991;83:356–62.
87. Muiesan MI, Salvetti M, Paini A, et al. Inappropriate left-ventricular mass changes during treatment adversely affects cardiovascular prognosis in hypertensive patients. Hypertension 2007;49:1077–83.
88. Sugishita Y, Iida K, Ohtsuka S, Yamaguchi I. Ventricular wall stress revisited. A keystone of cardiology. Jpn Heart J 1994;35:577–87.
89. Burns J, Sivananthan MV, Ball SG, et al. Relationship between central sympathetic drive and MRI imaging-determined left-ventricular mass in essential hypertension. Circulation 2007;115:1999–2005.
90. Kelm M, Schafer S, Mingers S, et al. Left-ventricular mass is linked to cardiac noradrenaline in normotensive and hypertensive patients. J Hypertens 1996;14:1365–7.
91. Schlaich MP, Kaye DM, Lambert E, et al. Relation between cardiac sympathetic activity and hypertensive left-ventricular hypertrophy. Circulation 2003;108:560–5.
92. Seeland V, Selejan S, Engelhardt S, et al. Interstitial remodelling in beta-1 adrenergic receptor transgenic mice. Basic Res Cardiol 2007; 102:183–93.
93. Asai K, Yang EP, Geng YJ, et al. Beta adrenergic blockade arrests myocyte damage and preserves cardiac function in the transgenic G(salpha) mouse. J Clin Invest 1999;104:551–8.
94. Tallaj J, Wei C-C, Hankes GH, et al. Beta-1 adrenergic receptor blockade attenuates angiotensin II-mediated catecholamine release into the cardiac interstitium in mitral regurgitation. Circulation 2003;1089:225–30.
95. Franklin SS, Pio JR, Wong ND, et al. Predictors of new-onset diastolic and systolic hypertension. The Framingham Heart Study. Circulation 2005;111:1121–7.
96. Agabiti-Rosei E, Marcia G, O'Rourke MF, et al. Central blood pressure measurements and antihypertensive therapy. A consensus document. Hypertension 2007;50:154–60.
97. Cruickshank JM, Lewis J, Moore V, Dodd C. Reversibility of left-ventricular hypertrophy by differing types of antihypertensive therapy. J Hum Hypertens 1992;6:85–90.
98. Schulman SP, Weiss JL, Becker LC, et al. Effect of antihypertensive therapy on left-ventricular mass in elderly patients. N Engl J Med 1990;322:1350–6.

99. Offili EO, Cohen JP, Vrain JA, et al. Effect of treatment of isolated systolic hypertension on left-ventricular mass. JAMA 1998;279:778–80.
100. Cruickshank JM, Higgins TJ, Pennart K, et al. The efficacy and tolerability of antihypertensive treatment based on atenolol in the prevention of stroke and the regression of left-ventricular hypertrophy. J Hum Hypertens 1987;1:87–93.
101. Otterstad JE, Froeland G, Soeyland AK, et al. Changes in left-ventricular dimensions and systolic function in 100 mildly hypertensive men during one year's treatment with atenolol vs hydrochlorthiazide and amiloride. J Intern Med 1992;231:493–501.
102. Franz IW, Behr V, Ketelhut R, Tonnesmann V. Decreasing the antihypertensive dosage during long-term treatment and complete regression of left-ventricular hypertrophy. Dtsch Med Wochenschr 1996;121:472–7.
103. de Teresa E, Gonzalez M, Camacho-Vasquez C, Tabuenca MJ. Effects of bisoprolol on left-ventricular hypertrophy in essential hypertension. Cardivasc Drugs Ther 1994;8:837–43.
104. Matuszewska G, Marek B, Kajdanink D, et al. The importance of bisoprolol in prevention of left-ventricular hypertrophy in patients with long-term L-thyroxin suppressive therapy. Endokrynol Pol 2007;58:384–96.
105. Motz W, Vogt M, Scheler S, et al. Improvement in coronary reserve following regression of hypertrophy resulting from blood pressure lowering with a beta-blocker. Dtsch Med Wochenschr 1993;118:535–40.
106. Goss P, Routaut R, Herreo G, Dallochio M. Beta-blockers vs ACE-inhibition: effects on left-ventricular hypertrophy. J Cardiovasc Pharmacol 1990;16:S145–50.
107. Adams KF. Which beta-blocker for heart failure? Am Heart J 2001;141:884–8.
108. Cintron G, Johnson G, Francis G, et al. Prognostic significance of serial changes in left-ventricular ejection fraction in patients with congestive heart failure. The V-HeFT VA Cooperative Studies Group. Circulation 1993;87(suppl 6):V117–23.
109. Dhaliwal AS, Habib G, Deswal A, et al. Impact of alpha-1 blockade use for benign prostatic hypertrophy on outcomes in patients with heart failure. Am J Cardiol 2009;104:270–5.
110. Thomas D, Bloehs R, Koschny R, et al. Doxazosin induces apoptosis of cells expressing hERG K+ channels. Eur J Pharmacol 2008;579:98–103.
111. Waldo AL, Camm AJ, deRuyter H, et al. Effect of D-sotalol on mortality in patients with left ventricular dysfunction after recent and remote myocardial infarction. The SWORD Investigators. Survival With Oral D-Sotalol. Lancet 1996;348:7-12.
112. Cruickshank JM. Beta-blockers and heart failure. Indian Heart J 2010;62:101-10.

CHAPTER 6

Adverse Reactions

INTRODUCTION

This topic has been well reviewed.[1] β-blockers have a high benefit/risk ratio, though inevitably some patients will experience adverse reactions. Because β-blockers are not a homogeneous class of drugs, efficacy and adverse reactions will vary greatly depending on (a) the degree of $β_1$-selectivity, (b) the presence of intrinsic sympathomimetic activity (ISA), (c) the presence of additional properties such as α-blocking activity (labetalol and carvedilol) or class III antiarrhythmic activity (sotalol), (d) the degree of lipophilicity (lipid solubility), and (e) unpredictable metabolism due to polymorphic variation (e.g., metoprolol).

As a general rule, side effects diminish with time, are more common at higher doses, and tend to be more frequent in the elderly.[2] All β-blockers share the core property of $β_1$-blockade; thus, all β-blockers will share (to a greater or lesser extent) the adverse reactions linked to $β_1$-blockade that may occur in some patients, that is

1. Bradycardia, which is seldom symptomatic.
2. Fatigue in some patients, which tends to diminish with time ($β_2$-blockade, via direct action on muscle, may exacerbate the situation).
3. Cold peripheries, probably a reflection of diminished cardiac output (though $β_2$-blockade, via vasoconstriction, may worsen the situation).
4. In rare cases, in which cardiac function is critically dependent on high sympathetic nerve activity, heart failure.

5. In rare cases, symptomatic hypotension (more likely in the frail elderly or in those with severe myocardial infarction).

1. Quality of life

The term "quality of life" used to be synonymous with angiotensin-converting enzyme (ACE) inhibition, since the study of Croog and coworkers[3] in which propranolol and methyldopa compared poorly with captopril. These findings were confirmed[4] when propranolol again performed poorly compared with the ACE inhibitor enalapril but moderately β_1-selective atenolol was as good as enalapril, and superior to captopril, in improving quality of life—**Figure 6-1**. Similar results were observed with highly β_1-selective bisoprolol vs. ACE inhibitors.[5-7]

These findings are important in the sense that most patients with essential hypertension are asymptomatic and agents that impair quality of life would be unwelcome. The implication is that in the case of propranolol, either β_2-blockade or high lipophilicity, or both, impart worrisome symptoms to an otherwise fit and well patient. Thus, problems with one β-blocker should not be extrapolated to the whole class.[2]

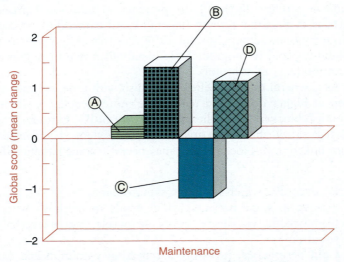

Fig. 6-1 Changes in global scores of the Life Satisfaction Questionnaire at maintenance relative to baseline. A, captopril; B, enalapril; C, propranolol; D, atenolol. (From Steiner SS, Friedhoff AJ, Wilson BL, et al. Antihypertensive therapy and quality of life: a comparison of atenolol, captopril, enalapril and propranolol. J Hum Hypertens 1990;4:217–25.)

2. Adverse reactions relating to the cardiovascular system

A) Bradycardia

Slow heart rates are not uncommon in the normal population. In normal middle-aged men, asymptomatic resting heart rates between 40 and 50 beats/min are not uncommon[8]—**Table 6-1**.

i) Hypertensive patients

In this mainly asymptomatic group, only rarely is it necessary to withdraw the β-blocker due to symptomatic bradycardia; only 1 out of 610 patients on propranolol needed to be withdrawn.[9]

In a review of patients on atenolol in general practice and hospital care,[10] various symptoms (fatigue, cold extremities, and dizziness) were assessed in relation to resting heart rate—**Table 6-2**. It is apparent that hypertensive patients in both general practice and hospital care, and in post-myocardial infarction patients, do not experience a higher frequency of symptoms at very low heart rates (<40 beats/min) with the possible exception of dizziness. The elderly (≥70 yr) tolerated bradycardia as well as the younger patients.

ii) Patients with coronary artery disease

As noted in **Table 6-2**, post-infarct patients tolerated lower heart rates as well as higher heart rates.[8] However, there are reports of angina pectoris worsening at very low heart rates,[11] particularly in patients with severely impaired myocardial function.[12] By contrast, in a post-infarction study involving propranolol and atenolol,[13] episodes of angina were assessed in relation to heart rate—**Table 6-3**; slower heart rates were beneficial to the patients (Wilcox, personal communication).

TABLE 6-1 Frequency of slow heart rates in 2000 normal middle-aged men

HR (beats/min)	% Population
40-49	9
50-59	36
60+	55

HR, heart rate.
From Erikssen J, Rodhal K. Resting heart rate in apparently healthy middle-aged men. Eur J Appl Physiol 1979;42:61–4.

TABLE 6-2 Heart rates and adverse effects in hypertensive patients and post-myocardial infarction patients on β-blockers from general practice and consultant clinics

		HYPERTENSIVE PATIENTS (N = 6818)				Post-myocardial infarction patients (N = 165)	
		General practice (N = 6006)		Consultant (N = 812)			
Adverse effects	Heart rate (beats/min)	N	%	N	%	N	%
All adverse effects	<40	63/141	45	5/6	83	—	—
	41-50	36/91	40	24/73	33	10/16	63
	51-60	286/923	31	100/328	30	42/73	57
	>60	1092/4851	23	119/405	29	53/86	62
Fatigue	<40	14/141	10	2/6	33	—	—
	41-50	16/91	18	12/73	13	7/16	44
	51-60	122/923	13	25/328	8	13/73	18
	>60	332/4851	7	41/405	10	17/86	20
Cold extremities	<40	1/141	1	0/6	0	—	—
	41-50	5/91	6	7/73	10	4/16	25
	51-60	43/923	5	36/328	11	20/73	27
	>60	134/4851	3	32/405	8	27/86	31
Dizziness	<40	23/141	16	0/6	0	—	—
	41-50	4/91	4	1/73	0	0/16	0
	51-60	85/923	9	12/328	4	6/73	8
	>60	277/4851	6	21/405	5	5/86	6

From Cruickshank JM. Beta-blockers, bradycardia and adverse effects. Acta Ther 1981;7:309–21.

TABLE 6-3 Relation of heart rate to anginal episodes in post-infarction patients on atenolol or propranolol

HR (beats/min)	% Patients—anginal episodes
41-50	6.3
51-60	9.5
60+	14.1

HR, heart rate.
From Wilcox RG, Roland JM, Banks DC, et al. Randomised trial comparing propranolol and atenolol in immediate treatment of suspected myocardial infarction. Br Med J 1980;280:885–8.

iii) Others

Patients with sinus node dysfunction (sick sinus syndrome) can experience troublesome bradycardia and should not be given β-blockers.[14] Likewise, elderly patients with the hyperactive carotid sinus reflex syndrome can also experience profound bradycardia if given a β-blocker.[15]

Heart block (second- and third-degree) can rarely be precipitated by intravenous propranolol given for arrhythmias.[11] In post-myocardial infarction patients, acute intravenous β-blockade was not associated with the appearance of heart block.[16] However, in the large ISIS-1 (First International Study of Infarct Survival) study,[17] patients with a pretreatment long PR interval (first-degree heart block) were more likely to develop complete heart block after intravenous atenolol. Patients with uncomplicated bundle-based block are not at risk.[18]

In the large hypertension trials involving β-blockers, there were no problems concerning heart block.[1]

B) Heart failure

Heart failure is extremely rare with β-blockers.[1] However, frail patients, usually elderly, with poor left ventricular function—ischemia—have experienced heart failure with low-dose oral propranolol.[19,20] Such elderly, frail patients receiving timolol eyedrops for glaucoma can also experience heart failure requiring drug withdrawal.[21]

The post-infarction period can occasionally be problematic. In the classic late intervention timolol post-infarct study, there was an excess of pulmonary edema in the β-blocker group vs. placebo.[22] More dramatic were the results of the large, early-intervention post-infarction study, COMMIT (Clopidogrel and Metoprolol in

Myocardial Infarction Trial), with intravenous followed by oral metoprolol,[23] in which there was a 30% excess of cardiogenic shock vs. placebo. Thus β-blockade post-infarction should be given only when the hemodynamic situation is stable.

In patients receiving β-blockers for treatment of heart failure, if the heart failure worsens at some later time point, it is important not to stop the β-blocker because such an action is linked to a worse prognosis for the patient.[24]

C) Hypotension

Symptomatic hypotension associated with β-blockade (provided α-blockade is not present) is very rare.[1] In hypertensive patients, marked hypotension with β-blockade can occur in the presence of renal artery stenosis or very high renin levels,[25] and in a case of malignant hypertension blindness was induced.[26]

Elderly, normotensive patients with glaucoma who are taking timolol eyedrops can occasionally experience marked hypotension causing dizziness and syncope, which resolves on stopping the eyedrops.[27]

Postural hypotension is not uncommon with agents containing both β-blocking and α-blocking properties (i.e., labetalol and carvedilol).[1] Though carvedilol is less likely than guanethidine, prazosin, and labetalol to induce postural hypotension,[28] dizziness and occasional syncope remain one of the most common side effects with carvedilol.[29] In a study involving elderly hypertensive patients, 25% were unable to stand after the first dose of carvedilol.[30]

β-Blocker-induced hypotension in the post-infarction period is more common, though usually asymptomatic;[1] however, withdrawal of the β-blocker is sometimes necessary.[1]

D) Fatigue

i) Symptom of fatigue/tiredness/lethargy

In the Medical Research Council (MRC) mild hypertension study, propranolol (vs. placebo) was responsible for significant increases in slowed walking and effort dyspnea[31]—**Table 6-4**—and lethargy was the main reason for withdrawal from the study in both men and women—**Table 6-5**. Fatigue is also the most common adverse reaction for moderately $β_1$-selective atenolol[10]—**Table 6-6**. Though such symptoms diminish with time, they are more common at higher doses and in the elderly.[2] Particularly vulnerable to fatigue are slow metabolizers of metoprolol, who experience up to three

TABLE 6-4 Prevalence of symptoms at 12 weeks and at 2 years after entry

Complaint	MEN: PERCENTAGE OF AFFIRMATIVE ANSWERS ($N = 1130$)						WOMEN: PERCENTAGE OF AFFIRMATIVE ANSWERS ($N = 958$)					
	Bendrofluazide		Propranolol		Placebos		Bendrofluazide		Propranolol		Placebos	
	12 wk	2 yr	12 wk	2 yr	12 wk	2 yr	12 wk	2 yr	12 wk	2 yr	12 wk	2 yr
Dizziness	13.7*	9.3	6.9	9.0	5.9	8.4	25.3‡	19.4	18.1	17.8	16.8	16.1
Muscle pain	13.5	22.2	15.7	14.1	14.6	16.8	25.2	14.6‡	21.6	17.2	22.5	26.8
Slowed walking	2.6	9.9	7.9	11.0	6.6	7.6	10.0	7.1	12.6‡	10.6	6.2	6.9
Exertional dyspnea	16.1	23.8	19.4	27.9‡	14.0	16.4	20.9	25.8	18.4	26.1	21.0	21.1
Headaches	19.6	16.5	21.9	19.7	27.1	26.2	31.9‡	36.0	33.1	29.8	42.4	37.8
Cold/numb digits	8.4	15.8	14.2	12.6	11.5	10.7	18.8	16.1	18.3	29.3‡‡	16.3	15.6
Paresthesia	11.6	14.9	14.7	14.3	14.7	11.2	28.9‡	28.9	19.7	25.0	18.4	17.5
Dry mouth	13.7	12.4	11.2	7.5	7.7	7.7	26.6	28.1‡	18.8	18.2	21.3	13.6
Blocked or runny nose	13.7	14.7	23.2†	26.8	12.5	18.2	11.5	18.3	20.1	22.6	19.2	12.9
Vomiting/nausea	3.9	5.0	7.9‡	3.7	3.2	4.5	13.4	5.1	6.3	4.3	8.2	10.3
Impotence	16.2‡	22.6‡	13.8	13.2	8.9	10.1	—	—	—	—	—	—

Reported in questionnaire. *$P < .001$; †$P < .01$; ‡$P < .05$. Significance levels refer to prevalence rates for each active drug separately compared with those for all control patients. The figures do not indicate comparisons between the two active drugs.
From Medical Research Council Working Party. Adverse reactions to bendrofluazide and propranolol for the treatment of mild hypertension. Lancet 1981;2:539–43.

TABLE 6-5 Principal reasons for withdrawal of randomized treatment rates per 1000 patient-years (number of reports)

	MEN				WOMEN		
Reasons for withdrawal	Bendrofluazide (2452 patient-years)	Propranolol (2738 patient-years)	Placebo (6776 patient-years)		Bendrofluazide (2827 patient-years)	Propranolol (2667 patient-years)	Placebo (6122 patient-years)
Impaired glucose tolerance	9.38* (23)	3.65 (10)	2.51 (17)		6.01* (17)	1.12 (3)	0.82 (5)
Gout (symptoms and serum uric acid ≥ 501 umol/L	12.23* (30)	2.56 (7)	1.03 (7)		1.06 (3)	0	0
Impotence	19.58* (48)	5.48 (15)	0.89 (6)		—	—	—
Raynaud's phenomenon	0	5.48* (15)	0.15 (1)		0.35 (1)	5.62 (15)	0
Skin disorder	0.41 (1)	2.19† (6)	0.15 (1)		0.35 (1)	1.87‡ (5)	0
Dyspnea	0	8.04* (22)	0.15 (1)		0	6.37* (17)	0.33 (2)
Constipation	1.63† (4)	0.37 (1)	0		2.12† (6)	0	0
Lethargy	6.93† (17)	10.23** (28)	0.30 (2)		2.12‡ (6)	15.00 (40)	0.33 (2)
Nausea, dizziness, or headache	8.56* (21)	6.57* (18)	1.18 (8)		16.27* (46)	13.87 (37)	2.12 (13)

*$P < .001$; †$P < .01$; ‡$P < .05$. Significance levels refer to incidence figures for each active drug separately compared with those for all control patients. The figures do not indicate comparisons between the two active drugs.
A small number of patients appear more than once in the table.
From Medical Research Council Working Party. Adverse reactions to bendrofluazide and propranolol for the treatment of mild hypertension. Lancet 1981;2:539-43.

TABLE 6-6 Adverse effects on atenolol and placebo ($N = 482$)

Side effects	PLACEBO		ATENOLOL	
	N	%	N	%
Cold extremities	47	9.8	75	15.6
Fatigue	82	17.0	107	22.2
Bronchospasm	27	5.6	30	6.2
Indigestion	16	3.3	16	3.3
Diarrhea	2	0.4	7	1.5
Constipation	24	5.0	13	2.7
Vivid dreams	17	3.5	14	2.9
Insomnia	12	2.5	9	1.9
Hallucinations	0	0	0	0
Dizziness	31	6.4	37	7.7
Depression	30	6.2	26	5.4
LV insufficiency	0	0	0	0
Impotence	12	2.5	13	2.7
Paresthesia	10	2.1	13	2.7
Skin rash	4	0.8	3	0.6
Ataxia	1	0.2	3	0.6
Total	315		366	

LV, left ventricular.
From Cruickshank JM. Beta-blockers, bradycardia and adverse effects. Acta Ther 1981;7: 309–21.

times normal peak blood levels[32] and over a 100% increase in fatigue score[33]—**Figure 6-2**.

The presence of ISA (e.g., pindolol) or α-blockade (e.g., labetalol) does not diminish the frequency of fatigue.[1]

ii) Effort tolerance

Effort tolerance can be impaired by β-blockers, particular nonselective agents.[1] In healthy volunteers, exercise tolerance was impaired more by propranolol than by atenolol,[34,35] but applied only to trained subjects.[36] These β-blocker differences are particularly noted in aerobic endurance exercise (e.g., long-distance runners).[37]

It thus appears sensible to avoid $β_2$-blockade in subjects involved in aerobic pursuits, as evidenced by the trend toward better exercise endurance with highly $β_1$-elective bisoprolol compared with moderately $β_1$-selective atenolol[38]—**Table 6-7**—and a lack of difference between bisoprolol and the calcium antagonist nitrendipine upon exercise capacity and the patients' perception of effort.[39]

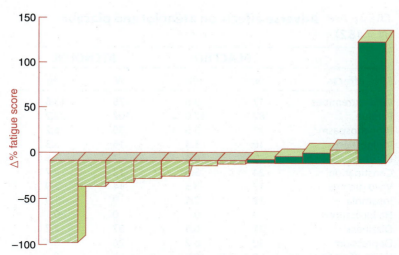

Fig. 6-2 Differences between metoprolol 100 mg and atenolol 100 mg in fatigue scores after exercise, expressed as percentage change. Negative values indicate less fatigue with metoprolol. Results for 9 extensive metabolizers (*hatched bars*) and 3 poor metabolizers (*solid bars*). (From Lewis RV, Ramsey LE, Jackson PR, et al. Influence of debrisoquine—oxidation phenotype on exercise tolerance and subjective fatigue after metoprolol and atenolol in healthy subjects. Br J Clin Pharmacol 1991;31:391–8.)

iii) Direct effects upon muscle

How β-blockers cause fatigue is clearly partly associated with the induced fall in cardiac output. However, there are powerful direct effects upon muscle arising not only from $β_2$-blockade but also from $β_2$-stimulation (via ISA) and also the combination β-/α-blockade.

As already mentioned in the chapter on Pharmacology, both labetalol (β-/α-blockade) and pindolol (high $β_2$ ISA), unlike a β-blocker without these properties, significantly reduced pain-free

TABLE 6-7 Effects of bisoprolol (10 mg) and atenolol (100 mg), vs. placebo, over 3 weeks, upon endurance exercise capacity in healthy men (double-blind, cross-over)

	Bisoprolol	Atenolol
Reduction in exercise duration (min)	−19.4 to 6.7%	−29.8 to 6.6%
P value (vs. placebo)	<.01	<.001

From Vanhees L, Defoor JG, Schepers D, et al. Effects of bisoprolol and atenolol on endurance exercise capacity in healthy men. J Hypertens 2000;18:35–43.

walking distance in hypertensive patients with intermittent claudication.[40] This unexpected effect is likely to be due to a "vasodilatory vascular steal" action within the leg muscles arising from α-blockade in the presence of β-blockade.

Pindolol, with its high level of $β_2$ ISA, has another detrimental effect upon muscle, resulting in muscle cramps[41] usually accompanied by increased creatine phosphokinase (CPK) levels[42]—**Figure 6-3**. The myotoxicity effects of $β_2$-stimulation can be abolished by the specific $β_2$-blocker ICI 118,551.[43]

$β_2$-Blockade has several direct effects upon the muscle, particularly on slow-twitch fibers, which predominate in aerobically fit muscle[44]—**Figure 6-4**. Thus, propranolol causes fatigue in the triceps muscle, which contains a high percentage of slow-twitch

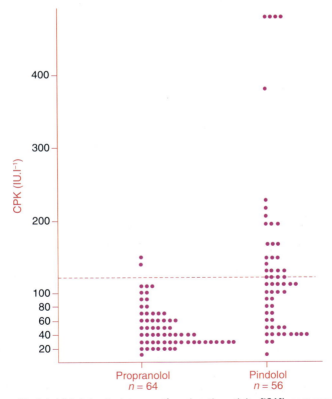

Fig. 6-3 Pindolol (high intrinsic sympathomimetic activity [ISA]), compared with propranolol, has the potential to increase plasma creatine phosphokinase (CPK) levels in hypertensive patients. *Dashed line* indicates upper limit of normal levels for CPK. (From Imataka K, Seki A, Takahashi N, et al. Elevation of serum creatine phosphokinase during pinololo treatment. J Jap Soc Int Med 1981;70:580–5.)

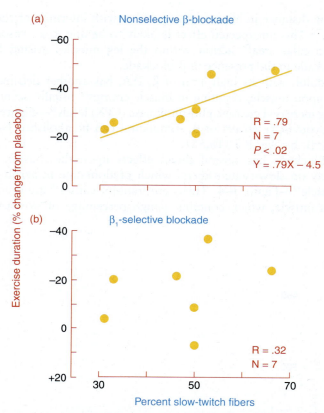

Fig. 6-4 Relationship between change in exercise endurance level with nonselective (a) and β_1-selective (b) blockade, and skeletal muscle fiber composition. There was a greater decrease in exercise duration with nonselective agents in patients with a high percentage of slow-twitch fibers. (From Cleroux J, van Nguyen P, Taylor AW, Leenen FH. Long duration exercise with beta-blockade: endurance versus skeletal muscle fibre composition. J Hypertens 1987;5[supp 5]:S197–9.)

fibers in contrast to the tibialis anterior muscle, which does not.[45] Relevant may be (a) the blocking action of the β_2-receptor upon the Na^+/K^+ pump in the muscle cell membrane[46] and (b) that propranolol, but not atenolol, inhibits muscle glycolysis resulting in a fall in muscle glucose levels[47] and impaired lactic acid release.[48] Indeed, propranolol (compared with other β-blockers like atenolol and metoprolol) can induce frank myopathy.[49]

All of these actions within muscle (particularly slow-twitch fibers) could explain why effort tolerance is best preserved, and fatigue diminished, by the avoidance of β_2-blockade.

E) Cold peripheries

Alongside fatigue cold peripheries is the most common side effect of classic β-blockers like atenolol and propranolol,[10] occurring in 15%-20% of patients vs. 10% on placebo—(see Table 6-6). In the MRC mild hypertension study,[31] the frequency of cold peripheries was significantly increased in women taking propranolol (vs. placebo)—(see Table 6-4)—and significant numbers of both men and women had to be withdrawn due to the Raynaud phenomenon—(see Table 6-5). Cold peripheries appear to be less common with $β_1$-selective agents and those with ISA or additional α-blocking properties.[50] Switching to labetalol from classic β-blockers results in fewer cold peripheries.[51] Avoidance of $β_2$-blockade results in fewer cold peripheries; thus, highly $β_1$-selective bisoprolol was better tolerated than nifedipine in 40 elderly hypertensive patients, with cold peripheries occurring in only 10% of patients on bisoprolol[52]—**Table 6-8**.

A very rare adverse reaction associated with cold peripheries is patchy skin necrosis[1,53], which heals rapidly on classic β-blocker withdrawal.

β-Blocker-induced cold peripheries are associated with a local fall in temperature, which is greater on a nonselective β-blocker.[54] In patients with peripheral vascular disease, the local temperature fall can be greater, particularly if the β-blocker (atenolol) is combined with a vasodilating calcium antagonist—presumably

TABLE 6-8 Adverse events with bisoprolol and sustained-release (SR) nifedipine

Adverse events	Bisoprolol	Nifedipine SR
Number of patients with adverse event	6	12
Total number of adverse events reported	20	51
Headache	2	9
Dizziness, weakness, asthenia, anxiety	3	8
Sleep disturbances	3	7
Gastrointestinal complaints	2	6
Palpitations	2	2
Dyspnea	2	2
Peripheral edemas	1	5
Cold extremities	2	0
Flush	1	6
Other	2	6

From Oliván Martinez J, Garcia MJ, Rodriguez Botaro A, et al. Bisoprolol and nifedipine SR in the treatment of hypertension in the elderly. J Cardiovasc Pharmacol 1990; 16(suppl 5):S95–9.

due to a "vascular steal" effect.[55] Reassuring, though, were the data from the U.K. Prospective Diabetes Study (UKPDS 39),[56] in which diabetic patients with peripheral artery disease had fewer amputations in the atenolol than in the captopril group.

3. Adverse reactions relating to renal function

$β_2$-Blockade is potentially harmful to renal function.[57] Nonselective β-blockers reduce renal blood flow[58]—**Figure 6-5**—and reduce glomerular filtration rate (GFR),[58,59] which contrasts with the renoprotective (increase in GFR) effects of $β_2$-stimulation (blocked by specific $β_2$-blockade).[60]

By contrast, moderately $β_1$-selective agents like atenolol[61] and metoprolol[62] have only minor effects upon renal blood flow/GFR. However, metoprolol is inferior to carvedilol in reducing albuminuria in type 2 diabetics,[63] and carvedilol in turn is inferior to ACE inhibitors and angiotensin receptor blockers (ARBs) in reducing proteinuria in patients with nephritis.[64]

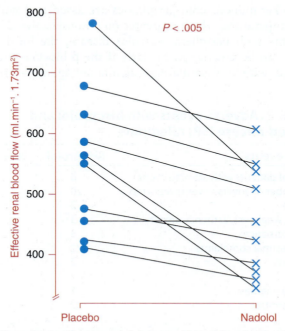

Fig. 6-5 Effect of nonselective nadolol on renal blood flow in 10 elderly hypertensive patients. (From O'Malley K, O'Callagham WG, Laher MS, et al. Beta-adrenoceptor blocking drugs and renal blood flow with special reference to the elderly. Drugs 1983;25[suppl Z]:103–7.)

Highly β_1-selective bisoprolol has proved as effective as the ARB losartan in its "renoprotective effects" (change in creatinine clearance over 1 yr) in middle-aged hypertensive patients[65]—**Table 6-9 and Figure 6-6**—that is, there is no evidence of special ARB renoprotective action.

Renal failure associated with malignant hypertension can respond exceedingly well to β-blockade; not only does blood pressure respond well (to atenolol), but also blood urea levels of 340 mg% were reduced to levels below 100 mg%[66]—**Figure 6-7**.

What does this mean in terms of "hard" end-points. Certainly, in UKPDS study 38,[67] tight control of blood pressure (with either atenolol or captopril) resulted in a significant 37% reduction in microvascular (including kidney) end-points vs. less-tight control of blood pressure (difference of 10/5 mm Hg). In UKPDS 39,[68] there was a 29% positive trend in terms of microvascular end-point reduction favoring atenolol over captopril after 9 to 10 years follow-up. **Table 6-10** illustrates the change in albumin urea over the 9- to 10-year follow up on the UKPDS study; the conclusion of the investigators was "the suggestion the angiotensin converting enzyme inhibitors have special renal protective effects in the treatment of type-2 diabetes is not supported."

Patients with chronic renal failure have very high sympathetic nerve activity, which is correlated with eventual cardiovascular end-points and fatal outcome.[69] This theoretically should favor β-blockade, though the debate, to date, remains unresolved.[70,71]

It is worth noting that in heart failure patients with chronic renal impairment, β-blockers vs. control improve renal function as assessed by creatinine clearance[72]—**Table 6-11**. Certainly, patients with systolic heart failure with moderate/severe renal dysfunction have a significantly higher (almost twofold) mortality than those with adequate renal function as shown in the MERIT (Metoprolol Randomised Intervention Trial) heart failure study;[73] in such patients, metoprolol was at least as effective in reducing death and hospitalization as in those patients with adequate renal function.

4. Adverse reactions relating to the respiratory system

A) Chronic obstructive pulmonary disease

Patients with conditions such as chronic bronchitis or emphysema tend to have fixed airways obstruction and, therefore, in theory, should tolerate even nonselective β-blockers.[74] Indeed, such patients

TABLE 6-9 Effects of bisoprolol 5 mg and losartan over 1 year upon renal hemodynamic parameters in middle-aged hypertensive patients

Parameter	LOSARTAN			BISOPROLOL		
	Baseline	1 yr	P value	Baseline	1 yr	P value
GFR (ml/mm)	131.3 ± 38	119.1 ± 39	NS	129.2 ± 32	119.5 ± 30	NS
Effective renal blood flow (ml/min)	757 ± 214	787 ± 265	NS	747 ± 125	753 ± 167	NS
Filtration fraction (%)	25.2 ± 5	20.9 ± 6	<.001	24.8 ± 5	22.7 ± 4	<.05
Renal vascular resistance (dynes/sec/cm^5)	13.4 ± 3.2	12.2 ± 301	NS	12.8 ± 1.9	12.1 ± 2.1	NS

GFR, glomerular filtration rate; NS, not significant.
From Parrinello G, Paterna S, Torres D, et al. One year renal and cardiac effects of bisoprolol versus losartan in recently diagnosed hypertensive patients. Clin Drug Invest 2009;29:591–600.

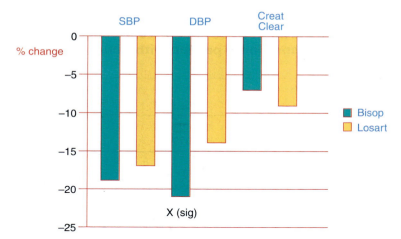

Fig. 6-6 In a comparison over 1 year of highly β_1-selective bisoprolol (Bisop) and losartan (Losar) in middle-aged hypertensive patients, there was no evidence of "special" renoprotective properties of the angiotensin receptor antagonist—that is, there was a similar small fall in creatinine clearance (Creat Clear) over 1 year with both agents. DBP, diastolic blood pressure; SBP, systolic blood pressure; sig, significant. (From Parrinello G, Paterna S, Torres D, et al. One year renal and cardiac effects of bisoprolol versus losartan in recently diagnosed hypertensive patients. Clin Drug Invest 2009;29:591–600.)

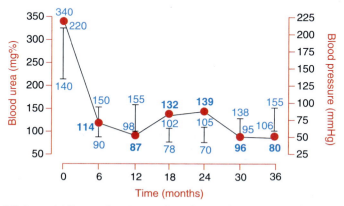

Fig. 6-7 In a middle-aged patient with malignant hypertension and marked renal dysfunction, control of blood pressure with atenolol-based therapy resulted in a dramatic fall in blood urea levels. (From Zacharias FJ. Long-term clinical experience with atenolol. Royal Society of Medicine, International Congress and Symposium Series N19. 1979, pp 75–91.)

TABLE 6-10 UKPDS 39—Renoprotection in hypertensive type 2 diabetics (in study 38 tight BP control significantly reduced the proportion of patients with albuminuria by 29%)

% of patients with albuminuria (50 mg/L)	Captopril	Atenolol
Baseline	16%	20%
After 9 yr follow-up	31%	26%

BP, blood pressure.
From U.K. Prospective Diabetes Study Group. Efficacy of atenolol and captopril in reducing risk of macro-vascular and microvascular complications in type 2 diabetes: UKPDS 39. BMJ 1998;317:713–20.

have been shown to tolerate even propranolol well[75] and differ little in terms of hospitalization from more selective β-blockers,[76] with no reduction of quality of life.[77] However, nonselective agents can reduce forced expiratory volume in 1 second (FEV_1) and inhibit $β_2$-stimulant action in such cases;[78] thus, the use of $β_1$-selective agents is to be recommended.[79,80] Certainly, in the MRC mild hypertension study, one of the most common side effects, and reason for patient withdrawal, was shortness of breath at rest and during exercise.[31]

B) Reversible, labile, reactive airway disease—asthma

Such patients have hyperreactive bronchi and can respond adversely to β-blockers, particularly nonselective agents.[1] Timolol eyedrops have been the cause of death.[81] Nonselective agents like timolol can reduce FEV_1 by over 50% in labile asthmatics and totally inhibit the benefits of $β_2$-stimulation[82]—(see **Chapter 1, Figure 1-36**). By contrast, more selective agents like atenolol effect a lesser fall in FEV_1 and permit $β_2$-stimulatory bronchodilatation.

TABLE 6-11 Heart failure patients with chronic renal impairment experience improved renal function on β-blockade for 1 year

	% Change in creatinine clearance over 1 yr
On β-blockers	+8.1
Control	−17.7

From Khan W, Deepak SM, Coppinger T. Beta-blocker treatment is associated with improvement in renal function and anaemia in patients with heart failure. Heart 2006;92:1856–7.

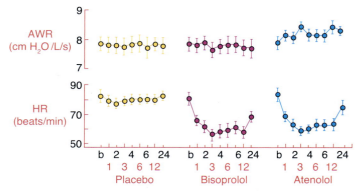

Fig. 6-8 In patients with chronic obstructive pulmonary disease (COPD), highly β$_1$-selective bisoprolol, in contrast to moderately β$_1$-selective atenolol, had no effect upon airways resistance (AWR). HR, heart rate. (Dorow P, Bethge M, Tonnesmann V. Effects of single oral doses of bisoprolol and atenolol on airways function in non-asthmatic chronic obstructive lung disease and angina pectoris. Eur J Clin Pharmacol 1986; 31: 143–7.)

However, even atenolol is only modestly β$_1$-selective, and one of the most common reasons for patient withdrawal in the UKPDS 39 study[68] was bronchoconstriction. Thus, not only should highly nonselective β-blockers like timolol, propranolol, and carvedilol[83] be avoided in vulnerable patients, but moderately β$_1$-selective β-blockers like metoprolol and atenolol should also be avoided, even though they are associated with fewer hospital admissions and emergency department visits than nonselective agents.[76]

The best choice for vulnerable patients with obstructive airways disease in need of a β-blocker is undoubtedly low-dose, highly β$_1$-selective bisoprolol. In patients with either chronic obstructive bronchitis[84]—Figure 6-8—or labile asthma[85]—Figure 6-9—there is, in contrast to atenolol, no change in airways resistance with bisoprolol.

C) Alveolar permeability

Alveoli are rich in β$_2$-receptors, which control alveolar fluid reabsorption and gas diffusion. In patients with heart failure, the effects of nonselective carvedilol and highly β$_1$-selective bisoprolol have been compared.[86] Carvedilol inhibited not only the bronchodilator effect of salbutamol but also, compared with bisoprolol, reduced carbon monoxide diffusion and peak oxygen volume (VO$_2$)—(see Table 1-2a in Chapter 1). This potentially negative effect of carvediolol, by reducing exercise-induced hyperventilation, bizarrely

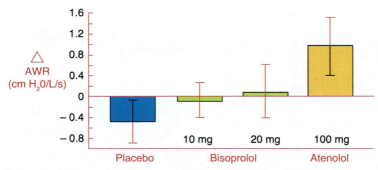

Fig. 6-9 In hypertensive patients with bronchial asthma, bisoprolol 10-20 mg, in contrast to atenolol 100 mg, had no effect upon airways resistance (AWR). (From Chatterjee SS. The cardioselective and hypotensive effects of bisoprolol in hypertensive asthmatics. J Cardiovasc Pharmacol 1986;8 [suppl 11]:S74–77.)

improves quality of life. However, at altitude, 2000 m, oxygen pressure (PO_2) is reduced by carvediolol, increasing the risk of anoxia.

D) Mucocilary action

The tracheobronchial tree, including the nasal cavity, is lined with ciliated cells down to the terminal bronchioles. These ciliated cells are responsible for the clearance of excess secretions, which are an important defense mechanism of the airways against bacterial infection.

Human tracheal ciliated epithelial cells are under the control of β_2-receptors.[87] In patients with airways infection with *Pseudomonas aeruginosa*, nasal mucociliary clearance is markedly impaired.[88] This action is benefited by β_2-stimulation, the action of which is inhibited by the β_2-blocker ICI 118551 and propranolol, and less so by atenolol.[88] Others have confirmed these findings with atenolol and propranolol upon tracheobronchial mucociliary clearance.[89] Modestly β_1-selective metoprolol, in contrast to nonselective propranolol, did not differ from placebo on tracheobronchial clearance[90]—**Figure 6-10**.

In terms of adverse reactions, nasal stuffiness and bronchorrhea appear to be relevant. Patients with chronic bronchitis or asthma have experienced bronchorrhea with nonselective timolol.[91] Nasal stuffiness is rarely checked for. However, this side effect has been noted with nonselective β-blockers, even with ISA or additional

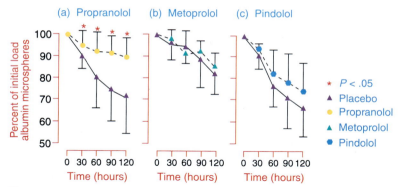

Fig. 6-10 In patients with coronary artery disease and normal lung function, only nonselective propranolol (a) significantly reduced tracheobronchial mucociliary clearance. Moderately β_1-selective metoprolol (b) and nonselective pindolol (c) with high ISA had no significant effects (From Dorow P, Weiss T, Felix R, et al. Influence of propranolol, metoprolol and pindolol on mucociliary clearance in patients with coronary heart disease. Respiration 1984;45:286–90.)

α-blocking properties.[1] Certainly, propranolol can induce watery nasal secretions.[92] In the MRC mild hypertension study[31]— (see Table 6-4,) there was an approximate twofold significant increase the frequency of a blocked or runny nose in men receiving propranolol compared with placebo.

5. Metabolic disturbance

As mentioned earlier (see the Hypertension chapter), various regulatory authorities are concerned about the ability of some β-blockers (particularly when co-prescribed with diuretics) to induce metabolic changes involving mainly blood sugar and lipids. As already indicated, the clinical significance of these changes are open to debate. However, most doctors would be happier using an agent that does not induce metabolic changes.

A) Blood sugar (and insulin)

Muscle glycogenolysis, liver glucose output, or secretion of insulin and glucagon are all modulated by the sympathetic nervous system via the β_2-receptor.[1] Thus, nonselective β-blockers would be expected to be the main culprits as regards changes in blood sugar.

i) Insulin-induced hypoglycemia

Insulin-induced hypoglycemia can, occasionally, lead to a loss of consciousness. The induced hypoglycemia can be prolonged by nonselective agents like propranolol, but not by relatively β_1-selective drugs like metoprolol and bisoprolol[93]—**Figure 6-12**. The hypoglycemic signs, other than tachycardia, are essentially unaffected, though sweating can be augmented.[1]

However, one important concern with nonselective β-blockers and insulin-induced hypoglycemia is the potential for serious hypertensive episodes (see the chapter on Pharmacology, plus later in this chapter). Hypoglycemia results in an outpouring of adrenaline;

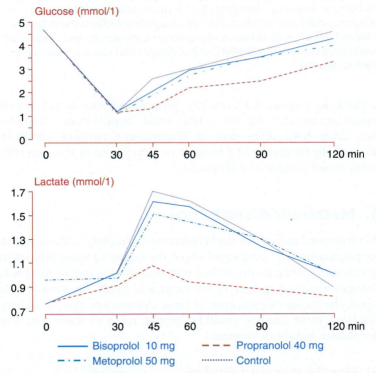

Fig. 6-11 In healthy volunteers, insulin-induced hypoglycemia is prolonged, and insulin-induced lactate release suppressed, by nonselective propranolol in contrast to highly β_1-selective bisoprolol that did not differ from control. (From Leopold G, Ungethum W, Pabst J, et al. Pharmacokinetic profile of bisoprolol, a new beta-1 selective beta-blocker. Br J Clin Pharmacol 1986;22:293–300.)

β_1- plus β_2-blockade results in unopposed α-stimulation, resulting in marked increases in blood pressure. This hypertensive phenomenon does not occur with high β_1-selectivity (i.e., bisoprolol).

ii) Hyperglycemia

Insulin sensitivity and release are reduced by both nonselective and moderately β_1-selective β-blockers.[94] This can result in marked increases in blood sugar with propranolol[95]—**Figure 6-12**. In the classic UKPDS study,[56] hemoglobin$_{A1c}$ (Hb$_{A1c}$) levels were increased by atenolol but not by captopril. In contrast, highly β_1-selective bisoprolol was similar to captopril in causing no change in blood sugar levels or insulin sensitivity[96] and did not differ from placebo in its effects upon blood sugar and Hb$_{A1}$[97,98]—**Table 6-12 and Figure 6-13**. β-Blockers with ISA (e.g., nebivolol)[99] or additional α-blockade (e.g., carvedilol)[100] also have minimal or absent effects on blood sugar and insulin sensitivity.

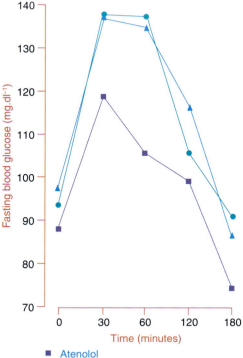

Fig. 6-12 In hypertensive patients on chronic antihypertensive therapy, both hydrochlorothiazide and nonselective propranolol impaired glucose tolerance. (From Nash DT. A comparison of long-term effects of hydrochlorthiazide, propranolol and atenolol on carbohydrate and lipid metabolism. J Cardiopulm Rehabil 1988;8:18–24.)

TABLE 6-12 Metabolic parameters in patients treated in a crossover design with placebo or bisoprolol 10 mg over a 6-week period: $N = 20$; means ± SEM

Treatment	Time (wk)	Glucose (mg/dl)	Hb_{A1} (%)	Cholesterol (mg/dl)	Triglycerides (mg/dl)
Baseline	0	161.8 ± 4.9	9.69 ± 0.19	250.9 ± 14.1	205.4 ± 18.8
Placebo	2	165.1 ± 5.9	9.65 ± 0.20	253.0 ± 12.0	207.8 ± 17.8
Bisoprolol	4	158.0 ± 4.7	9.64 ± 0.20	251.7 ± 13.3	210.8 ± 19.7
Placebo	6	158.6 ± 3.6	9.6 ± 0.20	253.3 ± 12.2	203.3 ± 5.1
Difference between wk 4 and 6		−0.6 to 3.3 (NS)	−0.01 ± 0.06 (NS)	−1.6 to 4.2 (NS)	7.5 ± 5.1 (NS)

Hb_{A1}, hemoglobin$_{A1}$; NS, not significant; SEM, standard error of the mean.
From Janka HU, Ziegler AG, Disselhoff G, Mehnert H. Influence of bisoprolol on blood glucose, glycosuria and haemoglobin A-1 in non-insulin dependent diabetics. J Cardiovasc Pharmacol 1986;8(suppl 11):S96–9.

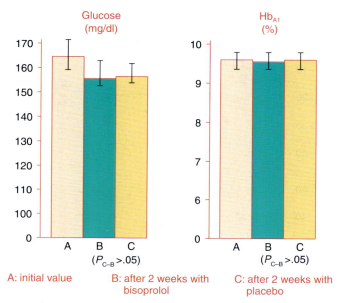

Fig. 6-13 In hypertensive patients with type 2 diabetes, highly β_1-selective bisoprolol did not differ from placebo in its effect upon fasting blood levels of blood sugar and hemoglobin$_{A1}$ (Hb$_{A1}$). (From Janka HU, Ziegler AG, Disselhoff G, Mehnert H. Influence of bisoprolol on blood glucose, glycosuria and haemoglobin A-1 in non-insulin dependent diabetics. J Cardiovasc Pharmacol 1986;8[suppl 11]:S96–9.)

The clinical relevance of the induced changes in blood sugar has been debated. In the UKPDS study,[56] in spite of atenolol increasing blood Hb$_{A1c}$ levels, all seven primary end-point trends favored the β-blocker over the ACE inhibitor (see the Hypertension chapter). Even more striking were the results of the SHEP (Systolic Hypertension in the Elderly Program) study (see the Hypertension chapter) involving placebo vs. first-line diuretic plus second-line atenolol. Over a 15-year follow-up, naturally occurring diabetes in the placebo arm was associated with significantly increased cardiovascular mortality, which contrasted with drug-induced diabetes in the treatment arm in which mortality was no different from those who had no diabetes (see Chapter 3, Table 3-9).

iii) Blood lipids

β-Blockers, including nonselective agents, have little or no effect upon total cholesterol.[1] Certainly, high β_1-selectivity causes no changes in blood cholesterol[98]—(**see Table 6-12.**)

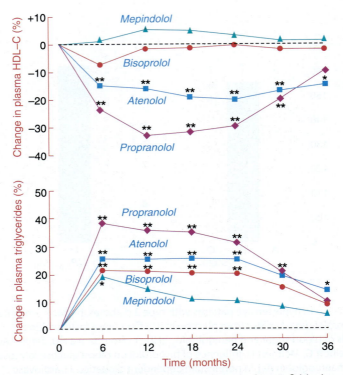

Fig. 6-14 In normocholesterolemic hypertensives on chronic β-blocker therapy, nonselective propranolol and moderately $β_1$-selective atenolol significantly reduced plasma high-density lipoprotein (HDL) levels and increased triglyceride levels, in contrast to highly $β_1$-selective bisoprolol and mepindolol with high ISA, which induced minor or no effects. (From Fogari R, Zoppi A. The clinical benefits of beta-1 selectivity. Rev Contemp Pharmacother 1997;8:45–54.)

In contrast, β-blockade can affect blood triglyceride and high-density lipoprotein (HDL) levels. Nonselective propranolol, and to a lesser extent moderately $β_1$-selective atenolol, can reduce HDL levels and increase triglyceride concentrates by 30%-40%[97]— Figure 6-14. High $β_1$-selectivity (bisoprolol) or ISA (mepindolol) ensured little or no change in HDL and triglyceride levels.[97,98]

Clearly, $β_2$-blockade is the cause of the lipid changes,[1,101] and the triglyceride changes could well be due to unopposed α-stimulatory affect inhibiting lipoprotein lipase.[102]

The β-blocker-induced changes in HDL and triglyceride levels can be avoided by low-dose, high-$β_1$-selectivity (i.e., bisoprolol),[97,98] ISA (e.g., mepindolol),[97] or α-blockade (e.g., carvedilol).[103]

6. Adverse reactions relating to the central nervous system

Many perceptions concerning β-blockers and central nervous system (CNS) problems, particularly depression, arose from old observational studies.[1] Only prospective, controlled, blind studies can supply the correct answers.

A) Depression

In the large placebo-controlled MRC mild hypertension study[31]—(see **Table 6-4**), depression was not a problem in the propranolol group. In an overview of seven placebo-controlled studies, depression occurred in 20.1% of the β-blocker group and 20.5% of the placebo group.[104]

B) Cognitive function and memory

In the MRC elderly study, over a 4½-year period, atenolol and placebo could not be separated in terms of cognitive function.[105] However, memory loss has been described with lipophilic metoprolol.[106] Lipophilic propranolol has likewise been linked to memory loss,[107] though not all agree.[108] It is possible that memory loss problems may be greater with propranolol than with highly water-soluble (low brain tissue levels) atenolol.[107]

C) Sleep disturbance (insomnia, dreams, and nightmares) and hallucinations

As noted in the chapter on Pharmacology (see **Fig. 1-24**), lipophilic agents like propranolol, oxprenolol, and metoprolol appear in human brain tissue at concentrations manyfold greater than levels of hydrophilic atenolol.

Accordingly, sleep problems and hallucinations occur at a greater frequency with lipophilic β-blockers including pindolol.[1] Under placebo-controlled conditions, in contrast to hydrophilic atenolol, lipophilic propranolol, metoprolol, and pindolol caused marked change on sleeping electroencephalograms, accompanied by disturbed sleep and dreaming.[109] In particular with pindolol, rapid eye movement sleep is disturbed.[110] Vivid dreams associated with lipophilic metoprolol have been reported to disappear on changing to hydrophilic atenolol.[111] The sleep disturbances described with metoprolol[112] can be accompanied by sleepwalking, or somnambulism.[113]

Hallucinations on lipophilic propranolol can disappear on changing to atenolol[114] or reappear upon rechallenge with propranolol.[115]

D) Motor performance and reaction times

It is possible that single (acute) doses of a β-blocker (e.g., propranolol)[116] can slow reaction times. However, such effects disappear on chronic dosing.[117] Chronic dosing results, which relate more to real-life situations, indicate that reaction times and general performance (e.g., driving motor vehicles) are not affected.[1,118]

7. Sexual dysfunction

In discussing this highly emotive topic, it is important to understand that (a) β-blockers are not a homogeneous class of drugs (1), (b) there is a powerful "placebo effect",[104] (c) patient "knowledge" of possible problems can increase the frequency of erectile dysfunction,[119] and (d) the frequency of erectile dysfunction is markedly increased in patients with coronary artery disease.[120]

The area of physiological mechanisms involved in penile smooth muscle/venous blood flow behavior in the flaccid/erect penis is complex.[1] We know that β_2- and α-receptors in particular[121] are involved in the process.

In six randomized, placebo-controlled studies involving almost 15,000 patients, there was a significant increase in sexual dysfunction in those receiving β-blockers[104]—**Table 6-13**. However, 17.4% experienced problems on placebo. In addition to the placebo effect that has to be taken into account, so does the so-called Hawthorne effect[122]—**Figure 6-15**. In this study involving metoprolol (given for 2 mo) and sexual dysfunction, if patients were told that they were to be given metoprolol, which causes sexual problems, 32% had dysfunction. If they were told it was metoprolol but not about

TABLE 6-13 The frequency of sexual dysfunction in those receiving randomized β-blockers or placebo

	β-blocker group	Placebo group	P value
Frequency of sexual dysfunction (%)	21.6	17.4	.05 (sig)

sig, significant.
From Ko DT, Hebert PR, Coffey CS, et al. Beta-blocker therapy and symptoms of depression, fatigue and sexual dysfunction. JAMA 2002;288:351–7.

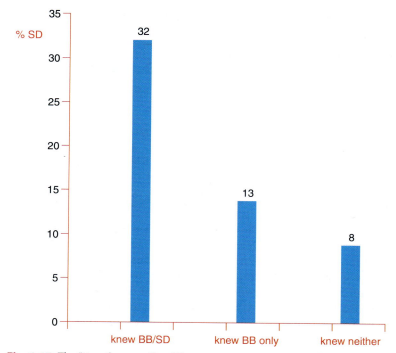

Fig. 6-15 The "Hawthorne effect." If a patient is ignorant of the fact that he is on a β-blocker (BB), or that β-blockers can cause sexual dysfunction (SD), the likelihood of impotence is low. Conversely, when he knows he was receiving a β-blocker or knew of the "problems" with β-blockers (BB/SD), the incidence of sexual dysfunction is high. (From Cocco G. Erectile dysfunction after therapy with metoprolol: the Hawthorne effect. Cardiology 2008;112:174–7.)

possible sexual dysfunction, 13% had problems. In those who knew neither, 8% had problems.

So to assess a β-blocker's adverse reaction pattern, the "placebo/Hawthorne effect" has to be subtracted, as shown in **Table 6-14**. It is clear that the biggest sexual dysfunction "problem" is with the combination of $β_1$-, $β_2$-, and α-blockade (i.e., carvedilol),[123] followed by nonselective propranolol,[31] followed by moderately $β_1$-selective atenolol,[119] with highly $β_1$-selective bisoprolol having sexual dysfunction problems at placebo level.[124] Certainly, in the MRC mild hypertension study, impotence with propranolol was a major cause of patient withdrawal—(see **Table 6-4**). With labetalol, with $β_1$-, $β_2$-, and α-blocking properties (stronger α-blocker than carvedilol), failure to ejaculate is a major cause of patient withdrawal.[125] Labetalol can also cause retrograde ejaculation[126] and urinary retention[127] and reduce vaginal lubrication.[128]

TABLE 6-14 Different β-blockers and sexual dysfunction vs. placebo

β-blocker	Sexual dysfunction— % increase vs. placebo	Reference
Carvedilol (nonselective + α-blockade)	13.5	Fogari et al, 2001[123]
Propranolol (nonselective)	5.0	MRC—Mild Hypertension, 1985[31]
Atenolol (moderately β$_1$-selective)	3.0	Silvestri et al, 2003[119]
Bisoprolol (highly β$_1$-selective)	0.0	Broekman et al, 1992[124]

Of possible relevance is, in animal studies, the ability of agents like propranolol, atenolol, and metoprolol to reduce sperm mobility and reduce testosterone levels,[129] noted also in humans.[130] By contrast, high β$_1$-selectivity (i.e., bisoprolol and nebivolol) increase testosterone levels (and decrease estrogens) and have no adverse affects on penile blood flow in middle-aged men.[131]

8. Weight gain

Weight gain on traditional β-blockers is well-recognized.[1] The mean increase in weight is about 1.2 kg and occurs mainly in the first few months.[132]

The mechanism of this phenomenon is debatable. Of interest is the fact that certain genotypes of the β$_2$-receptor are linked to weight gain and central obesity and also development of hypertension and high sympathetic nerve activity).[133] Thus, β$_2$-blockade may be linked to weight gain, possibly via its depressive effect on thermogenesis . There is evidence for a β$_2$-mediated facultative thermogenic component in skeletal muscle, and there is also 25% reduction in thermogenic response to food.[132] It has been noted that propranolol can decrease shivering thermogenesis—only 1% of postoperative patients on propranolol, vs. 30% in control, shivered.[134]

In support of the β$_2$-receptor involvement in weight gain is the fact that low-dose, highly β$_1$-selective bisoprolol (compared with losartan) was associated with a small weight loss after 1 year of therapy[65]—Table 6-15. It is also possible that the presence of an α-blocking property may modify the effects of β$_2$-blockade; in

TABLE 6-15 Effect of low-dose (5-mg) bisoprolol and losartan upon weight over 1 year

	BISOPROLOL 5 MG		LOSARTAN 50 MG	
	Baseline	1 yr	Baseline	1 yr
Change in weight (kg)	77	76	78	77

From Parrinello G, Paterna S, Torres D, et al. One year renal and cardiac effects of bisoprolol versus losartan in recently diagnosed hypertensive patients. Clin Drug Invest 2009;29:591–600.

contrast to modestly β_1-selective metoprolol, which caused a 1.2 kg weight-gain, there was no change in weight with carvedilol.[135]

9. Skin and rashes

A) Occulomucocutaneous syndrome associated with practolol

The unique toxicity to one β-blocker—practolol—has been well described.[1] It comprised (a) a psoriasiform rash with hyperkeratosis of the palms and soles, (b) keratoconjunctivitis sicca leading to corneal ulceration and opacification, (c) otitis media, and (d) slerosing peritonitis. Immunological mechanisms were responsible.

No other β-blocker has produced these problems.

B) Skin lesions with other β-blockers

Skin lesions are uncommon with β-blockers but do occur more commonly than with diuretics for example—as evidenced by the significant numbers of withdrawals in the MRC mild hypertension study in those receiving propranolol[31]—(see **Table 6-5**).

β-Blockers can worsen psoriasis[136]—**Table 6-16**. Even in nonpsoriasis sufferers, they can induce psoriasiform-type lesions as well as other forms of rash[137]—**Table 6-17**.

Whether the β_2-receptors are associated with skin problems is unclear. Certainly, a lichenoid eruption has been described with β_1-selective nebivolol,[138] though no skin problems have been described with highly β_1-selective bisoprolol.

C) Scalp tingling

This problem has been described with labetalol[1] and may be a function of vasodilatation.

TABLE 6-16 Response of psoriasis to β-blocker therapy

Drug	EFFECT ON PSORIASIS		
	Worse	Stable	Better
Propranolol ($n = 14$)	8	6	0
Nadolol ($n = 4$)	4	0	0
Atenolol ($n = 8$)	6	2	0
Metoprolol ($n = 3$)	2	0	1

From Gold MH, Holy AK, Roenigk HH. Beta-blocking drugs and psoriasis. J Am Acad Dermatol 1988;19:837–41.

TABLE 6-17 Cutaneous side effects (not common) of β-blockers

Oculumucocutaneous syndrome (practolol)
Lupus erythematosus
Psoriasiform eruptions
Lichenoid eruptions
Eczematous eruptions
Alopecia
Hyperpigmentation
Stevens-Johnson syndrome
Skin necrosis

From Richards S. Cutaneous side-effects of beta-adrenergic blockers. Aust J Dermatol 1985;26:25–8.

10. Arrhythmia induction

As indicated in Chapter 4 on arrhythmias, sotalol, which contains class III antiarrhythmic activity, can in 2%-4% of cases induce ventricular tachycardia (torsades de pointes")—see Figure 4-9.

SUMMARY AND CONCLUSIONS

1. β-Blockers are a heterogeneous class of drugs and adverse reactions will depend upon the mix of such properties as $β_1$-blockade (shared by all), $β_2$-blockade, ISA, additional α-blocking properties;, class III antiarrhythmic activity, degree of lipid solubility, and unpredictable metabolism due to polymorphic/genotype variation.
2. The shared property of $β_1$-blockade can cause symptoms in some patients (which tend to diminish in time and be dose-dependent and are more frequent in the elderly): (a) bradycardia (rarely symptomic), (b) fatigue (worse if accompanied by $β_2$-blockade,

which has direct muscle activity), (c) cold peripheries (again worse if accompanied by β_2-blockade), (d) rarely, heart failure (in high-risk hearts), and (e) rarely symptomatic hypotension (in the elderly).
3. Quality of-life is, compared with ACE inhibitors, impaired by nonselective agents like propranolol; high β_1-selectivity (e.g., bisoprolol) is associated with a quality of life similar to that with ACE inhibitors.
4. Adverse reactions relating to the cardiovascular system are
    a) Bradycardia and heart block—Heart rates of 40-50 beats/min are common in the normal population and are symptomless; such rates in hypertensive patients are also symptomless, only dizziness occurs in some with rates less than 40 beats/min. In patients with coronary heart disease, slow heart rates are linked to fewer anginal symptoms. Patients with sinus node dysfunction should avoid β-blockers, and post-myocardial infarction patients with a long PR interval are at increased risk of complete heart block with β-blockers.
    b) Heart failure—Induced heart failure is extremely rare with β-blockers, except in the frail elderly with poor cardiac function or some unstable patients in the post-infarct recovery period.
    c) Hypotension—Symptomatic hypotension is extremely rare, unless accompanying α-blockade is present (i.e., labetalol or carvediolol), in which postural hypotension (particularly after the first dose) can be troublesome in the elderly. Patients with very high plasma renin levels (e.g., renal artery stenosis or malignant hypertension) can experience marked, symptomatic falls in blood pressure.
    d) Fatigue—This is the most common symptom with β-blockade and is the most likely cause for withdrawal from nonselective agents (e.g., propranolol) or moderate β_1-selective agents (e.g., atenolol or metoprolol). Inhibition of both β_1 (cardiac) and β_2 (muscle slow-twitch fibers) are particularly troublesome for aerobic or long-distance exercises (or slow-metabolizers of metoprolol) in which effort tolerance and the training process are affected—low-dose, high β_1-selectivity is the best option for such individuals. With intermittent claudication sufferers, the combination of β- and α-blockade tends to reduce walking distance (vascular steal); a high degree of β_2 ISA (e.g., pindolol, which can sometimes induce myopathic symptoms, can induce inflammatory lesions in muscles (high C-reactive protein levels) resulting in painful muscle cramps.

e) Cold peripheries—This adverse reaction is a reflection of a fall in both cardiac output and vascular β_2-blockade (vasoconstriction) and is second only to fatigue as a cause of withdrawal from classic β-blockers like propranolol and atenolol. It is less common with high β_1-selectivity (e.g., bisoprolol) or high levels of ISA (e.g., pindolol) or accompanying α-blockade (e.g., labetalol). Very rarely, patchy skin necrosis has occurred with classic β-blockers.

5. Renal function —Renal dysfunction (i.e., fall in GFR or creatinine clearance) appears to be a function of β_2-blockade-induced falls in renal blood flow. In middle-aged, diabetic hypertensive patients, atenolol was at least as effective as ACE inhibition in preserving renal function (UKPDS) over a 10-year follow-up period and bisoprolol was at least as effective as angiotensin receptor blockade in preserving GFR in hypertensive patients over a 1-year period. Renal dysfunction associated with malignant hypertension improves on β-blocker therapy. Heart failure cases with renal dysfunction benefit from β-blockade in terms of fewer deaths and improved renal function.

6. Respiratory system
    a) Chronic obstructive airways disease (COPD)—Such patients with relatively "fixed" airways obstruction tend to tolerate β-blockers very well (even propranolol), though the action of β_2-stimulants are impaired by nonselectivity.
    b) Reversible, labile, reactive airways disease—Asthma patients have hyperreactive bronchi and even nonselective timolol eyedrops can precipitate marked bronchospasm and death. β_2-Blockade not only markedly reduces FEV_1 but also inhibits the salutary effects of β_2-stimulants. Even moderate β_1-selective agents (e.g., atenolol) can cause problems and the best approach for vulnerable patients in need of β-blockade is cautious low-dose, high-β_1-selective bisoprolol.
    c) Alveolar permeability—β_2-Receptors in the alveoli control fluid reabsorption and gas diffusion; avoidance of potential problems is possible by low-dose, high β_1-selectivity.
    d) Mucociliary action—The tracheobronchial tree and nasal passages are lined with ciliated cells that are important for clearance of excess secretions and act as a defense mechanism against bacterial infections. These cilia are under the control of β_2-receptors and their action is inhibited by β_2-blockade and, by implication, preserved by low-dose β_1-selective blockade.

7. Metabolic disturbance—This aspect of β-blockade is of particular concern to some regulatory authorities, especially when β-blockers are co-prescribed with diuretics.
   a) Blood sugar (and insulin) muscle glycogenolysis, liver glucose output, and secretion of insulin and glugagon are all modulated by the $β_2$-receptor; thus, "blood sugar problems" are a function of $β_2$-blockade.
      i) Insulin-induced hypoglycemia—This state can be prolonged by nonselective blockade, though symptoms are not usually worsened and (other than tachycardia) can still be recognized. Hypoglycemia–induced adrenalemia can be a problem for nonselective β-blockers with marked hypertensive reactions occurring, which are easily avoided by high $β_1$-selectivity.
      ii) Hyperglycemia—Insulin sensitivity and release is reduced by nonselective and moderately $β_1$-selective agents, resulting in marked increases in blood sugar and Hb_{A1c} levels; these problems are avoided by high $β_1$-selectivity (e.g., bisoprolol), ISA (e.g., nebivolol), or α-blockade (e.g., carvedilol). The clinical relevance of these $β_2$-blocking-induced changes is debatable.
   b) Blood lipids—Nonselective β-blockers have little or no effect on blood total cholesterol, but do affect blood triglycerides and HDL levels (possibly via unopposed α-stimulation). As with blood sugar changes, the "lipid-effects" can be avoided by low-dose, highly $β_1$-selective bisoprolol, ISA (e.g., mepindolol), or α-blockade (e.g., carvedilol). As for blood sugar changes, the clinical relevance of induced lipid changes is debatable.
8. Central nervous system
   a) Depression—The old belief that β-blockers cause depression is not confirmed under blind, placebo-controlled conditions, even for lipophilic agents like propranolol.
   b) Cognitive function and memory—β-Blockers do not impair cognitive function, even in the elderly; memory loss, though not all agree, may be a factor with lipophilic agents.
   c) Sleep disturbance, dreams, nightmares, and hallucinations—Lipophilic agents, like propranolol and metoprolol, appear in human brain tissue at high concentrations; such β-blockers, including pindolol, cause marked changes in the electroencephalogram and are linked to insomnia, dreams, nightmares, and occasionally hallucinations, which disappear on change to more hydrophilic drugs such as atenolol.

d) Motor performance and reaction times—Chronic dosing with β-blockers does not affect motor performance or reaction times (e.g., driving).
9. Sexual dysfunction in men. In this emotive topic there exists a powerful "placebo effect" that needs to be taken into account. When the placebo effect is subtracted, it is apparent that β-blockers that antagonize $β_1$- plus $β_2$- plus α receptors (e.g., labetalol and carvedilol) have the greatest detrimental effect, followed by nonselective and modestly $β_1$-selective agents (e.g., propranolol, atenolol and metoprolol), whereas high $β_1$-selectivity (e.g., bisoprolol) causes "problems" at placebo level.
10. Weight gain. Weight gain of 1 to 2 kg with traditional β-blockers is well recognized, possibly via the effect of $β_2$-blockade on thermogenesis. High $β_1$-selectivity or the addition of α-blocking properties appears to negate the weight gain factor.
11. Skin and rashes. Skin lesions are uncommon with β-blockers, though classic β-blockers can exacerbate psoriasis or, in nonpsoriasis patients, cause "psoriasiform-type" lesions. The role of the $β_2$-receptor in this process is unclear, but skin lesions are extremely rare with high $β_1$-selectivity The presence of α-blockade can cause scalp tingling.
12. The possession of class III antiarrhythmic activity (i.e., sotalol) can induce ventricular tachycardia ("torsades de pointes") in 2%-4% of cases.
13. Overall, the risk/benefit and cost/benefit ratios of β-blockers in cardiovascular medicine strongly favor high $β_1$-selectivity—i.e., optimal efficacy—with the least risk of adverse reactions.

REFERENCES

1. Cruickshank J, Prichard BP. Beta-blockers in Clinical Practice. 2nd ed. Edinburgh: Churchill Livingstone; 1994 pp. 907–1053.
2. Cruickshank JM, Higgins TJ, Pennart K, et al. The efficacy and tolerability of antihypertensive treatment based on atenolol in the prevention of stroke and regression of left ventricular hypertrophy. J Hum Hypertens 1987;1:87–93.
3. Croog SH, Levine S, Testa MA, et al. The effects of antihypertensive therapy on the quality of life. N Engl J Med 1986;314:1657–64.
4. Steiner SS, Friedhoff AJ, Wilson BL, et al. Antihypertensive therapy and quality of life: a comparison of atenolol, captopril, enalapril and propranolol. J Hum Hypertens 1990;4:217–25.
5. Prichard BN, Saul PA. Comparison of beta-blockade and ACE-inhibition in the treatment of hypertension. J Cardiovasc Pharmacol 1990;16(suppl 5):81–5.

6. Bracchetti D, Gradnick R, Alberti A, et al. A double-blind comparison of bisoprolol and captopril for treatment of essential hypertension in the elderly. Cardiovasc Drugs Therap 1990;4:261–4.
7. Breed JG, Ciampricotti S, Byington R, et al. Quality of life perception during antihypertensive treatment: a comparative study of bisoprolol and enalapril. J Cariovasc Pharmacol 1992;20:750–5.
8. Erikssen J, Rodhal K. Resting heart rate in apparently healthy middle-aged men. Eur J Appl Physiol 1979;42:61–4.
9. Andersson O, Berglund G. Hansson L, et al. Organisation and efficacy of an out-patient hypertension clinic. Acta Med Scand 1978;203:391–8.
10. Cruickshank JM. Beta-blockers, bradycardia and adverse effects. Acta Ther 1981;7:309–21.
11. Greenblatt DJ, Koch-Weser J. Adverse reactions of propranolol in hospitalized medical patients. Am heart J 1973;86:478–84.
12. Swanson H, Beauchamp GD, Bell H, Kindred L. Reversible cardiogenic shock. J Kans Med Soc 1975;76:2600.
13. Wilcox RG, Roland JM, Banks DC, et al. Randomised trial comparing propranolol and atenolol in immediate treatment of suspected myocardial infarction. Br Med J 1980;280:885–8.
14. Scheinman MM, Strauss HC, Evans GT, et al. Adverse effects of sympatholytic agents in patients with hypertension and sinus node dysfunction. Am J Med 1978;64:1013–20.
15. Reyes AJ. Propranolol and the hyperactive carotid sinus reflex syndrome. Br Med J 1973;2:662.
16. Yusuf S, Peto R, Bennett D, et al. Early intravenous atenolol treatment in suspected acute myocardial infarction. Lancet 1980;2:273–6.
17. ISIS-1 Collaborative Group. Randomised trial of intra-venous atenolol among 16,027 cases of suspected acute myocardial infarction. Lancet 1986;2:57–66.
18. Kirkorian G, Touboul P, Atallah G. Electrophysiological effects of propranolol in intraventricular conduction disturbance. Am J Cardiol 1988;61:341–5.
19. Greenblatt DJ, Koch-Weser J. Adverse reactions with propranolol in hospitalised medical patients. Am Heart J 1973;86:478–84.
20. Gillam PM, Prichard BN. Use of propranolol in angina pectoris. Br Med J 1965;2:337–9.
21. Linkwich JA, Herling JM. Bradycardia and heart failure associated with ocular timolol maleate. Am J Hosp Pharmacol 1981;38:699–701.
22. Norwegian Multi-centre Study Group. Timolol-induced reduction in mortality and re-infarction in patients surviving acute myocardial infarction. N Engl J Med 1981;304:801–7.
23. COMMIT. Early intravenous and oral metoprolol in 45,852 patients with acute myocardial infarctin. Lancet 2005;366:1622–32.
24. Swedberg K. Beta-blockers in worsening heart failure: good or bad? Eur Heart J 2009;30:2177–9.
25. Kohleif M, Isles C. Profound hypotension after atenolol in severe hypertension. Br Med J 1989;298:161–2.

26. Prior JS, Davies PD, Hamilton DV. Blindness and malignant hypertension. Lancet 1979;1:803.
27. Muller ME, van der Velde N, Kruder JW, ven der Cammen TJ. Syncope and falls due to timolol eye-drops. BMJ 2006;332:960–1.
28. Bartsch W, Sponer G, Strein K, et al. Evaluation of the risk for drug-induced postural hypotension in an experimental model: investigations with carvedilol, prazosin, labetalol and guanethidine. J Cardiovasc Pharmacol 1987;10(suppl):S49–51.
29. Dunn CJ, Lea AP, Wagstaff AJ. Carvedilol. A reappraisal of its pharmacological properties and therapeutic use in cardio-vascular disorders. Drugs 1997;54:161–85.
30. Krum H, Conway EL, Broadbear JH, et al. Postural hypotension in elderly patients given carvediolol. BMJ 1994;309:775–6.
31. Medical Research Council Working Party. Adverse reactions to bendrofluazide and propranolol for the treatment of mild hypertension. Lancet 1981;2:539–43.
32. Lennard MS, Silas JH, Freestone S, et al. Oxidation phenotype—a major determinant of metoprolol metabolism and response. N Engl J Med 1982;307:1558–60.
33. Lewis RV, Ramsey LE, Jackson PR, et al. Influence of debrisoquine—oxidation phenotype on exercise tolerance and subjective fatigue after metoprolol and atenolol in healthy subjects. Br J Clin Pharmacol 1991;31:391–8.
34. McLeod AA, Kraus WE, Williams RS. Effects of beta-1 selective and non-selective beta-blockade during exercise conditioning in healthy adults. Am J Cardiol 1984;53:1656–61.
35. Wilmore JH, Ewy GA, Freund BJ, et al. Cardiorespiratory alterations consequent to endurance exercise training during chronic beta-blockade with atenolol and propranolol. Am J Cardiol 1985; 55:D142–8.
36. Wilmore JH, Freund BJ, et al. Beta-blockade and response to exercise: influence of training. Physician Sportsmed 1985;13:60–9.
37. Kaiser P. Physical performance and muscle metabolism during beta-blockade in man. Acta Physiol Scand 1984;526(suppl):1–53.
38. Vanhees L, Defoor JG, Schepers D, et al. Effects of bisoprolol and atenolol on endurance exercise capacity in healthy men. J Hypertens 2000;18:35–43.
39. Brion R, Carre F, Verdier JC, et al. Comparative effects of bisoprolol and nitrendipine on exercise capacity in hypertensive patients with regular physical activity. J Cardiovasc Pharmacol 2000;35:78–83.
40. Roberts DH, Tsao Y, McLaughlin GA, Breckenridge A. Placebo-controlled comparison of captopril, atenolol, labetalol and pindolol in hypertension complicated by intermittent claudication. Lancet 1987;2:650–3.
41. Gonasun L, Langrall H. Adverse reactions to pindolol administration. Am Heart J 1982;104:482–6.

42. Imataka K, Seki A, Takahashi N, et al. Elevation of serum creatine phosphokinase during pinololo treatment. J Jap Soc Int Med 1981;70: 580–5.
43. Tan LB, Burniston JG, Clark WA, et al. Characterisation of adrenoceptors involvement in skeletal and cardiac myotoxicity induced by sympathomimetic agents. J Cardiovasc Pharmacol 2003;41:518–25.
44. Cleroux J, van Nguyen P, Taylor AW, Leenen FH. Long duration exercise with beta-blockade: endurance versus skeletal muscle fibre composition. J Hypertens 1987;5(supp 5):S197–9.
45. Alway SE, Hughson RL, Green HJ, Patla AE. Human tibialis anterior contractile responses following fatiguing exercise with and without beta-blockade. Clin Physiol 1988;8:215–25.
46. Clausen T, Flatman JA. Beta-2 adrenoceptors mediate the stimulating effect of adrenaline on active electronic Na-K-transport in rat soleus muscle. Br J Pharmacol 1980;68:749–55.
47. Kaiser P, Tesch PA, Frisk-Holmerg M, et al. Effect of beta-1 selective and non-selective beta-blockade on work capacity and muscle metabolism. Clin Physiol 1986;6:197–207.
48. Frisk-Holmberg M, Jorfeldt L, Juhlin-Dannfelt A. Metabolic effects in muscle during anti-hypertensive therapy with beta-1 and beta-1/beta-2 adrenoceptor blockers. Clin Pharmacol Ther 1981;30:611–8.
49. Setoguchi S, Higgins JM, Mogan H, et al. Propranolol and the risk of hospitalized myopahty. Am Heart J 2010;159:428–33.
50. Marshall AJ, Roberts CJ, Barritt DW. Raynauds phenomenon as side effects of beta-blockers in hypertension. Br Med J 1976;1:1498–9.
51. Eliasson K, Danilson M, Hylander B, Lindblad LE. Raynaud's phenomenon caused by beta-blockers. Acta Med Scand 1984;215:333–9.
52. Oliván Martinez J, Garcia MJ, Rodriguez Botaro A, et al. Bisoprolol and nifedipine SR in the treatment of hypertension in the elderly. J Cardiovasc Pharmacol 1990;16(suppl 5):S95–9.
53. Gokal R, Dornan TL, Ledingham JG. Peripheral skin necrosis complicating beta-blockade. Br Med J 1979;1:721–2.
54. Warren DJ, McSorley P, Naik RB. Effects of beta-adrenergic blocking drugs on peripheral blood flow (abstract). VIII World Congress of Cardiology, Tokyo, September 17-23, 1978.
55. Solomon SA, Ramsey LE, Yeo WW, et al. Beta-blockade and intermittent claudication. BMJ 1991;303:1100–4.
56. U.K. Prospective Diabetes Study Group. Efficacy of atenolol and captopril in reducing risk of macrovascular and microvascular complications in type 2 diabetes: UKPDS 39. BMJ 1998;317:713–20.
57. Wilkinson R. Beta-blockers and renal function. Drugs 1982;23:195–206.
58. O'Malley K, O'Callagham WG, Laher MS, et al. Beta-adrenoceptor blocking drugs and renal blood flow with special reference to the elderly. Drugs 1983;25(suppl Z):103–7.
59. Schermeister J, Decot M, Hallauer W, Willmann H. Beta-receptoren und renal hamodynamick des menschen. Arzneim Forsch 1966;16:847.

60. Nakamura A, Imaizumi A, Yanagawa Y, et al. Beta-2 adrenoceptor activation attenuates endotoxin-induced acute renal failure. J Am Soc Nephrol 2004;15:316–25.
61. De Leeuw PW, Birkenhager WH. Renal effects of beta-blockade in essential hypertension. Eur Heart J 1983;4(suppl D):13–7.
62. Lameyer LP, Hesse CJ. Metoprolol in high renin hypertension. A comparison with propranolol. Ann Clin Res 1981;13(suppl 30):16–22.
63. Bakris GL, Fonseca V, Katholi RE, et al. Differential effects of beta-blockers on albuminurea in patients with type-2 diabetes. Hypertension 2005;46:1309–15.
64. Kahvecioglu S, Akdag I, Gullulu M, et al. Comparison of higher dose of losartan treatment with losartan plus carvedilol and losartan plus ramipril in patients with glomerulonephritis and proteinuria. Ren Fail 2007;29:169–75.
65. Parrinello G, Paterna S, Torres D, et al. One year renal and cardiac effects of bisoprolol versus losartan in recently diagnosed hypertensive patients. Clin Drug Invest 2009;29:591–600.
66. Zacharias FJ. Long-term clinical experience with atenolol. Royal Society of Medicine, International Congress and Symposium Series N19. 1979, pp 75–91.
67. U.K. Prospective Diabetes Study Group. Tight blood pressure control and risk of macrovascular and microvascular complications in type-2 diabetes: UKPDS 38. BMJ 1998;317:703–13.
68. U.K. Prospective Diabetes Study Group. Efficacy of atenolol and captopril in reducing the risk of macrovascular and microvascular complications in type 2 diabetes; UKPDS 39. BMJ 1998;317:713–20.
69. Penne EL, Neumann J, Klein IH, et al. Sympathetic hyperactivity and clinical outcome in chronic kidney disease patients during standard treatment. J Nephrol 2009;22:208–15.
70. Norris K, Bourgoigne J, Gassman J, et al. Cardiovascular outcomes in the African American Study of Kidney Disease and hypertension (AASK) Trial. Am J Kidney Dis 2006;48:739–51.
71. Agarwal R, Sinha AD. Cardiovascular protection with anti hypertensive drugs in dialysis patients; systematic review and meta-analysis. Hypertension 2009;53:860–6.
72. Ghali JK, Wikstrand J, Van Veldhuisen DJ, et al. The influence of renal function on clinical outcome and response to beta-blockade in systolic heart failure (MERIT-HF). J Card Fail 2009;15:310–8.
73. Khan W, Deepak SM, Coppinger T. Beta-blocker treatment is associated with improvement in renal function and anaemia in patients with heart failure. Heart 2006;92:1856–7.
74. Andeson G, Jariwalla AG, Al-Zaibak M. A comparison of oral metoprolol and propranolol in patients with chronic bronchitis. J Int Med Res 1980;8:136–8.
75. Nordstrom LA, MacDonald F, Gobel FL. Effect of propranolol on respiratory function and exercise-tolerance in patients with chronic obstructive lung disease. Chest 1975;67:287–92.

76. Brooks TW, Greekmore FM, Young DC, et al. Rates of hospitalisations and emergency department visits in patients with asthma and chronic obstructive pulmonary disease taking beta-blockers. Pharmacotherapy 2007;27:684–90.
77. van Gestel YR, Holks SE, Sin DD, et al. Beta-blockers and health-related quality of life in patients with peripheral arterial disease and COPD. Int J Chron Obstr Pulm Dis 2009;4:177–83.
78. van der Woude, Zaagsma J, Postma DS, et al. Detrimental effects of beta-blockers in COPD: a concern for non-selective beta-blockers. Chest 2005;127:818–20.
79. Andrus MR, Holloway KP, Clark DS. Use of beta-blockers in patients with COPD. Ann Pharmacother 2004;38:142–5.
80. Andrus MR, Loyed JV. Use of beta-blockers in older patients with COPD and cardiovascular co-morbidity: safety issues. Drugs Aging 2008;25:131–4.
81. Fraunfelder FT, Barker AF. Respiratory effects of timolol. N Engl J Med 1984;311:1441.
82. Decalmer PB, Chetterjee SS, Cruickshank JM, et al. Beta-blockers and asthma. Br Heart J 1978;40:184–9.
83. Dunn CJ, Lea AP, Wagstaff AJ, Carvedilol. A reappraisal of all its pharmacological properties and therapeutic use in cardiovascular disorders. Drugs 1997;54:161–85.
84. Dorow P, Bethge M, Tonnesmann V. Effects of single oral doses of bisoprolol and atenolol on airways function in non-asthmatic chronic obstructive lung disease and angina pectoris. Eur J Clin Pharmacol 1986;31:143–7.
85. Chatterjee SS. The cardioselective and hypotensive effects of bisoprolol in hypertensive asthmatics. J Cardiovasc Pharmacol 1986;8 (suppl 11):S74–77.
86. Agostoni P, Contini M, Cattadori G, et al. Lung function with carvedilol and bisoprolol in chronic heart failure: is beta selectivity relevant? Eur J Heart Fail 2007;9:827–33.
87. Davis PB, Silski CL, Kercsmar CM, Infeld M. Beta-adrenergic receptors on human tracheal epithelial cells in primary culture. Am J Physiol Cell Physiol 1990;258:C71–6.
88. Kanthakumar K, Cundell DR, Johnson M, et al. Effect of salmeterol on human nasal epithelial cell ciliary beating: inhibition of the ciliotoxin pyocyanin. Br J Pharmacol 1994;112:493–8.
89. Pavia D, Bateman JR, Lennard-Jones AM, et al. Effect of selective and non-selective beta-blockade on pulmonary function and tracheobronchial mucociliary clearance in healthy subjects. Thorax 1986;41:301–5.
90. Dorow P, Weiss T, Felix R, et al. Influence of propranolol, metoprolol and pindolol on mucociliary clearance in patients with coronary heart disease. Respiration 1984;45:286–90.
91. Guzman CA. Exacerbation of bronchorrhea induced by topical timolol. Am Rev Resp Dis 1980;121:899–900.

92. Malm L. Propranolol as cause of watery nasal secretions. Lancet 1981;1:1006.
93. Leopold G, Ungethum W, Pabst J, et al. Pharmacokinetic profile of bisoprolol, a new beta-1 selective beta-blocker. Br J Clin Pharmacol 1986;22:293–300.
94. Berne C, Pollare T, Lithell H. Effects of antihypertensive treatments on insulin sensitivity with special reference to ACE-inhibitors. Diabetes Care 1991;14 (suppl 4):39–47.
95. Nash DT. A comparison of long-term effects of hydrochlorthiazide, propranolol and atenolol on carbohydrate and lipid metabolism. J Cardiopulm Rehabil 1988;8:18–24.
96. Dominguez LJ, Barbagallo M, Jacober SJ, et al. Bisoprolol and captopril effects on insulin receptor tyrosine kinase activity in essential hypertension. Am J Hypertens 1997;10:1349–55.
97. Fogari R, Zoppi A. The clinical benefits of beta-1 selectivity. Rev Contemp Pharmacother 1997;8:45–54.
98. Janka HU, Ziegler AG, Disselhoff G, Mehnert H. Influence of bisoprolol on blood glucose, glycosuria and haemoglobin A-1 in non-insulin dependent diabetics. J Cardiovasc Pharmacol 1986;8(suppl 11):S96–9.
99. Poirier L, Cleroux J, Nadeau A, Lacourciere Y. Effects of nebivolol and atenolol on insulin sensitivity and haemodynamics in hypertensive patients. J Hypertens 2001;19:1429–35.
100. Ehmer B, van der Does R, Rudorf J. Influence of carvedilol on blood glucose and Hb A 1-c in non-insulin-dependent diabetes. Drugs 1988;36(suppl 6):136–40.
101. Lijnen P. Biochemical mechanisms involved in the beta-blocker-induced changes in serum lipoproteins. Am Heart J 1992;124:549–56.
102. Day JL, Metcalf J, Simpson CN. Adrenergic mechanisms in control of plasma lipid concentrations. Br Med J 1982;284:1145–8.
103. Seguchi H, Nekamura H, Aosaki N, et al. Effects of carvedilol on serum lipids in hypertensive and normotensive subjects. Eur J Clin Pharmacol 1990;38(suppl 2):S139–42.
104. Ko DT, Hebert PR, Coffey CS, et al. Beta-blocker therapy and symptoms of depression, fatigue and sexual dysfunction. JAMA 2002;288:351–7.
105. Prince MJ, Bird AS, Blizzard RA, Mann AH. Is the cognitive function of older patients affected by antihypertensive treatment? Results of the MRC trial of hypertension in older adults. BMJ 1996; 312:801–5.
106. Krauseneck T., Padberg F, Roozendaal B, et al. A beta-adrenergic antagonist reduces traumatic memories and post-traumatic stress disorder symptoms in female but not male patients after cardiac surgery. Psychol Med 2010;40:861–9.
107. Fricka G, Lader M. Psychotropic effects of repeated doses of enalapril, propranolol and atenolol in normal subjects. Br J Clin Pharmacol 1988;25:67–73.

108. Madden DJ, Blumenthal JA, Ekelund L-G, et al. Memory performance by mild hypertensives following beta-blockade. Psychopharmacology 1986;89:20–4.
109. Betts TA, Alford C. Beta-blocking drugs and sleep a controlled trial. Drugs 1983;25(suppl 2):268–72.
110. Kostis JB, Rosen RC. Central nervous system effect of beta-blockers: the role of ancilliary properties. Circulation 1987;75:204–12.
111. Bellamy D. Letter to editor. Br Med J 1983;286:1439–40.
112. Yilmaz MB, Erdem, A, Yalta K, et al. Impact of beta-blockers on sleep in patients with mild hypertension. Adv Ther 2008;25:871–83.
113. Hensel J, Pillmann F. Late-life somnambulism after therapy with metoprolol. Clin Neuropharmacol 2008;31:248–50.
114. Fraser HS, Carr AC. Propranolol psychosis. Br J Psychiatr 1976;129:508–9.
115. Patterson JF. Propranolol induced mania. South Med J 1984;77:1603.
116. Salem SA, McDevitt DG. Central effects of single doses of propranolol in man. Br J Clin Pharmacol 1984;17:31–6.
117. Broadhurst AD. The effect of propranolol on human psychomotor performance. Aviat Space Environ Med 1980;51:176–9.
118. Betts TA, Blake A. The psychotropic affects of atenolol in normal subjects. Postgrad Med J 1977;53(suppl 3):151–6.
119. Silvestri A, Galetta P, Cerquetani E, et al. Report of erectile dysfunction after therapy with beta-blockers is related to patient knowledge of side effects and is reversed by placebo. Eur Heart J 2003;24:1928–32.
120. Foroutan SK, Rajabi M. Erectile dysfunction in men with angiographically documented coronary artery disease. Urol J 2007;4:28–32.
121. McVary KT. Erectile dysfunction. N Engl J Med 2007;357:2472–81.
122. Cocco G. Erectile dysfunction after therapy with metoprolol: the Hawthorne Effect. Cardiology 2008;112:174–7.
123. Fogari R, Zoppi A, Poletti L, et al. Sexual activity in hypertensive men treated with valsartan or carvedilol: a cross-over study. Am J Hypertens 2001;14:27–31.
124. Broekman CP, Haensel SM, van den Ven LL, Slob AK. Bisoprolol and hypertension: effects on sexual dysfunction in men. J Sex Marital Ther 1992;18:325–31.
125. Carter BL. Labetalol. New drug evaluations. Drug Intell Clin Pharm 1983;17:704–12.
126. Ohman KP, Asplund J. Labetalol in primary hypertension: a long-term effect and tolerance study. Curr Ther Res 1984;35:277–86.
127. Dargie HJ, Dollery CT, Daniel J. Labetalol in resistant hypertension. Br J Clin Pharmacol 1976;3(suppl 3):751–5.
128. Duncan L, Bateman DN. Sexual function in women. Do antihypertensive drugs have an impact? Drug Saf 1993;8:225–34.
129. el-Sayed MG, el Sayed MT, Elazab A-S, et al. Effects of some beta-blockers on male fertility parameters in rats. Dtsch Tierartzl Wochenschr 1998;105:10–2.

130. Fogari R, Preti P, Derosa G, et al. Effect of antihypertensive treatment with valsartan and atenolol on sexual activity and plasma testosterone in hypertensive men. Eur J Clin Pharmacol 2002;58:177–80.
131. Nurmamedova GS, Gumbatov NB, Muststafaev IF. [Level of hormones of pituitary-gonadal axis, penile blood-flow and sexual function in men with hypertension during mono-therapy with bisoprolol and nebivolol] (Russian). Kardiologiia 2007;47:50–3.
132. Sharma AM, Pischon T, Hardt S, et al. Beta-adrenergic receptor blockers and weight gain. A systematic analysis. Hypertension 2001;37:250–4.
133. Masuo K, Katsuya T, Fu Y, et al. Beta-2 and beta-3 adrenergic receptor polymorphisms are related to the onset of weight gain and blood pressure elevation over 5 years. Circulation 2005;111:3429–34.
134. Lee DS, Shaffer MJ. Low incidence of shivering with chronic propranolol therapy. Lancet 1986;1:500.
135. Messerli FH, Bell DS, Fonseea V, et al. Body weight changes with beta-blocker use: results from GEMINI. Am J Med 2007;120:610–5.
136. Gold MH, Holy AK, Roenigk HH. Beta-blocking drugs and psoriasis. J Am Acad Dermatol 1988;19:837–41.
137. Richards S. Cutaneous side-effects of beta-adrenergic blockers. Aust J Dermatol 1985;26:25–8.
138. Bodmer M, Egger SS, Hohenstein E, et al. Lichenord eruption associated with nebivolol. Ann Pharmacother 2006;40:1688–90.

Index

Note: Page references in *f* and *t* indicate figures and tables, respectively.

A

Acebutolol
  airway function effects, 18*f*, 19
  hemodynamic effects, 14*f*
  neurohumeral effects, 26*f*
Adenosine triphosphate, 3*f*
Adipokinins, 84
Adrenaline
  α-adrenoceptor-stimulating effect, 12
  β-adrenoceptor-stimulating effect, 12
  interaction with β-blockers, 12, 12*f*, 19, 20*f*, 21, 21*f*, 25, 28, 39, 92*f*, 119–120
  in pheochomocytoma, 119–120
  smoking-related secretion, 91, 92*f*, 125
β-Adrenergic receptor kinase, 3
Adrenergic receptors. *See* Adrenoceptors
Adrenoceptors, 1–5
  distribution, 1, 2*t*, 37
  structure, 1, 3
$α_1$-Adrenoceptors, distribution, 1, 2*t*
$α_2$-Adrenoceptors, distribution, 1, 2*t*
β-Adrenoceptors
  alveolar, 9–10
  down-regulation, 3
  inhibition, 4, 4*f*, 5*f*
  stimulation, 4
$β_1$-Adrenoceptors
  distribution, 1, 2*t*
  effector enzyme coupling, 3*f*
  genetic polymorphisms, 4
  genotype CB, 12
  genotype CC, 12
$β_2$-Adrenoceptors
  distribution, 1, 2*t*
  effector enzyme coupling, 3*f*
  genetic polymorphisms, 4, 5
$β_3$-Adrenoceptors
  distribution, 1, 2*t*
  as therapeutic targets, 22
Adverse reactions, to β-blockers, 207–250. *See also under specific β-blockers*
  cardiovascular system-related, 207, 209–220
    bradycardia, 209–211, 209*t*, 210*t*, 211*t*, 238–239
    cold extremities, 207, 209, 210*t*, 213*t*, 214*t*, 215*t*, 218–219, 240
    heart failure, 207, 211–212, 239
    hypotension, 208, 212, 239
  central nervous system-related, 233–234
  cutaneous disorders, 214*t*, 237, 238*t*
  impaired quality of life, 208, 208*f*

Adverse reactions, to β-blockers (*Continued*)
  metabolic disturbances, 24, 112–115, 114*f*, 114*t*, 116*f*, 227–232
  renal function impairment, 220–221, 220*f*, 224*f*, 240
  respiratory system-related, 221, 224–227, 240
  sexual dysfunction, 234–236, 234*t*, 235*f*, 236*t*
  weight gain, 236–237, 237*t*
Airway resistance, 7, 9, 9*f*, 16, 18*f*, 19, 23, 240
Albuminuria, 220, 224*t*
Aldosterone, 10, 11*t*, 19, 24
ALLHAT (Antihypertensive and Lipid-Lowering Treatment to Prevent Heart Attack Trial), 109, 109*t*, 115–116, 116*f*, 192, 193*t*, 199
Alpha-blockade
  antiarrhythmic activity, 163–164
  contraindication as heart failure treatment, 198
Alprenolol
  hemodynamic effects, 14*f*
  in myocardial infarction patients, 52, 55*f*
  neurohumeral effects, 26*f*
Alveolar permeability, 38, 225–226, 240
Amiodarone, antiarrhythmic activity, 66–67, 162
  in atrial fibrillation, 149, 150*t*
Amlodipine
  antihypertensive activity
    comparison with bisoprolol, 121–122, 122*t*, 123*f*
    comparison with fixed, low-dose β-blockers, 110, 111*f*
    in elderly patients, 98, 101*t*
    systolic blood pressure effects, 97
  as heart failure prophylaxis, 192, 193*f*, 193*t*
  pro-atherogenic activity, 71, 72*f*
  as syndrome X treatment, 58
Anesthesia, as ventricular arrhythmia cause, 160, 161*t*
Aneurysms, aortic, 67–68, 68*t*, 74
Angina. *See also* Myocardial ischemia
  β-blocker treatment for, 51, 56–58, 57*f*, 209, 211*t*
Angiotensin, 10, 11*t*
Angiotensin-converting enzyme inhibitors (ACEIs)
  as atrial fibrillation prophylaxis, 148, 148*t*
  as cardiac fibrosis treatment, 194
  comparison with atenolol, 231
  C-reactive protein level effects, 70, 70*f*
  in diabetic patients
    as heart failure prophylaxis, 93–94, 94*f*
    as peripheral arterial disease prophylaxis, 93–94, 94*f*
    as stroke prophylaxis, 93–94, 94*f*
  as heart failure treatment, 189, 198
  as left ventricular hypertrophy treatment, 195
  as myocardial infarction prophylaxis, 117*t*
  quality of life effects, 208, 208*f*
  renal effects, 220
  therapeutic guidelines for, 82
  U.K. NICE Committee recommendations regarding, 116, 118–119
Angiotensin II, 10, 11*t*, 85
Angiotensin receptor blockers (ARBs)
  as atrial fibrillation prophylaxis, 148, 148*t*
  C-reactive protein level effects, 70, 70*f*

ineffectiveness as myocardial infarction prophylaxis, 115–116, 117t, 118f
U.K. NICE Committee recommendations regarding, 116, 118–119
Anglo-Scandinavian Cardiac Output Trial (ASCOT), 97, 100, 101t
Antiarrhythmic activity, of β-blockers
  with $β_1$-blockade, 162, 165
  with $β_2$-blockade, 162, 165
  with α-β-blockade, 163–164, 165
  with intrinsic sympathomimetic activity, 162–163
  in supraventricular arrhythmias, 143–154, 164
  in ventricular arrhythmias, 155–162
    catecholaminergic mono-/polymorphic ventricular tachycardia, 162
    digitalis toxicity-related, 158, 165
    hypertrophic obstructive cardiomyopathy, 160, 165
    idiopathic arrhythmia, 155–156
    intraoperative, 160, 161t
    long QT syndrome, 159–160, 165
    mitral valve prolapse-related, 158–159, 165
    pacemaker-induced arrhythmia, 160
    post-myocardial infarction, 155, 156–158, 165
  in ventricular fibrillation, 85, 89f
    defibrillation-refractory, 155t
    digitalis toxicity-related, 155t
    exercise-induced, in children, 156
    mitral valve prolapse-related, 159
    post-myocardial infarction, 156–157
    stress-induced, in children, 156
    as sudden death cause, 155
    sympathomimetic amines-related, 155t
    threshold for, 141
  in ventricular tachycardia
    digitalis toxicity, 155t
    exercise-induced, 155, 155t
    long QT syndrome, 156t
    sustained, 155, 155t
Antiarrhythmic drugs. *See also names of specific drugs*
  action mechanism, 141, 164
  action site, 143t
  classification, 141–142, 142t, 164
Antiatherogenic activity, of β-blockers, 68–72, 70f, 72f, 74
Antihypertensive activity, of β-blockers
  AB/CD rule for, 82
  age factors in, 15, 16f
  as $β_2$-blockade, 126
  as bradycardia cause, 209, 210t
  disadvantages, 81–82
  efficacy, 121–126
    in elderly patients, 124–125, 125f
    in young/middle-aged patients, 121–124, 122f, 122t, 123f, 124f
  in elderly patients, 96–107
    central (aortic) hemodynamic effects, 100, 105f, 124, 125
    in coronary artery disease, 98–101, 100f, 102f
    effect on left ventricular hypertrophy, 102, 105, 106f, 107
    efficacy of, 124–125, 125f
    as first-line therapy, 96–107, 98–100, 100f, 101t, 102f

Antihypertensive activity, of
β-blockers (*Continued*)
  as fixed, low-dose β-blocker/
    diuretics combination, 110–
    112, 111*f*, 112*f*
  interaction with smoking, 107,
    107*f*
  J-curve phenomenon in,
    98–100, 100*f*, 102*f*, 104*t*
  as second-line therapy, 108–
    112, 113*f*
  without coronary artery disease, 98, 101*t*
  as first-line therapy, 88–99, 89*t*,
    96–107, 100*f*, 101*t*, 102*f*
  guidelines for, 81–82
  as heart failure prophylaxis,
    191–196
  in hemodialysis patients, 119
  interaction with smoking, 88–93,
    90*f*, 91*f*, 92*f*, 107, 107*f*
  with intrinsic sympathomimetic
    activity, 22–23, 23*f*
  of nonselective β-blockers, 13, 15
  in obese diabetic patients, 93–94
  of partial beta$_1$-selective
    β-blockers, 13, 15
  pharmacodynamics of, 13,
    15–16, 16*f*, 17*f*
  in pregnancy-related hypertension, 120–121, 120*f*
  racial factors in, 15–16, 17*f*
  in renal failure patients, 119
  in secondary hypertension,
    119–121
  smoking-related impairment of,
    90–93, 90*f*, 91*f*, 92*f*, 107*f*,
    125–126
  in young/middle-aged patients,
    84–96, 121–124, 122*f*, 122*t*,
    123*f*, 124*f*
  efficacy of, 121–124, 122*f*,
    122*t*, 123*f*, 124*f*
  inflammatory mechanism,
    84–88, 88*f*, 89*f*
  smoking-related impairment
    of, 90–93, 90*f*, 91*f*, 92*f*

Antihypertensive and Lipid-
  Lowering Treatment to Prevent
  Heart Attack Trial (ALLHAT),
  109, 109*t*, 115–116, 116*f*, 192,
  193*t*, 199
Arginine, 125, 183
Arrhythmia. *See also*
  Antiarrhythmic activity,
  of β-blockers
  β-blocker-related, 238
ASCOT (Anglo-Scandinavian
  Cardiac Output Trial), 97, 100,
  101*t*
Asthma, β-blocker use in, 224–
  225, 226, 226*f*
  in heart failure patients, 190
Atenolol
  absorption and bioavailability,
    30*t*, 31
  adverse reactions to
    cardiovascular, 209, 211,
      211*t*
    cold extremities, 215*t*,
      219–220
    exercise tolerance impairment,
      215, 216*t*
    fatigue, 212, 215*t*
    psoriasis, 238*t*
    sexual dysfunction, 235–236,
      236*f*
    sleep disturbances, 233
  airway function effects, 7, 9, 9*f*,
    18*f*, 19
  as angina treatment, 58
  antiarrhythmic activity, 162
    in paroxysmal supraventricular tachycardia, 144
    in pediatric ventricular tachycardia, 155
    in post-myocardial infarction
      ventricular antiarrhythmia,
      156, 157
    in supraventricular tachycardia, 153, 153*f*
  antihypertensive activity, 15, 15*f*
    central (aortic) hemodynamic
      effects, 100, 105*f*, 124, 125

in combination with diuretics, 93–94, 94f, 108, 108t, 113, 114f
  comparison with bisoprolol, 121, 122f
  comparison with propranolol, 121
  effect of adrenaline on, 21, 21f
  effect on augmentation index, 125f
  in elderly patients, 98, 100, 101t, 102, 105–107
  as heart failure prophylaxis, 93–94, 94f, 191, 192t
  in pregnancy-related hypertension, 120–121, 120f
  racial factors in, 15
  systolic blood pressure effects, 97
 in asthmatic patients, 224, 225
 as atrial fibrillation prophylaxis, 148
 β_1-/β_2-selectivity ratios, 5, 6f
 brain concentration, 31, 33f, 233
 in combination with diuretics, 93–94, 94f
   in diabetic patients, 113, 114f
   in elderly patients, 108, 108t
   as second-line therapy, 108, 108t
 in combination with nifedipine, 109–110
 in diabetic patients, 220
 drug interactions, 31
 hemodynamic effects, 13, 14f
 hepatic metabolism, 32
 in intermittent claudication patients, 24f, 27
 left ventricular hypertrophy effects, 102, 105, 107
 as left ventricular hypertrophy treatment, 105, 107, 195–196, 196f
 metabolic disturbances associated with, 11f, 19, 232
 mucociliary action, 226
 in myocardial infarction patients, 50, 51f, 52f, 54f
 as myocardial ischemia treatment, 61
 neurohumeral effects, 10, 20f, 25, 26f
 as peripheral arterial disease treatment, 62, 65f
 pharmacokinetic profile, 30t
 quality of life effects, 208, 208f
 renal effects, 220, 223f
 renal elimination, 31, 34f
 as silent myocardial ischemia treatment, 58, 59f, 73
 as syndrome X treatment, 58
 water-solubility, 29, 31t
Atheromatous process
 effect of β-blockers on, 68–72, 72f, 74
 inflammatory mechanisms, 85
Atrial fibrillation, 147–152
 β-blocker prophylaxis and treatment for, 162–163
 electroconversion treatment for, 149, 149t
 heart failure-related, 151–152, 151f, 152t, 181, 182f
 paroxysmal, 148, 164
 post-coronary artery bypass grafting, 66–67, 149–150, 150t
 post-myocardial infarction, 153
 propranolol treatment for, 146t
 sustained, 149
Atrial flutter, 145t, 146t, 152t
Atrial natriuretic peptide (ANP), 11–12, 20, 28

B

Bendrofluazide, antihypertensive activity of
 comparison with bisoprolol, 121, 122t, 123f
 comparison with propranolol, 90f, 96t, 214t
BEST (Beta-blocker Evaluation of Survival Trial), 178f, 180t, 182

Beta$_1$-blockade, in young/middle-aged diastolic hypertension patients, 121–124, 122*f*, 123*f*, 124*f*
Beta$_2$-blockade
  as bronchospasm cause, 198
  contraindication as heart failure treatment, 198
Beta-blocker(s). *See also names of specific β-blockers*
  development of, 50
  with intrinsic sympathomimetic activity
    as angina treatment, 58
    antiarrhythmic activity, 162–163, 165
    contraindication as heart failure treatment, 180*t*, 196
    as myocardial infarction treatment, 52–53, 55*f*, 73
    as myocardial ischemia treatment, 58, 59*f*
    pharmacodynamics, 22–26
  lipophilic, brain concentrations of, 233
  sudden perioperative withdrawal of, 65
  vasodilatory, 24*f*
    as peripheral vascular disease treatment, 62
  without intrinsic sympathomimetic activity
    as angina treatment, 56, 57*f*
    as heart failure treatment, 180*t*, 196, 198
Beta-blocker Heart Attack Trial (BHAT), 156–157, 158*f*, 178*f*
Beta$_1$-selective β-blockers, antihypertensive activity of, 13, 15
Betaxolol, 5, 6*f*, 150
BHAT (Beta-blocker Heart Attack Trial), 156–157, 158*f*, 178*f*
Bisoprolol
  absorption and bioavailability, 30*t*, 31
  adverse reactions to
    comparison with nifedipine, 219, 219*t*
    sexual dysfunction, 235–236, 236*f*
  airway function effects, 7, 9, 9*f*, 19
  alveolar permeability effects, 28
  as angina treatment, 56
  antiarrhythmic activity, 141, 162
    in atrial fibrillation, 148, 149, 149*t*, 150, 150*t*
  antihypertensive activity, 13, 15, 15*f*, 38
    in combination with hydrochlorothiazide, 110, 111*f*, 112*f*
    comparison with amlodipine, 121–122, 122*t*, 123*f*
    comparison with atenolol, 121, 122*f*
    comparison with bendrofluazide, 121, 122*t*, 123*f*
    comparison with doxazosin, 121, 122*t*, 123*f*
    comparison with linisopril, 121, 122*t*, 123*f*
    comparison with losartan, 121–122, 123*f*
    fixed, low-dose, 110, 111*f*, 112*f*
    neurological changes associated with, 15*f*, 22–23
    in smokers, 121, 122*f*, 126
    in young/middle-aged patients, 121–124, 122*f*, 123*f*, 124*f*
  exercise tolerance effects, 215, 216*t*
  as heart failure treatment, 176, 178, 178*t*, 179, 180*t*, 181–182, 184*f*, 185–186, 190, 196, 198
    comparison with enalapril, 184, 184*f*
    in end-stage heart failure, 187–188, 188*f*
  respiratory effects, 225

hemodynamic effects, 5, 7, 8t, 13
high $β_1$-selectivity ratio, 5, 7–12
in idiopathic dilated cardiomyopathy, 174
interaction with
  adrenaline, 92f
  losartan, 7, 8t
  natriuretic peptides, 11–12
as left ventricular hypertrophy treatment, 105, 106f, 196, 197f
metabolic disturbances associated with
  blood glucose changes, 229, 230t, 231f
  blood lipid level changes, 10, 11f, 230t, 232
  insulin sensitivity, 229, 230t
as myocardial ischemia treatment, 61, 61f
in silent myocardial ischemia, 58–59, 60f, 73
neurohumeral effects, 10, 11t
as peripheral arterial disease treatment
  in coronary artery bypass graft surgery patients, 66–67
  in noncardiac surgery patients, 62, 63–65, 63f, 65f, 66f
pharmacokinetic profile, 30t
pulmonary effects, 10, 10t
renal/hepatic elimination, 32, 35f, 36
renoprotective effects, 124, 221, 222t, 223f
in respiratory disorder patients, 225, 225f, 226f
as weight loss cause, 236–237, 237t
Black, James, 50
α-Blockade
  antiarrhythmic activity, 163–164
  contraindication as heart failure treatment, 198
$β_1$-Blockade, in young/middle-aged patients, 121–124, 122f, 123f, 124f

$β_2$-Blockade
  as bronchospasm cause, 198
  contraindication as heart failure treatment, 198
Blood-brain barrier, 31
Blood flow
  arterial, in atheromatous plaque formation, 68, 69f, 70–71, 71t
  muscular, 7, 13, 22, 26–27
  renal, 220, 220f
Blood glucose levels. *See also* Hyperglycemia; Hypoglycemia
  β-blocker-related changes in, 227, 228–231, 229, 241
  effect of $β_2$-blockade on, 19
Bopindolol, 22
Bradycardia, β-blocker-related, 97, 207, 209–211, 209t, 210t, 211t, 238–239
Brain natriuretic peptide (BNP), 11–12, 20, 28
British Hypertension Society, 82
Bronchospasm, 28, 198
Bucindolol
  contraindication as heart failure treatment, 180t, 196
  as systolic heart failure treatment, 179f, 180t, 181–182

C
CAFE (Conduit Artery Function Evaluation) substudy, 100
Calcium antagonists
  as atrial fibrillation prophylaxis, 148, 148t
  C-reactive protein level effects, 70, 70f
  ineffectiveness as myocardial infarction prophylaxis, 116
Calcium antagonists/β-blocker combinations, as first-line therapy, 108–110
CAMELOT (Comparison of Amlodipine to Enalapril to Limit Occurrences of Thrombosis) study, 72f

Candesartan, 189
Candesartan in Heart Failure-Failure Assessment of Reduction in Mortality and Morbidity (CHARM) program, 189
CAPRICORN (Carvedilol Post-Infarction Survival Control) study, 183
Captopril
  antihypertensive activity
    in combination with diuretics, 93–94, 94f
    as heart failure prophylaxis, 93–94, 94f, 191, 192t
  atheromatous plaque formation effects, 71t
  comparison with atenolol, 113, 114f
  in diabetic patients, 220
  insulin sensitivity and, 229
  as left ventricular hypertrophy treatment, 105, 107
  quality of life effects, 208, 208f
Cardiac Insufficiency Bisoprolol Study (CIBIS), 179, 180t, 181, 184, 184f
Cardiac output
  effect of β-blockers on, 7, 8t, 13, 14f, 22
  effect of nonselective β/α-blockers on, 26, 27f
  in hypertension, 83, 86f
Cardiac surgery patients, β-blocker treatment in, 66–67
Cardiomyopathy
  arrhythmogenic right, 162
  hypertrophic obstructive, 153
  idiopathic dilated, 173–174, 178
Cardiovascular system, effect of β-blockers on, 207, 209–220
  bradycardia, 209–211, 209t, 210t, 211t, 238–24
  cold extremities, 207, 209, 210t, 213t, 214t, 215t, 218–219, 240
  heart failure, 207, 211–212, 239
  hypotension, 208, 212, 239

Carvedilol
  adverse reactions to
    bronchospasm, 28
    hypertension, 212
    respiratory disorders, 225
    sexual dysfunction, 235, 236f
    syncope, 27
  alveolar permeability effects, 28
  antiarrhythmic activity
    in atrial fibrillation, 150
    in post-CABG atrial fibrillation, 163
    in post-myocardial infarction arrhythmias, 156, 164
  body weight and, 236–237, 237t
  as heart failure treatment, 179, 179f, 180t, 181, 183–184, 196, 198
    in end-stage heart failure, 187–188
    respiratory effects, 225–226
  lipid level effects, 232
  neurohumeral effects, 28
  pharmacokinetic profile, 30t
  pharmacology, 26
  pulmonary effects, 10, 10t
  renal effects, 220
Carvedilol Or Metoprolol European Trial (COMET), 183–184
Carvedilol Post-Infarction Survival Control (CAPRICORN) study, 183
Catecholaminergic mono-/polymorphic ventricular tachycardia, 162
Catecholamines, plasma concentration of, 4, 4f, 5f, 19, 20f, 24, 28
Celiprolol, 22, 124
Central nervous system disorders, β-blocker–related, 233–234, 241
CHARM (Candesartan in Heart Failure-Failure Assessment of Reduction in Mortality and Morbidity) program, 189

Children
  arrhythmia treatment in, 144, 147, 147t
  catecholaminergic mono-/polymorphic ventricular tachycardia in, 162
  ectopic supraventricular arrhythmia treatment in, 143
  exercise-induced ventricular tachycardia in, 155
  heart failure treatment in, 183
  stress-induced ventricular fibrillation in, 156
  ventricular fibrillation in, 156
Chlorthalidone, 17f, 109, 109t
  comparison with angiotensin-converting enzyme inhibitors, 116f
Cholesterol levels, effect of β-blockers on, 230t, 231–232
Chronic obstructive pulmonary disease (COPD), 221, 224, 225, 225f, 240
CIBIS (Cardiac Insufficiency Bisoprolol Study), 179, 180t, 181, 184, 184f, 184f
Cimetidine, 31
Cirrhosis, 34f, 35f
Claudication, intermittent, 7, 13, 22, 24f, 27, 216–217
Clenbuterol, 187–188, 188f
Clonidine, 105, 107, 182
Clopidogrel and Metoprolol in Myocardial Infarction Trial (COMMIT), 156
Cognitive function, 233, 241
Cold extremities, 207, 209, 210t, 213t, 214t, 215t, 218–219, 232–233, 234
COMET (Carvedilol Or Metoprolol European Trial), 183–184
COMMIT (Clopidogrel and Metoprolol in Myocardial Infarction Trial), 50, 52, 156, 190, 211–212

Comparison of Amlodipine to Enalapril to Limit Occurrences of Thrombosis (CAMELOT) study, 72f
Conduit Artery Function Evaluation (CAFE), 100
COPERNICUS (Carvedilol Prospective Randomized Cumulative Survival) Trial, 180t, 181
Coronary artery bypass graft surgery patients
  atrial fibrillation in, 149–150, 150t
  $β_1$-blockade in, 66–67
  ventricular arrhythmia in, 161t
Coronary artery disease
  antihypertensive therapy in, 98–101, 100f, 102f
  as heart failure cause, 173, 198–199
C-reactive protein, 68, 70, 70f, 84, 88f
Creatinine phosphokinase, 216, 216f
Creatinine phosphokinase-MB, 195
Cutaneous disorders, 214t, 237, 238t

D

DECREASE (Dutch Echocardiographic Cardiac Risk Evaluation Applying Stress Echo) studies, 62, 63–65, 63f, 66t
Depression, 233
Dermatologic disorders, 214t, 237, 238t, 241
Diabetes mellitus
  albuminuria in, 220, 224t
  antihypertensive therapy in
    as heart failure prophylaxis, 191, 192t
    in obese patients, 93–94
  β-blocker-induced hypertension in, 21

Diabetes mellitus (*Continued*)
　diuretic/β-blocker-induced, 113–115, 114*f*
　diuretic/β-blocker therapy in, 113–115, 114*f*
　obesity-related, 83
　peripheral arterial disease associated with, 220
　sympathetic nerve activity in, 83, 87*f*
　tight hypertension control in, 93–94, 93*f*, 94*f*
Diazepam, 31
Diazoxide, 27*f*
Digitalis toxicity, 158
Digoxin
　as atrial fibrillation treatment, 149, 151–152
　　in heart failure patients, 151*f*
　as heart failure treatment, 181, 182*f*
　toxicity, 144
Dilevalol, 124–125
Diltiazem
　as left ventricular hypertrophy treatment, 105, 107
　as syndrome X treatment, 58
Disopyramide, 160
Diuretics. *See also names of specific diuretics*
　co-administration with β-blockers, 241
　C-reactive protein level effects, 70, 70*f*
　in elderly patients, 98, 101*t*
　ineffectiveness as myocardial infarction prophylaxis, 116, 116*f*
　metabolic disturbances associated with, 112–113
　as stroke prophylaxis, 95–96
　　as first-line therapy, 108–109, 108*t*, 109*t*
Diuretics/β-blocker combinations
　as diabetes mellitus cause, 113–115, 114*f*
　as first-line therapy, 108–110, 108*t*, 109*t*, 110*f*
　fixed, low-dose, 110–112, 111*f*
　as heart failure prophylaxis, 192, 193*f*, 193*t*
　metabolic disturbances associated with, 112–115, 114*f*, 114*t*, 116*f*
Dizziness, 209, 210*t*
Doxazosin, 109
　cardiac apoptosis effects, 198
　comparison with bisoprolol, 121, 122*t*, 123*f*
　as heart failure prophylaxis, 193*t*
　in ventricular fibrillation, 163
Drug metabolism phenotypes, 36, 37*f*
Dutch Echocardiographic Cardiac Risk Evaluation Applying Stress Echo (DECREASE) studies, 62, 63–65, 63*f*, 66*t*

E
Edema, pulmonary, 9–10, 119, 211
Ejection fraction, effect of bisoprolol on, 8*t*
Elderly patients
　drug clearance in, 32, 36, 36*f*
　systolic hypertension in
　　β-blocker treatment for, 96–107
　　enalapril treatment for, 124
　　hemodynamics of, 97–98, 98*f*, 99*f*
Enalapril, 208, 208*f*
　antihypertensive activity
　　central (aortic) hemodynamic effects, 124
　　comparison with fixed, low-dose β-blockers, 110, 111*f*
　　in elderly patients, 124
　as heart failure treatment, 198
　　comparison with bisoprolol, 184, 184*f*

as left ventricular hypertrophy treatment, 196, 197f
pro-atherogenic activity, 71, 72f
Epinephrine. *See* Adrenaline
ESH/ESC (European Society of Hypertension/European Society of Cardiology) Guidelines, for hypertension management, 82
Estrogen-receptor stimulation, 22
European Society of Hypertension/European Society of Cardiology (ESH/ESC) Guidelines, for hypertension management, 82
Exercise tolerance, β-blocker-related impairment, 215, 216–217, 216t, 217f

F

Fatigue, β-blocker-related, 207, 209, 210t, 212, 214t, 215–218, 215t, 238–239
Flubastin, 63–64, 66f
Fractures, 109, 110f
Framingham Heart Study, 82–83, 83t, 158–159, 194t
Frusimide, 31

G

Genetic polymorphisms, 4–5, 5f
drug metabolism phenotypes, 36, 37f
Glomerular filtration rate (GFR), 220
Glyceryl trinitrate, 56, 57f, 73
G-proteins, 3
Guanine nucleotide triphosphate, 3

H

Hallucinations, 233, 234
Halothane, 160
HAPPHY (Heart Attack Primary Prevention in Hypertension), 88–89
Hawthorne effect, 234, 235f

Head injury patients
atenolol therapy in, 185, 186f
supraventricular tachycardia in, 153, 153f, 164
Heart Attack Primary Prevention in Hypertension (HAPPHY), 88–89
Heart block, 190, 211, 239
Heart failure, 173–206
angiotensin-converting enzyme inhibitor treatment for, 181
atrial fibrillation associated with, 151–152, 151f, 162–163
β-blocker-related, 207, 211–212, 238–39
β-blocker treatment/prophylaxis for, 10, 10t, 11, 11t, 12, 190–196, 192t, 193f, 193t, 194f, 194t, 195f, 196f, 199, 212
action mechanisms, 185–187, 186f, 187f
contraindications to, 189–190
in diabetic patients, 93–94, 94f
effect on left ventricular hypertrophy, 194, 194f
in end-stage heart failure, 187–188, 188f
with intrinsic sympathomimetic activity, 181–183, 182f
without intrinsic sympathomimetic activity, 179–181, 183–187
in women, 181
diastolic, 188–189
angiotensin-converting enzyme inhibitor treatment for, 189
β-blocker treatment for, 189, 189t
left ventricular hypertrophy-related, 195, 196f
pathophysiology, 175–176, 175t, 177t
gender differences, 173, 174f

Heart failure (*Continued*)
  in hypertensive patients, development of, 195*f*
  incidence, 173, 174*f*
  lung function in, 1*f*, 10
  systolic
    β-blocker treatment for, 176, 178–187, 196, 198
    pathophysiology, 173–176, 175*t*, 177*t*
  in women, 181
Heart malformations, 121
Heart rate. *See also* Bradycardia
  effect of β-blockers on, 4*f*, 5, 11*f*, 22, 23*f*, 38
    with intrinsic sympathomimetic activity, 14*f*
    nonselective β-blockers, 13, 14*f*
    selective β-blockers, 13, 14*f*
  in hypertension, 83, 86*f*
Heart transplantation, 187, 188
Hemodialysis patients, antihypertensive therapy in, 119
Hemoglobin$_{A1C}$, 113, 229, 230*t*, 231, 231*f*, 241
HEP (Hypertension in Primary Care) study, 101*t*
High-density lipoprotein (HDL), 232, 232*f*
HINT (Holland Interuniversity Nifedipine Trial), 61
HOT (Hypertension Optimal Treatment) study, 99, 103*t*, 104*t*
Hydralazine
  atheromatous plaque formation effects, 70–71, 71*t*
  in combination with propranolol, 27*f*
Hydrochlorothiazide, 229
  in combination with atenolol, 109–110
  as first-line therapy, 109–110
  as left ventricular hypertrophy treatment, 105, 107
  metabolic disturbances associated with, 112–113

Hyperactive carotid sinus reflex syndrome, 211
Hyperglycemia, 229, 230*t*, 231, 231*f*
Hypertension, 81–140. *See also* Antihypertensive activity, of β-blockers
  as cardiovascular disease risk factor, 81
  C-reactive protein levels in, 70
  essential, 81
  Gly/Gly genotype in, 5
  as heart failure risk factor, 198–199
  hypoglycemia-related, 228–229, 241
  obesity-related, 82–88, 83*t*, 84*f*, 85*f*, 86*f*
  primary, pathophysiology of, 82–84, 83*t*, 84*f*
  smoking-related, 82–83
  systolic, pulse pressure in, 97–98, 98*f*, 99*f*
Hypertension in Primary Care (HEP) study, 101*t*
Hypertension Optimal Treatment (HOT) study, 99, 103*t*, 104*t*
Hypertensive crises, 27, 29*f*, 119–120
Hypoglycemia
  fetal, 121
  insulin-independent, 228–229, 228*f*, 229*f*, 241
Hypotension
  β-blocker-related, 208, 212, 239
  in heart failure patients, 190

I

Ibesartan, 105, 105*f*
ICI 118, 551, 38, 121, 126, 185–186, 216, 226
Impotence. *See* Sexual dysfunction
Inderal, 147*f*
INSIGHT (International Nifedipine GITS Study: Intervention as a Goal in Hypertension Treatment), 109–110

Insulin resistance, 19, 84, 88*f*, 89*f*
Insulin sensitivity, 229, 241
Interleukin-6, 84, 88*f*
International Nifedipine GITS Study: Intervention as a Goal in Hypertension Treatment (INSIGHT), 109–110
International Prospective Primary Prevention Study in Hypertension (IPPSH), 88–89, 89*t*, 90, 91*f*, 94–95, 95*t*
International Study of Infarct Survival (ISIS-1), 50, 156, 211
International Verapamil/ Trandolopril Study (INVEST), 98–99, 100*f*
Intrinsic sympathomimetic activity (ISA), 4, 4*f*, 5*f*, 22–26. See also under specific β-blockers
INVEST (International Verapamil/ Trandolopril Study), 98–99, 100*f*
IPPPSH (The International Prospective Primary Prevention Study in Hypertension), 88–89, 89*t*, 90, 91*f*, 94–95, 95*t*
Ischemic heart disease. See also Myocardial ischemia
C-reactive protein levels in, 70
ISIS-1 (First International Study of Infarct Survival), 50, 156, 211

J

J-curve phenomenon, 98–100, 100*f*, 102*f*, 104*t*

L

Labetalol
adverse reactions to, 27
bronchospasm, 28
hypertension, 212
in intermittent claudication, 216–217
metabolic disturbances, 28
myotoxicity, 216–217
scalp tingling, 237
sexual dysfunction, 235
antihypertensive activity, 27, 27*f*
in intermittent claudication, 24*f*
hemodynamic effects, 26–27, 27*f*
interaction with adrenaline, 28, 29*f*
neurohumeral effects, 28
as peripheral arterial disease treatment, 62
pharmacokinetic profile, 30*t*
pharmacology, 26–29
Left ventricular hypertrophy, 85, 192, 194–196
β-blocker-related reversal of, 195–196, 196*f*, 197*f*, 199
age factors in, 102–105, 106*f*, 107
noradrenaline in, 194, 194*f*
relationship to heart failure, 192, 194*t*, 195, 195*f*
Left ventricular remodeling, post-myocardial infarction, 173, 174*f*, 176*f*
Leptin, 84–85, 89*f*
LIFE (Losartan Intervention for Endpoint Reduction), 98, 101*t*, 105, 107, 148
Life Satisfaction Questionnaire, 208*f*
Lipids, plasma levels of
effect of β_2-blockade on, 19
effect of β-blockers on, 10, 11*f*, 230*t*, 231–232, 232*f*
Lipid solubility (lipophilicity), 29, 30*t*, 31, 39
Lisinopril
antihypertensive activity, 116*f*, 122*t*
comparison with bisoprolol, 121, 122*t*, 123*f*
in young/middle-aged patients, 122*t*
in combination with β-blockers, 192, 193*f*, 193*t*
as heart failure prophylaxis, 192, 193*f*, 193*t*
Liver failure, 32, 40

Long QT syndrome, 159–160, 159f, 162
Losartan
  antihypertensive activity, 7, 8t2
    in combination with diuretics, 110, 112
    comparison with bisoprolol, 121–122, 123f, 124
    in elderly patients, 98, 101t
    in young/middle-aged patients, 124
  as atrial fibrillation prophylaxis, 148
  interaction with bisoprolol, 7, 8t
  renal effects, 222t, 223f
Losartan Intervention for Endpoint Reduction (LIFE), 98, 101t, 105, 107, 148
Low birth weight, 120

M

MAPHY (Metoprolol in Patients with Hypertension), 88–89, 89t, 90, 91f
Marfan's syndrome, 67, 68
Mean arterial pressure (MAP), 14f
Medical Research Council (MRC) mild hypertension study, 88–89, 89t, 90, 90f, 91, 91f, 94–96, 95f, 95t, 96t, 101t, 109, 212, 213t, 214t, 224, 233, 235, 237
Medical Research Council (MRC) trial of treatment of hypertension in older adults, 101t, 107, 107f, 108–109, 108t
Memory loss, 233
Mepindolol, 11f, 232
MERIT (Metoprolol Randomized Intervention Trial), 180t, 181, 184, 221
Metabolic disturbances, β-blocker-related, 39, 227–232, 241
  $β_2$-blockade-related, 2t
  diuretics/β-blocker combinations-related, 112–115, 114f, 114t, 116f, 227
  intrinsic sympathomimetic activity-related, 24
Metabolic syndrome, 82, 83, 87f, 115, 116f
Methyldopa, 208
Metoprolol
  absorption and bioavailability, 30t, 31
  adverse reactions to
    fatigue, 212, 215
    memory loss, 233
    psoriasis, 238t
    respiratory disorders, 225
    sexual dysfunction, 234–235, 236
    sleep disturbances, 233
  airway function effects, 18f, 19
  antiarrhythmic activity
    in paroxysmal supraventricular tachycardia, 144
    in post-CABG atrial fibrillation, 163
    in post-myocardial infarction ventricular arrhythmia, 156
    in supraventricular arrhythmias, 145t
  antihypertensive activity
    effect of adrenaline on, 21, 21f
    interaction with smoking, 89, 90, 91f, 92f
    racial factors in, 15
  atheromatous plaque formation effects, 71t
  $β_1$-/$β_2$-selectivity ratios, 5, 6f
  brain concentration, 31, 33f, 233
  drug interactions, 31, 33f
  as heart failure treatment, 180t, 196, 198
  hemodynamic effects, 13, 14f
  hepatic metabolism, 32, 34f
  interaction with smoking, 89, 90, 91f, 92f, 107

as left ventricular hypertrophy treatment, 195–196
lipid solubility (lipophilicity), 29, 30t, 31
metabolic disturbances associated with, 19
metabolism, 36, 37f
mucociliary action, 226
in myocardial infarction patients, 50, 52, 52f, 54f, 55f
adverse cardiovascular reactions to, 211–212
as myocardial ischemia treatment, 61
in silent myocardial ischemia, 58–59
neurohumeral effects, 20, 20f, 25, 26f
as peripheral arterial disease treatment, 62–63, 64–65, 64f, 65f, 74
pharmacokinetic profile, 30t
poor metabolizers of, 212, 215
renal effects, 220
as systolic heart failure treatment, 179, 179f, 180t, 181–183
as weight loss cause, 236–237, 237t
Metoprolol in Acute Myocardial Infarction (MIAMI), 50, 156
Metoprolol in Patients with Hypertension (MAPHY), 88–89, 89t, 90, 91f
Metoprolol Randomized Intervention Trial (MERIT), 180t, 181, 184, 221
MIAMI (Metoprolol in Acute Myocardial Infarction), 50, 156
Mitral valve prolapse, as ventricular arrhythmia cause, 158–159
Motor performance impairment, 234
Mucociliary action, 213t, 226–227, 227f, 240
Muscle, effect of β-blockers on, 216–218, 239

Myocardial infarction
angiotensin-receptor blocker prophylaxis for, 115–116, 117t, 118f
atheromatous plaque rupture-related, 68, 69f
β-blocker treatment/prophylaxis for, 50–53
adverse reactions to, 209, 210t, 211–212, 211t
as early intervention, 50–52, 51f, 52f, 73, 190
in heart failure, 178, 178f, 190–191, 191t
infarct size and reinfarction effects, 52f, 53f, 73
with intrinsic sympathomimetic activity, 52–53, 55f, 73
as late intervention, 52–53, 55f, 56f, 73, 190–191, 191t
mortality rate effects, 50, 52, 73
for pain relief, 50, 51f
in smokers *versus* nonsmokers, 90–91, 90f, 91f
diuretics as risk factor for, 95–96
as supraventricular arrhythmia cause, 152–153, 152t, 164
as systolic heart failure cause, 173, 174f
with treated diastolic blood pressure, 99–100, 102f, 103t, 104t
ventricular arrhythmias associated with
acute treatment for, 156, 157f
late-intervention prophylaxis for, 156–158, 158f
Myocardial ischemia
β-blocker treatment for, 53, 56–62, 73
action mechanism, 61–62
cardiac event risk effects, 61, 61f
with ECG ST segment depression, 51, 58–59

Myocardial ischemia (*Continued*)
   in painful ischemia, 56–58, 57f, 73
   in silent ischemia, 53, 58–61, 73
  silent
    smoking-related exacerbation, 59, 61
    "vulnerable period" for, 53, 59, 60f, 73

N

Nadolol
  as angina treatment/prophylaxis, 56, 57f
  antiarrhythmic activity
    in paroxysmal supraventricular tachycardia, 144
    in pediatric ventricular fibrillation, 156
  metabolic disturbances associated with, 112–113
  neurohumeral effects, 19
  as psoriasis cause, 238t
  water-solubility, 29, 31t
National Institute for Clinical Excellence (NICE), 82, 116, 118–119
Nebivolol
  antihypertensive activity
    effect on augmentation index, 125, 125f
    in intermittent claudication, 24f
  as atrial fibrillation prophylaxis, 151, 162–163, 165
  contraindication as heart failure treatment, 180t, 196
  as cutaneous disorders cause, 237
  as heart failure treatment, 179f, 180t, 181–183
  intrinsic sympathomimetic activity of, 22
  neurological effects, 22
  pharmacokinetic profile, 30t
Nephritis, 220

Neurohumeral effects, of β-blockers, 10–12, 11t, 19–20, 39
Nifedipine
  adverse reactions to, 219, 219t
  as angina treatment, 56, 57f
  antiatherogenic activity, 71
  atheromatous plaque formation effects, 70–71, 71t
  in combination with atenolol, 109–110
  comparison with bisoprolol, 219, 219t
  in intermittent claudication, 27
  as myocardial ischemia treatment, 59, 61, 61f
    in silent myocardial ischemia, 58, 73
  as peripheral arterial disease treatment, 62
Nitrates, as syndrome X treatment, 58
Nitric oxide, 22, 125, 182–183
Noradrenaline
  in heart failure, 28, 182
  in hypertension, 85, 89f
  interaction with β-blockers, 10, 11, 11t, 19, 20f, 25
  in left ventricular hypertrophy, 194, 194f
  in pheochomocytoma, 119

O

Obesity
  as diabetes mellitus risk factor, 83
  as hypertension risk factor, 82–88, 83t, 84f, 85f, 86f
  mechanisms of, 84–88, 87f
  as systolic heart failure risk factor, 173
Oculomucocutaneous syndrome, 237
Oslo Study, 96
Oxprenolol
  airway function effects, 18f, 19
  antiarrhythmic activity, 24
  antihypertensive activity

interaction with smoking, 89, 90, 91f, 107
neurological effects, 14f, 22–23
brain concentration, 31, 33f, 233
hemodynamic effects, 14f
hepatic metabolism, 32
intrinsic sympathomimetic activity, 22
in myocardial infarction patients, 52, 55f
neurohumeral effects, 22, 26f
pharmacokinetic profile, 30t
renin level effects, 24

P

Pacemakers, as arrhythmia cause, 153, 164
Penbutolol
hemodynamic effects, 14f
neurohumeral effects, 20f, 26f
Perindopril, 105, 105f
Peri-Operative Ischaemic Evaluation (POISE) trial, 62–63, 64–65, 64f, 66t
Peripheral arterial disease
β-blocker treatment/prophylaxis for, 62–68
in diabetic patients, 93–94, 94f
effect on pain-free walking distance, 62, 73–74
in high-risk noncardiac surgery patients, 62–68, 63f, 64f, 65f, 66f, 66t, 74
sudden perioperative withdrawal of, 65
as contraindication to β-blockers, 190
Pharmacodynamics, of β-blockers, 5–29
β_1-/β_2-selectivity ratios, 5, 6f
intrinsic sympathomimetic activity, 22–26
moderate β_1-selectivity without intrinsic sympathomimetic activity, 13–21
nonselective β/α blockade, 26–29
nonselectivity without intrinsic sympathomimetic activity, 13–21
Pharmacogenetics, of β-blockers, 4–5, 5f
Pharmacokinetics, of β-blockers, 29–37
absorption and bioavailability, 30t, 31, 34f
elimination and metabolism, 30t, 31–37
lipid solubility (lipophilicity), 29, 30t, 31
plasma half-life, 30t, 35f
Phenoxybenzamine, 120
Phenytoin, 144
Pheochromocytoma, 28, 29f, 119–120
Pindolol
adverse reactions to
myotoxicity, 216–217
sleep disturbances, 233
airway function effects, 15f, 18f, 19, 23
antiarrhythmic activity, 24, 25f, 26f
antihypertensive activity
in intermittent claudication, 24f
neurological effects, 14f, 22–23
hemodynamic effects, 14f
intrinsic sympathomimetic activity, 22
in myocardial infarction patients, 52, 55f
neurohumeral effects, 20f, 22–23, 26f
neurological effects, 22
as peripheral arterial disease treatment, 62
pharmacokinetic profile, 30t

Pindolol (*Continued*)
  as silent myocardial ischemia treatment, 58, 59f, 73
  as vascular steal cause, 27
  ventricular fibrillation threshold effects, 162
Plasma renin/angiotensin/aldosterone axis, 10, 11t, 17f, 19, 24, 26f, 28
POISE (Peri-Operative Ischaemic Evaluation) trial, 62–63, 64–65, 64f, 66t
Postural tachycardia syndrome (POTS), 154, 154f
Practolol
  antiarrhythmic activity, 152, 152t, 156
  as cutaneous disorders cause, 237
  hemodynamic effects, 14f
  in myocardial infarction patients, 55f
  neurohumeral effects, 26f
  neurological effects, 22
Prazosin
  contraindication as heart failure treatment, 198
  as left ventricular hypertrophy treatment, 105, 107
Pregnancy, hypertension of, 120–121, 120f
Prichard, Brian, 81
Prolonged QT syndrome, 159–160, 159f, 162
Propafenone, 31
Propranolol
  absorption and bioavailability, 30t, 31
  adverse reactions to
    cardiovascular, 209, 211, 211t, 214t, 219
    cold extremities, 214t, 219
    cutaneous disorders, 214t, 237
    fatigue, 212, 214t, 216–217, 217f
    glucose tolerance impairment, 229f
    hallucinations, 234
    hypoglycemia, 228
    impaired quality of life, 208, 208f
    impaired thermogenesis, 236
    memory loss, 233
    motor performance impairment, 234
    mucociliary, 213t, 227
    myotoxicity, 216–217, 217f
    psoriasis, 238t
    respiratory disorders, 225
    sexual dysfunction, 235–236, 236f
    sleep disturbances, 233
  airway function effects, 18f
  as angina treatment, 56, 57f
  antiarrhythmic activity, 142, 165
    in ectopic supraventricular tachycardia, 144
    in hypertrophic obstructive cardiomyopathy, 160
    in long QT syndrome, 159–160, 159f
    in pediatric ventricular fibrillation, 156
    in perioperative ventricular arrhythmias, 160, 161t
    in post-myocardial infarction arrhythmias, 156–157, 158f
    in postural tachycardia syndrome (POTS), 154, 154f
    in supraventricular arrhythmias, 144
    in ventricular arrhythmias, 158, 159–160
    in ventricular tachycardia, 155
  antiatherogenic activity, 68
  antihypertensive activity, 15
    comparison with atenolol, 121
    effect of adrenaline on, 21, 21f
    interaction with smoking, 89, 90–91, 90f, 91f

as myocardial infarction prophylaxis, 95, 96t
racial factors in, 15, 17f
relationship to plasma renin status, 15, 17f
as stroke prophylaxis, 94
as sudden death prophylaxis, 96t
β_1-/β_2-selectivity ratios, 5, 6f
brain concentration, 31, 33f
in combination with hydralazine, 27f
drug interactions, 31, 32f
as heart failure treatment, 178, 178f
hemodynamic effects, 13, 14f, 27f
hepatic metabolism, 32, 36
in the elderly, 36, 36f
interaction with smoking, 107
lipid solubility (lipophilicity), 29, 30t, 31
metabolic disturbances associated with, 11f, 19, 112–113, 229f, 232
mucociliary action, 213t, 226
in myocardial infarction patients, 52f
as myocardial ischemia treatment, 59, 60f
neurohumeral effects, 19, 20f, 26f
pharmacokinetic profile, 30t
as syndrome X treatment, 58
Protein kinase A, 3
Pseudomonas aeruginosa, 226
Psoriasis, 237, 238t
Pulse pressure, in systolic hypertension, 97–98, 98f, 99f

Q
Quality of life, 208, 208f, 225–226, 233
Quinidine, 31, 33f

R
Rashes, 237, 238t
Raynaud phenomenon, 214t, 219
Renal failure, 32, 35f, 40, 116, 119, 221
Renal function
β-blocker-related impairment, 220–221, 220f, 224f, 240
β-blocker-related improvement, 221, 224t
Renin/angiotensin/aldosterone axis, 10, 11t, 17f, 19, 24, 26f, 28
Renin/blood pressure relationship, 15, 17f, 24, 26f
Respiratory system, effect of β-blockers on, 221, 224–227, 234, 238–239
Ryanodine receptors, in heart failure, 185–186

S
Salbutamol, 9, 225
Scalp tingling, 237
SENIORS (Study of Effects of Nebivolol on Outcomes and Rehospitalization in Seniors with Heart Failure) trial, 151, 180t
Sexual dysfunction, 234–236, 234t, 235f, 236t
SHEP (Systolic Hypertension in the Elderly Program), 108t, 109, 113–115, 191–192, 195, 231
Shock, cardiogenic, 190, 211–212
Sick sinus syndrome, 211
Sinus bradycardia, 190
Skin disorders, 214t, 237, 238t
Sleep disturbances, 233, 241
Smoking
as hypertension risk factor, 82–83
interaction with β-blockers, 59, 61, 88–93, 90f, 91f, 92f, 107f, 125–126
in elderly patients, 107, 107f
Sotalol
adverse reactions to
torsades de pointes, 163, 163f
ventricular tachycardia, 238

Sotalol (*Continued*)
  antiarrhythmic activity, 141, 163, 165
    in atrial fibrillation, 149, 149*t*, 150
    in ectopic supraventricular arrhythmias, 143
    post-myocardial infarction, 157
    in supraventricular arrhythmias, 144, 147
    as torsades de pointes cause, 163, 163*f*
    in ventricular tachycardia, 155
  contraindication as heart failure treatment, 198
  hepatic metabolism, 32
  in myocardial infarction patients, 55*f*
  pharmacokinetics, 30*t*, 31
  renal elimination, 31
  water-solubility, 29, 31*t*
Stroke
  β-blocker prophylaxis for, 95–96
    comparison with diuretics, 95–96
    in diabetic patients, 93–94, 94*f*
    with first-line therapy, 108, 108*t*
    with second-line therapy, 108, 108*t*
  smoking as risk factor for, 90
  as supraventricular tachycardia cause, 153
Strong Heart Study, 86*f*
Sudden death, 85, 95, 96*t*
Supraventricular arrhythmias, 143–154
  atrial fibrillation, 147–152
    β-blocker prophylaxis and treatment for, 145*t*, 146*t*, 162–163
    electroconversion treatment for, 149, 149*t*

    heart failure-related, 151–152, 151*f*, 152*t*, 181, 182*f*
    paroxysmal, 148, 164
    post-coronary artery bypass grafting, 66–67, 149–150, 150*t*
    post-myocardial infarction, 153
    sustained, 149
  ectopic supraventricular tachycardia, 143–144
  paroxysmal supraventricular tachycardia, 144, 146*f*, 147
  post-myocardial infarction, 152–153, 152*t*
  preexcitation syndromes, 144, 146*f*, 147
Supraventricular tachycardia, myocardial infarction-related, 153, 164
SWORD (Survival With Oral D-Sotalol) study, 198
Syncope, 27
Syndrome X, 58
Systolic Hypertension in the Elderly Program (SHEP), 108*t*, 109, 113–115, 191–192, 195, 231

T

Thermogenesis, 236
TIBBS (Total Ischemic Burden Bisoprolol) study, 58–59, 61
Timolol
  adverse reactions to
    cardiovascular, 211
    mucociliary, 226
    respiratory effects, 224, 225
  airway function effects, 18*f*
  antiarrhythmic activity, 156–157
  as heart failure treatment, 178
  hemodynamic effects, 13, 14*f*
  metabolic disturbances associated with, 112–113

in myocardial infarction
patients, 52*f*, 211
neurohumeral effects, 19, 26*f*
pharmacokinetic profile, 30*t*
Timolol eyedrops, 212, 224
Torsade de pointes, 163, 163*f*, 238
Total Ischemic Burden Bisoprolol (TIBBS) study, 58–59, 61
Trandolopril, 98–99, 100*f*
Triglyceride levels, effect of β-blockers on, 230*t*, 232, 232*f*
Tumor necrosis factor-α, 84, 88*f*

U

United Kingdom National Institute for Clinical Excellence (NICE), 82, 116, 118–119
United Kingdom Prospective Diabetes Studies (UKPDS), 88–89, 89*t*, 93–94, 93*f*, 94*f*, 95*f*, 113, 191, 220, 221, 224*t*, 225, 229, 231
United States Carvedilol Trial Program, 183

V

Vascular resistance, 7, 13, 14*f*, 22, 24*f*, 26–27, 38
"Vascular steal" effect, 22, 27, 217, 219–220
Ventricular arrhythmias, 155–162
catecholaminergic mono-/polymorphic ventricular tachycardia, 162
hypertrophic obstructive cardiomyopathy, 160, 165
idiopathic arrhythmia, 155–156
intraoperative, 160, 161*t*
long QT syndrome-related, 159–160, 165
mitral valve prolapse-related, 158–159, 165
pacemaker-induced arrhythmia, 160
post-myocardial infarction, 155, 156–158, 165
Ventricular fibrillation, 85, 89*f*
defibrillation-refractory, 155*t*
digitalis toxicity-related, 155*t*
exercise-induced, in children, 156
mitral valve prolapse-related, 159
post-myocardial infarction, 156–157
stress-induced, in children, 156
as sudden death cause, 155
sympathominetic amines-related, 155*t*
threshold for, 141
Ventricular premature beats, 155, 155*t*, 159
Ventricular tachycardia
digitalis toxicity-related, 155*t*
exercise-related, 155, 155*t*
long QT syndrome-related, 156*t*
sustained, 155, 155*t*
Verapamil, 153, 160
as angina treatment, 56
in elderly patients, 98–99, 100*f*
as syndrome X treatment, 58

W

Warfarin, 31, 32*f*
Weight gain, 236–237, 237*t*
Wolff-Parkinson-White syndrome, 144, 146*t*, 147, 147*f*, 164

X

Xamoterol
contraindication as heart failure treatment, 180*t*, 196
as heart failure treatment, 179*f*, 180*t*, 181, 182*f*

Z

Ziac, 111*f*